HEPATITIS C

"It would be helpful to my patients with hepatitis C to read this book before we discuss the different treatment choices. They will find a lot of information from an unbiased source."

—Daniel R. Ganger, M.D.
Rush Presbyterian St. Luke's Medical Center
Chicago, Illinois

"Brings together information about the liver as well clarifying diet issues, diagnosis of hepatitis C, treatments (including alternative health options), and risk behavior in a very accessible way."

—Robert G. Gish, M.D.
Medical Director, Liver Transplant Program
California Pacific Medical Center

HEPATITIS C
A Personal Guide to Good Health

Beth Ann Petro Roybal, M.A.

Ulysses Press Berkeley, CA

1999

Published by: Ulysses Press
           P.O. Box 3440
           Berkeley, CA 94703-3440

Library of Congress Catalog Card Number: 99-60327

ISBN: 1-56975-183-8

Printed in Canada by Transcontinental Printing

10 9 8 7 6 5 4 3

Editor: Joanna Pearlman
Editorial and production staff: Steven Schwartz, David Wells, Lily Chou, Leslie Henriques
Cover Design: Leslie Henriques
Cover Illustration: Diana Ong (Crowd IV)/SuperStock
Indexer: Sayre Van Young

Distributed in the United States by Publishers Group West, in Canada by Raincoast Books, and in Great Britain and Europe by World Leisure Marketing.

This book has been written and published strictly for informational purposes, and in no way should it be used as a substitute for consultation with your medical doctor or health care professional. All facts in this book came from medical files, clinical journals, scientific publications, personal interviews, published trade books, self-published materials by experts, magazine articles, and the personal-practice experiences of the authorities quoted or sources cited. You should not consider educational material herein to be the practice of medicine or to replace consultation with a physician or other medical practitioner. The author and publisher are providing you with information in this work so that you can have the knowledge and can choose, at your own risk, to act on that knowledge. The author and publisher also urge all readers to be aware of their health status and to consult health professionals before beginning any health program, including changes in dietary habits.

The author welcomes your comments and suggestions for
future editions. We would also appreciate hearing how
this book has helped you. Please write us at Ulysses Press,
P.O. Box 3440, Berkeley, CA 94703-3440. You can e-mail us
at readermail@ulyssespress.com.

CONTENTS

FOREWORD

Viral hepatitis is a major public health concern in the United States and around the world. Globally, the hepatitis C virus (along with the less common hepatitis B virus) accounts for most cases of chronic hepatitis, cirrhosis, and primary liver cancer. In the United States, 3.9 million people are infected with the hepatitis C virus, or nearly 2 percent of the general population, and as many as 10,000 people die from it every year.

The hepatitis C virus was identified barely a decade ago in 1989, and only since 1990 have physicians had widely available diagnostic tests to confirm the infection. As the tests become more sophisticated, and efforts by many groups to educate the general public increase, a growing percentage of individuals infected with chronic hepatitis C are being diagnosed and seeking information and assistance.

In this setting of increasing recognition of the disease, Beth Ann Petro Roybal has summarized and updated the existing knowledge regarding all of the important aspects of hepatitis C in a readable and thorough fashion. This revised edition of *Hepatitis C: A Personal Guide to Good Health* provides background information on the discovery of the hepatitis C virus, modes of transmission, symptoms, diagnostic tests, treatment, and, most importantly, resources for coping with this chronic

disease. A glossary of common medical terminology assists the reader in understanding the medical aspects of hepatitis C. Practical issues, such as selecting a physician and seeking out information through local and national organizations, including addresses for web sites, are all provided in this comprehensive little book.

Treatment of chronic hepatitis C remains the greatest challenge for patients and physicians alike. Since the initial licensure of interferon for the treatment of chronic hepatitis C in 1991, there have been incremental improvements in therapy, even though less than half of treated patients have a sustained response or "cure." The details of interferon therapy and the newer combination treatments, including side effects, are outlined in this book, and some alternative treatments are also mentioned, with appropriate caution regarding the unproven nature of these alternative approaches. General practical advice regarding diet and exercise are also included.

If you or a close family member has chronic hepatitis C, this book will provide you all the information you need to understand what to expect, what treatment is available, and how to cope when treatment fails.

Emmet B. Keeffe, M.D.
Professor of Medicine
Stanford University Medical Center
June 1999

Acknowledgments

Thanks to Liz Webb for her inspiring dedication to hepatitis C education and support; to Dr. Emmet Keeffe for his thorough and timely answers to all my questions; and to all who shared their hard-earned wisdom about living with hepatitis C.

INTRODUCTION

"We are all here to help each other get over the bumps in life."

—Nutritional counselor who has hepatitis C,
Hixson, Tennessee

Is hepatitis C your own "bump in life"? Are you dealing with this disease yourself, or are you trying to help someone you love cope with hepatitis C? Or are you simply curious to know more about the disease and how you can protect yourself from it? This book is intended to help you become better informed about hepatitis C and more in control of your health and well-being.

When you first heard about hepatitis C, it probably sounded scary. Initial symptoms can be practically unnoticeable, yet long-term effects can be devastating. There is so little known about this disease, yet so many people seem to be affected by it. And so few traditional medical treatments are available.

How should you react to such a disease? Fortunately, there are many reasons not to panic or feel despair. For most people with hepatitis C, the disease usually progresses slowly. In the years before serious liver problems might occur, there are many things you can do to preserve your health and enjoy your life. Even if you already have signs of liver damage as the result of hepatitis C, you can work with your health care team to investigate options such as new medications or alternative therapies that may help you live a more normal life. If you do not have hepatitis C, you can take comfort in the fact that infection rates are stabilizing. There are steps you can take to protect yourself from this disease.

Whether or not you have hepatitis C, learning more about it can make you better prepared for dealing with it. Reading this book is a good start. The book describes the cause and course of hepatitis C. It provides information about how this disease is detected and monitored. It explains medical treatments and other steps you can take to stay healthy if you have hepatitis C. It also outlines current research into hepatitis C.

Several elements in this book are intended to help you put this information to practical use. Special boxes contain checklists, key information, risks and benefits, and questions for you to consider about hepatitis C. You'll find basic, critical information in the main body of the book. If you wish to learn more about particular aspects of hepatitis C, terms in *italic type* are explained in fuller detail in the *Glossary* at the back of this book. Perhaps most important, throughout this book you'll find statements from persons with hepatitis C and from health professionals who are knowledgeable about this disease.

Rather than simply overwhelming you with a lot of information, it is hoped that this book will both reassure and inform you, helping you navigate successfully through the "bumps" in your life that may be caused by hepatitis C.

PART I
UNDERSTANDING HEPATITIS C

"I was devastated. And when I tried to find out some information about it, nobody else seemed to have heard of it, either."

—Accountant, San Francisco, as reported in the
San Francisco Chronicle, May 31, 1997

In order to better understand treatment for any disease or condition, many people find it helpful to learn more about the disease itself. The benefits of knowing more about hepatitis C are many. Whether you have found out that you have hepatitis C or you know someone who has the disease, increasing your knowledge about hepatitis C can:

- Give you insight into why particular treatments may be helpful in controlling or combating hepatitis C.

- Help you prevent the spread of hepatitis C.

- Help you be prepared for what to expect over time if the disease progresses.

Part I of this book provides basic information about hepatitis C and the virus that causes it, *HCV* (hepatitis C virus). It describes how HCV was discovered. It explains how HCV is able to survive your body's defenses and cause damage to the liver. And it presents reasons why you should be concerned about HCV, whether or not you are infected with the virus.

If you would rather start by learning right away about the treatment for HCV, you may prefer to skip ahead to *PART II: Treating HCV* and *PART III: Other Steps to Take*. After reading the rest of the book, you can return to *PART I* or to the *Glossary* if you have specific questions about HCV and its development.

HEPATITIS C— A SURPRISING DISCOVERY

CHAPTER 1

"Although hepatitis C is a tough illness to fight and not exactly what anyone would care to experience, I have found it to have changed my life for the better."

—Nutritional counselor, Hixson, Tennessee

Perhaps it was just a routine physical, even though you did mumble something to your doctor about feeling a little rundown the last few weeks. The doctor probably nodded, handing you a page with boxes checked off for routine blood tests: complete blood count, cholesterol, glucose, liver function. As he guided you toward the door, the doctor said, "We'll call if there's anything wrong with any of these tests. See you next year." He then shook your hand, and was off to see his next patient.

The following week you got a phone call from a nurse at the office. "We got your blood tests back. Everything looks normal—except for the liver function. One of these numbers seems a little high and the doctor would like you to come in for some more blood work." You have already started to feel better, but decide it's probably worth having the extra tests just in case.

A few weeks later you're back in the doctor's office. You ask your doctor incredulously, "How can I have hepatitis C? I feel fine. Just had a touch of the flu or something." Your doctor shrugs. He tries to be helpful, but it seems like he's a little short on details about the disease and how it's treated.

If this sounds somewhat familiar to you, you're not alone. This scenario is typical of how many people find out they have hepatitis C. It's a disease that sneaks up on you while you're totally unaware. It's usually discovered as the result of blood tests for other reasons—such as during a routine physical or when donating blood. Many people never even figure out how they got the disease.

So what should you do about hepatitis C? Is it really a serious threat to your health? Should you worry about passing it on to others? Or should you follow the advice of some doctors and "just wait and see"?

Test Your Knowledge of Hepatitis C

When was hepatitis C discovered?

How many people have hepatitis C?

How many new cases of hepatitis C occur each year?

How many deaths each year are caused by hepatitis C?

Of the two diseases—hepatitis C and AIDS:

> Which one affects more people each year?
>
> Which one kills more people each year?
>
> Which one can go unnoticed for decades before health is seriously damaged?
>
> Which one is the leading cause for liver transplants in the U.S.?

The first step is to find out more about hepatitis C—the prevalence of this disease, how the virus that causes hepatitis C is acquired, and what it does once it is inside your body. Then we'll see how the virus spreads and what kind of damage can result from it. After that, we'll examine how hepatitis C is diagnosed and treated, and then give suggestions for what you can do to live well despite this disease.

Let's start by learning some hepatitis C facts. To warm up to the topic, try the short quiz on page 4. Heck, if you're feeling especially brave, ask your doctor these same questions (politely, of course) at your next appointment! Hepatitis C is still such a new and unknown disease, that many doctors are only beginning to understand the potential health threat of HCV. Unless they specialize in dealing with liver problems, they probably need to learn as much about hepatitis C as you do.

Discover the Facts About Hepatitis C

When was hepatitis C discovered? Hepatitis C was first suspected to exist in 1975, when it was named "non-A, non-B hepatitis." The actual virus that causes hepatitis C was not isolated until 1989.

How many people have hepatitis C? If you have hepatitis C, you're not alone. This disease affects about 4 million persons in the U.S. (almost two percent of the population) and perhaps up to 400 million people worldwide. In the U.S., this number may be slowly stabilizing as the primary sources of infection (infected blood and shared needles) are eliminated. Most new cases in the U.S. are in people between the ages of 20 and 45.

How many new cases of hepatitis C occur each year? Up to 150,000 new cases of hepatitis C occurred annually in recent years. Currently, there are approximately 33,000 new cases per year.

How many deaths each year are caused by hepatitis C? This disease causes about 10,000 deaths each year in the U.S. Unfortunately, the number of deaths is growing, and may triple within ten years, as people infected years ago are only now starting to show signs of serious liver damage and liver failure.

Of the two diseases—hepatitis C and AIDS—which affects more people? Believe it or not, hepatitis C affects far more people than does HIV/ AIDS. In fact, by the year 2000, more people will die each year from hepatitis C than from AIDS. Hepatitis C can go unnoticed for decades before a person's health is seriously damaged. And hepatitis C is the number-one cause of liver transplantation in the U.S. Take a look at these comparisons between HIV/AIDS and hepatitis C:

	HIV/AIDS	Hepatitis C
Infected in U.S.	700,000	4,000,000
Infected worldwide	20,000,000	400,000,000
New cases per year in U.S.	40,000	33,000

A Serious Threat to Your Health

Perhaps you were surprised by how prevalent hepatitis C is, especially when compared to HIV/AIDS. This comparison is not intended to trivialize the seriousness of HIV and AIDS. HIV/AIDS is a condition that almost everyone recognizes as a dangerous epidemic. Still, hepatitis C is an even greater threat to the public health. Yet many of us haven't ever heard of it. Many physicians know little about it. That's not surprising. Hepatitis C wasn't suspected until 1975 or named until 1989.

But how could such a widespread and catastrophic condition go unnoticed for so long? We can answer this by taking a closer look at the underlying cause of hepatitis C: the hepatitis C virus (HCV).

The Hepatitis C Virus
Tricks the Immune System

We'll start with general information about viruses and then get more specific about the hepatitis C virus. There are countless different viruses. A *virus* is an extremely small organism, invisible to the eye and even to all but the strongest microscopes. Unlike other living organisms, a virus cannot reproduce within its own body; it needs to "borrow" or, more appropriately, take over the reproduction mechanisms of cells. Once a virus invades a cell, it duplicates quickly, eventually bursting the cell and scattering new viruses. These new viruses search out and invade still other cells, repeating the duplication process over and over again.

Most viruses are harmless to humans. Some, upon invading cells in the body, cause relatively minor illnesses like colds and the flu. Others, such as the virus that causes hepatitis A, can make you pretty sick for a while, but you eventually recover. Still others, such as HIV (*human immunodeficiency virus*, the cause of AIDS) and the hepatitis C virus (HCV), can be very serious, even deadly.

The question is, why can you get over a cold in a week or so, but have hepatitis C for the rest of your life? And why might you get HCV and not even know it for years? It all has to do with how your body defends itself against "foreign invaders," a sophisticated mechanism called the *immune system*.

To better understand the role of the immune system, let's first take a look at some more obvious ways the body defends itself against viruses and other invaders. Simply by closing your mouth or blinking your eyes, you protect yourself from many potential invaders such as dust or gnats. And think of what would happen if you didn't have skin to prevent who-knows-what from entering your body. But sometimes some things do get past these initial lines of defense. For example, you could scrape your knee and get dirt and bacteria in the wound. You could accidentally get poked with a needle that you've used to inject medication into a patient who was a carrier of a contagious virus. You could use a friend's razor, not even noticing that you nicked your face as you shaved. You could have a hot, heavy, and condom-less lovemaking session with a new partner, not realizing that he or she had a disease that could be transmitted through sexual contact.

If any substance does enter the body through these or other means, the body initiates a coordinated response to disable or destroy the invader. First off, when any foreign substance, such as a virus, passes into the body, it becomes marked as an invader. This marked invader is called an *antigen*.

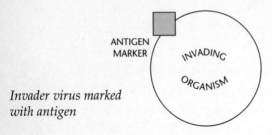

Invader virus marked with antigen

The body responds to an antigen in two ways:

1) Certain white blood cells (*B cells*) remember this particular antigen and manufacture a unique *antibody* to fight it. Each time these white blood cells encounter the antigen, they generate these specific antibodies, which attach to the antigen to help disable it. (This process is called the *humoral response*).

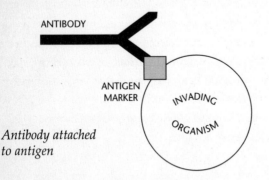

Antibody attached to antigen

2) Other white blood cells (*T cells*) also notice the antigen and get rid of it, either through a chemical assault or by "eating" or engulfing the antigen (*phagocytosis*). The remains of the antigen and the cell that ate it are then dragged off by other cells to the liver for disposal. (This process is called the *cell-mediated response*.)

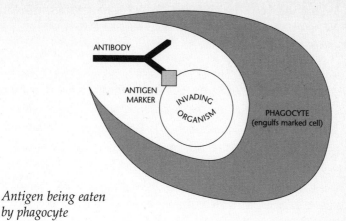

*Antigen being eaten
by phagocyte*

During the immune response, blood and other fluids (*lymph*) accumulate at the site of the invasion, bringing with them all the necessary cells, antibodies, and other chemicals needed to fight off the invading substance. With all this extra material at the site, the area becomes swollen, red, and maybe even warm, a reaction called *inflammation*. After the invader has been successfully overcome, the inflammation subsides.

The immune system usually works effectively to protect you from thousands of foreign substances, including viruses, bacteria, fungi, parasites, chemicals, and even any of your own cells that are abnormal or damaged (such as cancer cells).

Unfortunately, though, HCV seems to be able to "put one over" on the immune system. If HCV enters your body, the immune system response begins as it normally would:

- The virus is marked (creating antigen) and antibody is created (*anti-HCV*).

- Some of the HCV is ingested and destroyed.

- However, HCV is able to change its form frequently. As it continually changes, the body cannot keep up with identifying and destroying all of the *mutations*.

- This leaves much of the virus free to roam and multiply. As it multiplies, it changes slightly, which helps it to continue evading detection.

HCV can be found in blood, but its favorite hideout is the liver. As the body repeatedly attempts to destroy the virus in the liver, inflammation of the liver occurs. This inflammation is called *hepatitis* ("hepat" means "liver," while "itis" means "inflammation"). Sometimes the inflammation occurs for one episode, then disappears. This condition is called *acute hepatitis*. If the inflammation does not go away, it is called *chronic hepatitis* and gradually can lead to other liver problems. Most people who have been infected with HCV do not have a clinically recognized episode of acute hepatitis, but still go on to develop chronic hepatitis C.

Hepatitis and Your Liver

Now you know that hepatitis means inflammation of the liver. But what is the big deal about an inflamed liver? The second-largest organ in the body (just so you know, skin is considered an organ, making it the largest organ of the body), your liver normally performs a range of critical tasks. The liver is located behind the ribs, just below the diaphragm, on the right side. It weighs about three pounds.

Perhaps the easiest way to understand the liver's importance is to view the liver as the "central processing station" for your body. Some of its functions include:

- Processing all nutrients as they come out from the digestive tract.

- Storing excess amounts of carbohydrates, fat, protein, vitamins, and minerals (especially iron—that's why people with *anemia* are often encouraged to eat iron-rich cow's liver), so they can be readily available in case of a shortage.

- Manufacturing a digestive juice called *bile* as well as substances used to help your blood clot (*clotting factors*).

- Regulating chemical, hormonal, and cholesterol levels.

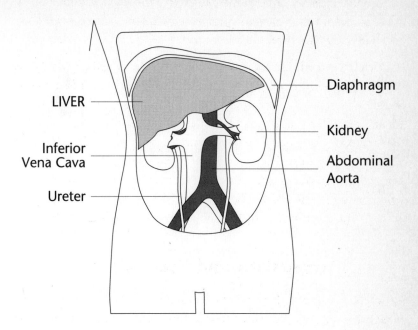

LIVER

Inferior
Vena Cava

Ureter

Diaphragm

Kidney

Abdominal
Aorta

- Destroying old blood cells.

- Breaking down toxic substances, including drugs (such as aspirin and prescription medications), alcohol, and bacteria.

- Cleaning waste products from the blood.

As if the liver weren't already amazing enough, it is also one of the few organs in your body that can normally regenerate its tissue if damaged.

This is how the liver works under normal conditions. But inflammation of the liver—hepatitis—can change all that. Hepatitis may be caused by any one of several viruses. The liver enlarges, becomes inflamed, and may become tender. In addition, you may get a fever, feel weak, or have nausea and vomiting. You may also develop *jaundice*, a condition in which a certain chemical *(bilirubin)* builds up and cannot be removed from the body by the liver. This results in a yellowing of the skin or eyes.

Hepatitis ranges in severity, depending somewhat on which virus caused it:

- Some people, approximately 15%, become ill with acute hepatitis but recover completely with no treatment; the other 85% have chronic infection.

- A few people have a severe acute illness and die.

- Among chronically infected individuals, some may carry the virus, but never develop the disease. Even if these *carriers* (persons whose bodies harbor a virus, whether or not they have the disease associated with the virus) have no symptoms of hepatitis, they can still infect others.

- The majority of people infected with HCV develop long-term chronic hepatitis—the inflammation never goes away completely. The liver, so resilient and self-healing, manages to remain healthy and perform its many critical functions for years. However, over time persistent inflammation may lead to a range of liver problems, including *cirrhosis* (liver scarring) and liver cancer.

Hepatitis C and Other Types of Hepatitis

Hepatitis C is a member of the *Flaviviridae* family of viruses. It is one of several types of hepatitis, including hepatitis A, B, D, E, and G. All these types of hepatitis are caused by different viruses. Hepatitis can also be caused by certain drugs. More types of viral hepatitis continue to be discovered and debated (there is some discussion, for instance, over whether hepatitis F actually exists). Hepatitis C was first recognized in 1975, when it was named *"non-A, non-B" (NANB)*. At that time, persons receiving blood transfusions were developing a type of hepatitis that could not be traced to either hepatitis A or hepatitis B, for which tests had already been developed. However, it wasn't until 1989 that scientists were able to isolate, clone, and name hepatitis C, the virus that caused NANB hepatitis. One year later, the first test for the HCV antibody was developed. Since then, other tests have been created to detect both the HCV antibody (anti-HCV) and even the virus itself.

Genotypes of HCV

HCV comes in many forms, making it harder to treat than other types of hepatitis. Known genotypes (distinct groupings) of HCV and where they are most common are as follows:

- Types 1, 2, 3: Worldwide, including the U.S.

- Type 4: Middle East and Africa

- Type 5: South Africa

- Type 6: Asia

Within each genotype are subgroups, such as genotype 1a and 1b. A quicker, easier way to classify HCV is *serotyping*, which groups HCV based on antibodies detected. Serotypes correlate with genotypes. This method of classifying HCV is not as accurate, however, as genotyping.

Hepatitis C is unlike the diseases caused by the other hepatitis viruses in that initial symptoms are often minor and frequently unrecognized, while long-term damage to the liver can be great. It is also unlike most other types of hepatitis viruses in that there are many *genotypes* of HCV. In addition, within a single individual, HCV can change into slightly different forms, called "quasispecies." This may be what makes it difficult for the body to detect and eliminate HCV and why people with HCV report such a variety of symptoms or no symptoms at all. All these various forms of HCV also pose problems for scientists trying to develop treatments and vaccines that can be effective against all mutations of HCV.

Why Worry About Hepatitis C?

If hepatitis C has few, if any, early symptoms and doesn't cause major health problems for many years, then why worry about it now? You

(Text continued on page 16)

Alphabet Soup: The Many Forms of Hepatitis

Hepatitis A was formerly called *infectious hepatitis* because its virus spreads through contaminated water and food. It is more common in developing countries, but is also found in the U.S., where outbreaks peak in approximately ten-year cycles. You may have heard of persons catching hepatitis A from strawberries and other fruit arriving in the U.S. from Mexico. Most people recover completely from hepatitis A, and no chronic infection remains. A vaccine that can protect from hepatitis A has been in use for several years. *Gamma globulin* can also be taken to protect against exposure for a shorter period of time. If you travel to less-developed areas of the world, it is recommended that you get vaccinated or receive gamma globulin before leaving on your trip.

Hepatitis B used to be called *serum hepatitis* because its virus, HBV, spreads through blood and other body fluids. It is often considered the most serious form of hepatitis. Hepatitis B can be transmitted from a pregnant woman to her baby. Most people (95 percent of adults) recover from hepatitis B, but some may retain chronic infection. There is a vaccine to prevent hepatitis B. A special gamma globulin can also be taken for protection after exposure.

Hepatitis C was originally named *non-A, non-B (NANB) hepatitis*. HCV spreads through blood and is the most common form of hepatitis. The initial illness is often so slight that most people don't even notice it, yet few people recover completely. Most people with HCV go on to develop chronic hepatitis infection. Currently, there is no vaccine to prevent hepatitis C. Gamma globulin does not seem to protect against hepatitis C.

Hepatitis D was previously called *delta hepatitis*. It is only found along with hepatitis B and is rare in the U.S., except in people who use contaminated needles or people who have had many blood transfusions. Like hepatitis B and hepatitis C, hepatitis D can cause both acute and chronic illness.

Hepatitis E used to be named *enteric* or *epidemic non-A, non-B hepatitis*. It is similar to hepatitis A and also does not result in chronic infection. It is most common in areas around the Indian Ocean and is rare in the U.S.

Hepatitis G has only recently been discovered. The HGV virus (there are at least three subtypes of this virus) spreads through blood and is often found along with HBV, HCV, and HIV (the virus that leads to AIDS). HGV's effect on the body is still being studied. Most people suffer no apparent symptoms from this virus.

Drug-induced hepatitis can result from long-term use of some prescription medications, including isoniazid (a tuberculosis-fighting drug), methyldopa (used to treat high blood pressure), nitrofurantoin (for urinary tract infections), and phenytoin (for seizures). Stopping the drug as soon as the problem is discovered usually prevents any long-term liver damage such as cirrhosis.

Herpes viruses (such as the virus that causes chickenpox) can induce acute hepatitis that usually does not become chronic.

Are You at Risk for HCV?

You may be at risk for having HCV or developing chronic hepatitis if:

- You received blood transfusions or any other blood products before 1990.

- You have ever injected drugs with a shared needle—even one time.

- You have ever used cocaine intranasally (sniffed).

- You are a hemophiliac.

- You are a health care worker, especially involved with patient contact or in laboratory work.

- You have had sex with many partners.

- You have had an STD *(sexually transmitted disease)*.

If you have any of these risks, you may want to ask your doctor to test your blood to see if you have HCV.

---

certainly could take your chances and hope that a cure is found before you develop serious liver problems. However, there are many reasons why you should start right now to be concerned about hepatitis C and its potential effect on your health and the health of those you love. Here are just a few reasons:

- Many people carry HCV and don't know it.

- HCV can easily be spread without your knowledge.

- You may have risks or behaviors you can do something about now to keep yourself from acquiring HCV or from spreading it to others.

- Although initially the symptoms may be negligible, it is now thought that some damage to the liver occurs in most cases (up to 85 percent). Long-term problems from the virus can include chronic hepatitis, cirrhosis, and liver cancer.

If you find you have HCV, there are things you can do now to maintain your health and prevent future damage to your liver. Pay close attention to *Parts II* and *III* of this book, which describe how you can live well despite being infected with HCV. If you are at risk for getting HCV, in many cases you can take action now to be sure you don't acquire this dangerous virus. These steps are described in *Chapter 8*. To find out more about how HCV is acquired and the effects of hepatitis C on the body, turn the page to *Chapter 2: The Course of HCV and Hepatitis C.*

THE COURSE OF HCV AND HEPATITIS C

"Even though I have had these symptoms for nearly six years, I was just diagnosed with hep-c in March of this year. I thought that I was just old, weak, crazy, or something."

—44-year-old man with hepatitis C

If you've found out that you have HCV, you probably have many more questions than answers. You may wonder how you got this virus and what you might expect in terms of symptoms and liver problems. Perhaps you have noticed symptoms already, but have been told that they probably have nothing to do with HCV. Or maybe you feel just fine. If your symptoms are insignificant, are you going to be okay in the long run? Have you somehow managed to rid yourself of HCV? A few lucky people—about 15 percent of people infected with HCV—do seem to clear the virus from their bodies spontaneously. For the rest of the folks with HCV, the news is mixed. The good news is that you may notice just a few symptoms over the course of several years. With a little bit of care, you can still lead an active, normal life. In fact, most statistics show that the death rate for people with HCV is no higher than the death rate for the general population. On a more sobering note, recent evidence suggests that even if you have only a few symptoms, you may still develop liver problems that can go undetected for many years.

Let's take some time here to review briefly the entire course of hepatitis C, starting with how people are infected, then looking at some of the symptoms associated with hepatitis C, and finally describing some of the liver problems that can arise from chronic hepatitis.

A Virus Transmitted Through Contact with Infected Blood

HCV is transmitted by contact with infected blood—contact that must be "percutaneous," that is, passing through the skin to enter into the body. Some common ways in which persons are potentially exposed to HCV-infected blood include the following:

• *Sharing of needles used for injected drugs.* This accounts for about half of all new cases of HCV. Some people who "did drugs" only once—while in college, for example—are surprised to find out years later that they probably contracted HCV in this manner. It is estimated that perhaps up to 90 percent of current injection drug users are infected with HCV. And if you use someone else's needle to inject drugs, the

---

"I presume I contracted hepatitis C through a blood transfusion in 1970, but I have had several surgeries, starting at age 3. I am now 50. I was diagnosed . . . as a result of blood tests done to determine the cause of my constant gastrointestinal complaints."

—Woman with hepatitis C

How You Could Be Exposed to HCV

- Sharing of injection-drug needles
- Blood transfusions, organ transplants, or receipt of blood components
- Hemodialysis
- On-the-job exposure to infected blood
- Exposure to infected personal care items
- Sexual intercourse with many partners
- Re-use of infected tools used for acupuncture, tattooing, and body piercing
- Sniffing or snorting cocaine
- From a pregnant woman to her child during birth

chances are fifty-fifty that you'll pick up up HCV. Bleach, which is effective against HIV, *won't* kill HCV.

• *Blood transfusions and receipt of other blood components or donated organs.* Blood and transplant organs in the U.S. and most other developed countries are now screened for HCV, so new transmission rates through this means are extremely low. However, many people who received blood products or organ transplants prior to 1990, when the donated blood supply began to be screened, may already have been exposed to HCV. Many people are just now finding out they have hepatitis C, years after having a transfusion during surgery, receiving a transplanted organ, or using clotting factor to combat *hemophilia*. As of March 1998, blood banks throughout the U.S. must review all their records from 1988 on to identify all blood donated by persons now known to have HCV. They must notify the hospitals that received tainted blood, who in turn must notify the physician or patient who received the blood.

• *Hemodialysis.* Persons with kidney problems (such as kidney failure or complications from diabetes or heart disease) who undergo hemo-

dialysis to cleanse the blood are more likely to acquire HCV. This may be due to the hemodialysis facility's failure to consistently follow proper procedures in cleaning and sterilizing equipment used by many people.

• *Exposure to infected blood on the job.* Health care workers may have needle-stick injuries or may be exposed to infected blood in other ways, such as spilled blood or a broken test tube in a pathology laboratory.

• *Exposure to infected personal care items, especially razors.* One likely scenario is spending the night at a buddy's house and using his razor the next morning, not realizing he is a carrier of HCV. The risk is low—but transmission of HCV still has been known to occur in this way.

• *Having had sexual intercourse with many partners.* This means of transmission is not nearly as common for HCV as it is for HIV and other sexually transmitted diseases (STDs). No one is completely sure how HCV is transmitted through sex. There is a low rate of transmission in people who are in monogamous relationships, while there is a higher rate of transmission in people who have had many partners. For example, people who have had more than 50 partners are 23 times more likely to get HCV. Also, it seems that it is easier for women to acquire HCV through sex than for men, perhaps because of the potential for irritation and breaks in the vaginal membrane.

• *Re-use of infected tools used for acupuncture, tattooing, and body piercing.* Reputable providers of these services should be using disposable or sterilized needles; HCV could be transmitted if needles have been re-used or improperly sterilized.

• *Intranasal use (sniffing or snorting) of cocaine.* A connection has been noted between HCV infection and snorting cocaine.

• *From a pregnant woman with HCV to her child.* This route of transmission appears to be relatively rare. Transmission probably occurs during birth. It has been noted that the chances of a baby acquiring HCV are greater if the mother has both HCV and HIV.

In many cases, persons with HCV have no idea how they acquired the virus. They may have forgotten the incident during which they were

exposed—perhaps a blood transfusion that was received while unconscious from anesthesia during surgery. They may simply be too
ashamed to tell their doctor about a short-term "slip-up," such as
having injected drugs a few times. Or, they may have been exposed
through a means which has not yet been linked to HCV transmission.
In any case, if you have HCV, knowing how you were exposed simply provides a small piece of a confusing puzzle—it doesn't change
your diagnosis or treatment. If you don't have HCV, understanding
the ways HCV is known to be transmitted can help keep you safe.

Once Infection Occurs

Luckily for most people, even upon exposure to HCV it is fairly difficult to acquire the virus. If infection does occur, usually between 3
and 20 weeks after exposure, you may have a few flu-like symptoms
(fatigue, nausea, fever) that are so slight they may not be noticed.
These symptoms usually go away in a few days or weeks. After initially acquiring the virus, the course of your disease could follow any
one of these paths:

- You may become totally free of HCV.

- You may still have the virus (be a carrier), but have no further symptoms or problems resulting from it.

- You may carry the virus with few accompanying symptoms
  for years, then later experience problems as a result of liver
  damage.

- You may carry the virus and have noticeable symptoms,
  which may progressively worsen over time.

It can be frustrating to see such a list of possibilities ranging from relatively innocuous to extremely serious, not knowing which of these
scenarios is most likely to happen to you. As researchers learn more
about this disease, they hope to be able to predict with better accuracy how the virus is likely to affect different people—and how to tailor
treatment programs to individual patients with HCV. For instance,
there is growing evidence to indicate which strains of HCV respond

best to interferon therapy (see *Chapter 4* for details on interferon). All the more reason to stay informed about this disease!

The Initial Symptoms of Hepatitis C

Doctors treating patients with HCV used to think most people had no initial symptoms or few symptoms associated with the virus unless they developed full-fledged chronic hepatitis. This may still be the case for many persons with HCV. However, persons infected with the virus commonly report a variety of symptoms, ranging from mild to severe.

Flu-like symptoms are the most frequent symptoms mentioned by persons with HCV. These symptoms include chills, fever, sweating, nausea, fatigue, and malaise (a general sense of not feeling well). These symptoms may be due to the body's immune response in trying to fight off the virus.

Pain in joints, muscles, the area around the liver, or the right shoulder (*referred pain*) have all been reported by people with hepatitis C. Pain can have a number of causes, including pressure on nerves from excess fluid, buildup of toxic substances that the liver can't remove, related immune system disorders such as rheumatoid arthritis, or tests such as liver biopsies.

Chronic fatigue or sudden exhaustion are common. These symptoms may come and go, and, as the flu-like symptoms, are probably due to the suppression of the immune system.

Gastrointestinal problems noted by persons with HCV include indigestion, *irritable bowel syndrome* (IBS), and diarrhea. Some of these prob-

---

"I used to have enough energy for ten [people]. I taught swimming, was a library mother, worked full time."

—Florida woman who developed liver failure 30 years after a blood transfusion, as reported in the *Lakeland Ledger*, June 1, 1997

Some Hepatitis C Symptoms

- Flu-like symptoms
- Chronic fatigue, exhaustion
- Sleep problems
- Adverse reactions to alcohol
- Frequent urination

- Headache, dizziness, "floaters"
- Jaundice

- Pain
- Gastrointestinal problems
- Psychological problems
- Fluid retention
- Loss of appetite, aversion to fatty foods
- Itchy skin
- Red spider veins

lems may be caused by the backup of fluid that can no longer flow from the digestive tract through the liver.

Psychological problems include depression, mood swings, *seasonal affective disorder, cognitive dysfunction,* and various sleep problems (vivid dreams, restless sleep, and not feeling rested after sleeping). Some of these problems may be caused by medication. Others may be linked to the buildup of toxins in the body. Still others may be associated with the stress (both physical and mental) of dealing with such a serious chronic illness.

Adverse reactions to alcohol and growing sensitivity to medications may occur as the liver becomes less able to process these substances.

Fluid retention—abdominal bloating, puffy face, and *edema* (fluid retention in the arms and legs)—and frequent urination can be caused by the backup of blood and fluid that can no longer flow readily through the liver.

Other symptoms felt by persons with HCV include loss of appetite, aversion to fatty foods, headache, dizziness, *"floaters"* (cobweb-like strands that appear to float in your visual field), and appearance of red spider veins.

Symptoms of serious liver damage include itchy skin, jaundice, and vomiting blood.

There are bound to be many other symptoms not listed here. Because most of these symptoms are so general in nature (the medical term for these general symptoms is *"nonspecific"*), often it's tempting for doctors and patients to attribute them to other causes: stress, hypochondria ("it's all in your head"), the flu, whatever. However, these symptoms can usually be linked to hepatitis C in some way:

• Certain symptoms, such as itchy skin and jaundice, are directly caused by liver damage brought on by hepatitis C. These are signs of serious liver failure that need immediate medical attention.

• Some symptoms may be due to medication used to treat hepatitis C. For instance, depression and suicidal feelings are relatively common side effects for people using interferon (see *Chapter 4* for more information about interferon).

• Symptoms such as chronic fatigue may not be caused by liver damage per se, but may be the result of HCV's assault on the immune system. Persons with other chronic health conditions caused by immune system problems, such as *rheumatoid arthritis* or *multiple sclerosis*, often experience similar symptoms.

The point of describing this range of symptoms is not to scare or overwhelm you. Rather, if you have hepatitis C, you may be relieved to learn that these symptoms are commonly associated with this condition —it's not simply "all in your head" as you may have been told by friends and family or even your physician. Furthermore, some of these symptoms may be signs that your liver is being damaged. Other symptoms can be treated so that you feel more comfortable. If you are aware of all these possible symptoms, rather than ignoring problems or feeling like you just have to learn to live with them, you can report them to your doctor and make sure there isn't something more you could be doing to preserve your health and feel better.

When Hepatitis C Becomes Chronic

For many people infected with HCV—up to 85 percent—hepatitis becomes chronic. This means that the liver inflammation does not go

Chronic HCV is typically an insidious process, progressing, if at all, at a slow rate without symptoms or physical signs in the majority of patients during the first two decades after infection. A small proportion of patients with chronic HCV hepatitis—perhaps less than 20 percent—develop nonspecific symptoms, including mild intermittent fatigue and malaise. Symptoms first appear in many patients with chronic HCV hepatitis at the time of development of advanced liver disease.

—National Institutes of Health *Consensus Development Statement on the Management of Hepatitis C*

away. It is now realized that even if you experience hardly any symptoms and your blood tests indicate "normal" liver function, your liver may still be inflamed. This inflammation may continue for 10 to 30 years or more. Previously, doctors took a "wait and see" approach if you were in this sort of "hepatitis holding pattern." However, now that it is known that liver damage is possibly occurring even when you don't have symptoms, many specialists (usually *gastroenterologists* or *hepatologists*) are doing whatever they can to monitor and treat this stage more aggressively. To keep your liver healthy, you may need to have regular exams and tests, take medication (such as interferon), and make changes in your diet and lifestyle (see *Part II* and *Part III* of this book for more information). The goal is to try to prevent or delay serious liver problems that otherwise are likely to develop. So that you understand the impact these problems can have on your health and your life, let's take a brief look at some of these conditions.

Liver Problems Caused by Chronic Hepatitis C

Chronic hepatitis C can lead to serious health problems including cirrhosis, liver failure, liver cancer, and general immune system problems.

Cirrhosis. Most people associate cirrhosis with alcoholics. And while it's true that alcohol use is the most common cause of cirrhosis, there are many other causes as well, including hepatitis C. In fact, at least 20 percent of persons with HCV develop cirrhosis within 20 years of being infected with the virus. Rarely, it can develop within the first two years after becoming infected.

But what exactly is cirrhosis? Earlier, we described how a healthy liver is able to regenerate itself when tissue is damaged. However, in cirrhosis, normal liver cells that become damaged are replaced by scar tissue. This useless tissue is unable to perform the various functions carried out by normal liver cells. Scar tissue also blocks blood from flowing through the liver, causing it to back up into surrounding veins (*portal hypertension*). As scar tissue builds, the liver enlarges and gradually performs fewer and fewer of its vital functions.

Many people do not have symptoms in the early stages of cirrhosis and only find out about the condition when they have blood tests for other purposes. However, there are several symptoms associated with cirrhosis:

- Loss of appetite and weight loss

- Nausea and vomiting (sometimes vomiting of blood)

- Jaundice

- Itching

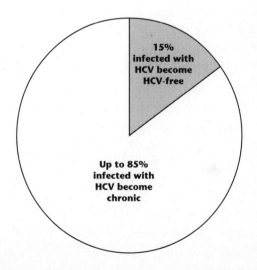

"I've not only survived—I've thrived."

—Naomi Judd, singer and spokeswoman for the
American Liver Foundation, as quoted in
the *San Jose Mercury News*, June 24, 1998

- Swelling of the abdomen (ascites)

- Increasing sensitivity to drugs

- Mental confusion leading to coma (encephalopathy)

People with cirrhosis are also more at risk for developing kidney failure, ulcers, gallstones, diabetes, liver cancer, and bacterial infections.

Treatment of cirrhosis involves treating any accompanying problems (such as bleeding or fluid accumulation) with medication or surgical procedures. Some medications, including interferon, may be used to treat the cirrhosis itself. If the liver completely fails to function (liver failure), transplantation may be an option to consider.

Liver cancer. There seems to be a strong connection between HCV and a certain kind of primary liver cancer called *hepatocellular carcinoma* (HCC). Not everyone with HCV gets HCC; in fact, probably only about 6 to 8 percent of people with chronic HCV will go on to develop liver cancer. However, more than half of all people who develop HCC are found to also have HCV. This is especially true in southern Europe and Japan. Cirrhosis can also progress to HCC. Even though these connections have been documented, doctors don't know yet exactly how HCV leads to cancer. It is thought that the constant inflammation, cell damage, and cell regrowth in the liver caused by HCV over time leads to growth of new abnormal (cancerous) cells. It's as if the liver eventually exhausts its ability to create new, healthy cells. It is known that HCC appears to develop only in persons with HCV who also have cirrhosis. Once cirrhosis from chronic HCV infection develops, the annual risk of HCC is 1 to 4 percent.

HCC is usually discovered during testing for other liver conditions such as cirrhosis. It may show up on an imaging test or blood test. It is thought that this form of liver cancer may be prevented or slowed with interferon treatment, whether or not the person's HCV responded well to the treatment. Currently, the best treatment for HCC is surgical removal of the cancerous portion of the liver *(hepatectomy)*. Larger tumors can be treated with other medications or *chemotherapy* (use of strong chemicals) to stop or slow the growth or spread of the cancer. Sometimes a liver transplant is also considered.

Immune system problems. Some people with chronic hepatitis C also develop other conditions as a result of their damaged immune systems. Some of these conditions include *essential mixed cryoglobulinemia* (EMS), rheumatoid arthritis, *lichen planus*, kidney disease *(glomerulonephritis)*, and other immune system disorders.

Using Your Knowledge to Protect Your Health

With such a litany of problems associated with hepatitis C, it may seem like the only option is to crawl into a corner and wait for the end to come. But many people with HCV have seen this challenge or "bump" in their lives as an opportunity to take charge of their health and well-being. The place to start is to learn more about the disease and how it can affect you. This knowledge can help keep you alive— and make your life more fulfilling. If you need more convincing, you have only to hop onto the Internet and visit one of hundreds of web sites devoted to hepatitis C (see *Chapter 7*) to realize that people with this disease have found power both in knowledge and in sharing their hard-learned experiences with others in hopes of empowering them as well. And once you know what you're up against, you can go on to the next step: taking control of your treatment.

PART II
TREATING HCV

"I try to teach others that they are the ones in control of their own life and that they can do anything they put their minds to. Of course I do not tell them they will be cured or a miracle will happen, but only make them aware that if they just sit back and wait to die, then that's probably what will happen. I want everyone to have the courage to fight for their health and well-being, and not to be afraid of what the future holds."

—Nutritional counselor, Tennessee

Whether you have hepatitis C or not, these words go to the heart of what treatment of HCV or any chronic health condition is all about. What do you normally think of when you hear the word "treatment"? Cure, perhaps? Probably medication. Maybe surgery. That's what most of us have in mind when thinking about the potential treatment for any given health problem. But for a condition such as hepatitis C where a "cure" is infrequent, treatment means more than that. When dealing with chronic conditions such as hepatitis C, treatment is a long-term proposition, more like a love–hate intimate relationship with the disease rather than an all-out assault in an attempt to overcome it. And the responsibility of confronting HCV rests primarily with you. A contingent of doctors, nurses, counselors, and other health care professionals can all assist you, of course, but in the end, it's up to you to take control of your own health. Perhaps that's why the National Institutes of Health wisely titled their consensus paper the *Management of Hepatitis C*. Everyone recognizes that treatment of this serious disease requires a broad-based approach.

Start along this path of controlling your own health by reshaping how you view your treatment. More than simply thinking about cures, medications, and procedures, remember that treatment (management) goals for hepatitis C include a range of possible options. Some goals may be more appropriate for you than others—and your goals may even change over time. Here are some typical treatment goals to keep in mind:

Cure of the disease. Of course, this is the one treatment goal everyone hopes for—and that researchers are striving to achieve as they try to develop vaccines and antiviral drugs to combat HCV (see *Chapter 4*). But even without ways to cure HCV, some fortunate people lose all signs of the hepatitis C virus within about six months of infection. These people may never even know that they were infected with the virus. Another group of people totally clear the virus from their systems after treatment with strong medications for up to two years.

Remission of HCV. For some people, treatments (such as interferon) may suppress the virus and eliminate symptoms (*remission*). In most cases, the virus doesn't completely leave your system, and in fact might

Hepatitis C Treatment Goals

- Cure
- Remission
- Prevention or delay of liver damage
- Maintaining adequate liver function
- Alleviation of symptoms
- Elimination of infectiousness
- General health maintenance

return if treatment is discontinued. However, suppression of the virus —even temporarily—can probably slow down liver damage.

Prevention or delay of liver damage. Even if some treatments don't rid your body of HCV as hoped, there is evidence that at least these treatments seem to slow down damage to the liver. In addition, there are many other steps you can take to keep unnecessary stress off your liver. These will be discussed in the chapters that follow.

Maintaining adequate liver function. If you're like many people with HCV, by the time the disease is discovered, some liver damage may have already occurred. Even so, a range of treatments can often help preserve adequate function of your liver for many years. If your liver fails, which happens in a small percentage of persons with chronic hepatitis C, a liver transplant is an option to consider.

Alleviating any symptoms. If you have noticeable symptoms from chronic hepatitis or related problems, there is a lot you can do to gain relief. This is where working closely with your doctor and other health care professionals is critical. Make sure they know about any symptoms you may be having. Don't simply assume that you have to live with symptoms.

Elimination of infectiousness. If treatment is effective in eliminating HCV from circulation in your blood, there should be no risk of infecting others.

General health maintenance. The healthier you are overall, the less strain you place on your liver. There are many steps you can take to maintain your health, including having regular exams by your doctor, eating a diet that encourages the health of your liver, and getting enough exercise. These steps are described in the following chapters.

It's Up to You

Knowledge about HCV and its treatment is changing constantly. And help in combating this disease comes from many sources, some traditional, some not. The only way to ensure that you are getting the best care possible is for you to personally take responsibility for your health.

Taking Charge of Your Health Means

- Learning as much as you can about HCV.

- Accepting responsibility to coordinate your health care.

- Investigating new and alternative treatments.

- Keeping your health care providers informed about all your symptoms and treatments.

This doesn't mean ignoring your doctor's advice or foregoing traditional medical treatment. Rather, it means staying on top of the latest information about HCV and pursuing all options to see if they are appropriate for you. It also means making sure you keep your doctor and any other health care professionals you see informed about your health, including any symptoms you notice and all the steps you are taking to improve your health.

These next few chapters can help. First, we'll describe briefly the ways HCV is diagnosed, confirmed, and monitored. Then we'll take a look at a range of treatments to consider, including medical, surgical, and so-called "alternative" therapies. Finally, we'll outline other steps you can take to maintain your health and list resources for support and more information.

DIAGNOSING AND MONITORING HCV

CHAPTER 3

"I'd given up on any real diagnosis. I went to a doctor for separated ribs a few months ago, and he suggested an ultrasound scan of the liver and the HCV tests, then referred me to a liver specialist."

—44-year-old man with hepatitis C

Many—if not most—people are surprised when they find out they have hepatitis C. After all, not many of us go into the doctor's office asking to be tested for this disease. Most people find out about the diagnosis by accident: from blood tests done for an annual physical or while donating blood, for example. Some people learn of their diagnosis after going to the doctor because of unusual symptoms such as a flu that doesn't seem to go away. Instead of finding out they have mononucleosis or are just under a lot of stress, they come away learning they have a serious, potentially life-threatening condition.

Blood Tests Are the Key to Diagnosis

Just how does a diagnosis of HCV arise in the first place? And how can you be sure the doctor is right about it? An initial, tentative diagnosis of liver problems or, specifically, of hepatitis C can result from the following blood tests:

• **EIA-2 and EIA-3 (second- and third-generation enzyme immunoassay) blood tests** are simple, inexpensive, sensitive and highly accurate. They check for antibodies to HCV (anti-HCV) and can detect them beginning at 8 to 9 weeks after exposure. Remember, antibodies are manufactured by your body in response to a foreign invader. If antibodies to HCV are found, this means that you were exposed in some way and may carry the virus. Note, though, that this test does not actually detect the hepatitis C virus itself. That's why follow-up testing should be done if the EIA comes back "positive" (that is, anti-HCV was found). There are several versions of the EIA test. Even more sensitive and accurate tests should be available soon.

• **ALT (alanine aminotransferase) levels** are often measured in routine blood testing and sometimes as part of a group of tests referred to as *liver function tests*. The test for ALT used to be called the SGPT. ALT is an *enzyme* found in liver cells. When the liver is damaged, ALT escapes out into the blood. Therefore, high ALT levels in the blood usually indicate some sort of liver problem. However, the opposite is not true—a low ALT does not mean the liver is healthy. Generally ALT levels rise 4 to 6 weeks after HCV infection. However, approximately one-third of people with HCV have normal ALT blood levels. Also,

Tests to Diagnose HCV Infection

- EIA and bDNA to detect HCV antibodies
- ALT or AST to help detect liver problems
- RIBA to confirm the presence of HCV antibodies
- HCV RNA to confirm the presence of HCV itself

the ALT level in the blood can dramatically shift from one time to the next, even from abnormal to normal levels. Therefore, ALT is one indication of liver problems, but other testing (such as the EIA test) needs to be done to confirm the problem and the extent of liver damage.

• **AST (aspartate aminotransferase) levels** are also measured in routine blood testing. This test used to be called the SGOT. Like ALT, AST is an enzyme found in liver cells. It can escape out into the blood when the liver is damaged. But it can also leak out from muscle tissue, including the heart. This means that a high AST level in and of itself does not necessarily mean there is a liver problem. It can signal other problems as well, such as a heart attack. If AST levels suggest a possible liver problem, additional testing should be done.

If an initial diagnosis of hepatitis C is made on the basis of one or more of these blood test results, follow-up testing should almost always be performed, especially if you are at low risk for becoming infected by HCV. One of the following is usually done to confirm the diagnosis:

• **RIBA-2 or RIBA-3 (recombinant immunoblot assay),** like EIA, detects antibodies to HCV, but does not detect the virus itself.

• **HCV RNA by RT-PCR (reverse transcription polymerase chain reaction)** tests blood for the presence of the hepatitis C virus itself, and can identify the virus starting 1 to 2 weeks after infection. RT-PCR is the most accurate way to check for HCV, but results vary greatly between labs.

• **HCV RNA by bDNA (branched chain DNA)** tests blood for the presence of HCV as well. It is easier to perform, but less sensitive to low levels of the virus than RT-PCR.

In addition to these initial blood tests, your doctor should conduct a thorough health evaluation. He or she will ask you questions about your health and behaviors to see if you have symptoms or risks associated with hepatitis C or problems with similar symptoms. You'll also receive a complete physical exam to assess your general health status.

If you have hepatitis C, your doctor should request genotype testing. Knowing the genotype helps guide treatment decisions, such as how long to continue interferon therapy.

Assessing the Health of Your Liver

Once your doctor has determined that you have hepatitis C, the next step is to assess your liver's health. This will help determine your treatment goals. A variety of tests are done to assess the liver. Your doctor may ask you to have some of these tests repeated periodically.

Liver function tests (LFTs) are a series of blood tests that measure a range of substances normally found in the liver. We'll describe the tests most likely to be given in order to monitor problems related to hepatitis C.

- **ALT and AST levels** may be measured routinely. High levels of these enzymes indicate possible liver damage. Remember, though, that you can have a normal ALT level and still have liver inflammation, and high AST levels can sometimes be signs of problems with the heart or muscles, not the liver.

- **Alkaline phosphatase and GGT or GGTP (gamma-glutamyltranspeptidase)** levels may also be measured routinely. Elevated levels of these enzymes may indicate some sort of blockage in the common bile duct or within the smaller bile ducts inside the liver itself. This blockage could be due to scarring (cirrhosis) or a tumor, for example.

- **Bilirubin** is the bile pigment that causes yellowing of the skin and eyes (jaundice). It is created when red blood cells break down. The liver processes these cells, then secretes the bilirubin into the bile. If the liver is unable to process bilirubin, it accumulates in the blood, where it can be measured by a blood test.

Tests to Assess Liver Health

- Liver function tests (blood tests)
- Imaging studies (ultrasound, CT, MRI)
- Liver biopsy

- **Albumin** is a protein synthesized in the liver. If the liver is damaged, it cannot produce enough albumin. Hence, lower levels of albumin in the blood are a sign of liver damage.

- **Prothrombin time (Protime or PT)** is a test to determine how long it takes for your blood to clot. Labs now often report results as an International Normalized Ratio (INR). The liver makes *clotting factors*, the proteins used for blood clotting. If the liver is damaged, fewer clotting factors are made and it takes longer for your blood to clot.

- **Other blood tests** may be done to assess your liver function, depending on your own situation. Ask your doctor to explain these tests to you.

Imaging studies (ultrasound, CT, or MRI scans) may be done to aid in the assessment of your liver health. These images can indicate whether the liver is enlarged and may show whether there is any scarring or sign of cancer.

Liver biopsy is still considered the best way to assess liver damage and determine the need for treatment. It can help determine how much inflammation and fibrosis (scar tissue) is present. But liver biopsy isn't to be considered lightly. It's costly, requires a skilled physician to get best results, and does have risks associated with it. To make matters worse, there aren't consistent guidelines for when a biopsy is most useful; however, the NIH's *Consensus Development Statement on the Management of Hepatitis C* recommends that biopsy be considered in these circumstances:

- In a person with high ALT levels, a positive EIA result, and a positive confirmatory testing result (RIBA-2 or HCV RNA)

- In a person with repeatedly high ALT levels and a positive EIA result

- In any person for whom therapy with interferon or other antiviral drugs is being considered

The biopsy should be done by an experienced physician. This is usually a gastroenterologist, hepatologist, surgeon, transplant surgeon, or

---

Questions to Ask Your Doctor About Biopsy

- How will the biopsy help you with my care?
- What technique do you use for the biopsy?
- How much experience do you have in performing biopsies?
- Where is the procedure done?
- What should I expect during the procedure?
- What should I expect after the procedure?
- Will I be able to go home the same day?
- What are the risks of this procedure?
- Will you give me medication for any pain?
- When will you discuss the results of the biopsy with me?

---

radiologist. The procedure is usually done at an outpatient surgical center or as an inpatient at the hospital. During the biopsy, a small tissue sample is obtained from the liver, then examined for signs of liver disease. Risks of biopsy vary, depending on the method used. General risks include bleeding, accidental puncture of other organs, and leakage of bile if the gallbladder is accidentally punctured. The risk of death ranges from 0.1% to 0.01%, making this a relatively low-risk procedure. Ask your doctor about other risks you should be aware of. Several biopsy methods can be used to obtain the sample:

- **Needle biopsy**. Most commonly, a needle is quickly inserted into the liver after the skin and underlying tissues have been anesthetized. Sometimes the physician uses ultrasound or CT (computed tomography) to help determine the ideal location for the needle.

- **Surgical biopsy**. The biopsy may be done through either traditional open surgery or laparoscopic surgery (where small instruments are inserted through tiny abdominal incisions).

- **Transvenous biopsy**. If you have problems with bleeding or if your abdomen is swollen, a transvenous (transjugular) biopsy may be done by a radiologist. A small tube (catheter) is inserted into the jugular vein in your neck and guided into the vein in the liver. Once in the liver, a needle is inserted through the catheter and a tissue sample is removed.

After the procedure, you will be monitored for a few hours to make sure there are no complications. In most cases, unless open surgery was performed or unless you are being monitored in the hospital, you can go home the same day as the procedure.

After the biopsy, you may have some pain at the site of the needle insertion or incision. You may also notice pain in your right shoulder, caused by the pressure on and disturbance of the nerves in the abdomen and liver. If the procedure was done laparoscopically, you may have bloating and gas afterward (gas is used to expand the abdominal cavity to provide for easier viewing of and access to the liver). Ask your doctor about medication for any pain you may feel.

Just because a biopsy sounds scary, don't write it off. Biopsies can be invaluable in assessing your liver status and planning your treatment. If you have been diagnosed with HCV, biopsy is worth considering. Talk to your doctor about your concerns. Weigh the risks and benefits. Find out how a biopsy can aid in planning your treatment. Then make your decision—an informed decision based on what's best for you.

Determining Your Treatment Plan

After diagnosing HCV and assessing the health of your liver, you and your doctor can work together to develop a treatment plan appropriate to your needs. Treatments may include medication, surgery, and "nonmedical" steps such as eating a well-balanced diet, getting regular exercise, and trying alternative therapies. Medical and surgical treatments are usually recommended if

- ALT levels are high for more than six months
- EIA results are positive

When Seeing Your Doctor

. . . or any other health care provider, follow these tips to get the
most out of your appointment:

- *Before the appointment, write down any questions you have.*
  There's nothing more frustrating than walking out of the
  office and suddenly remembering an important question
  you forgot to ask!

- *Take a pencil and paper with you.* Write down any instructions or information you want to remember. You can even
  ask the doctor or nurse to write it down for you.

- *Don't be afraid to ask questions.* If you don't understand
  something, ask the doctor to explain it again.

- *Consider bringing someone you trust with you.* This person
  can ask any questions you might have forgotten or can be
  a second set of ears to help you remember any instructions you're supposed to follow.

- HCV RNA testing, such as RT-PCR or bDNA tests that measure the actual amount of virus present, confirms the presence of HCV

- A liver biopsy shows chronic hepatitis

If you are interested in treatments your doctor has not mentioned, be
sure to ask about them. Provide as much information about alternative therapies to your doctor as possible, even if he or she does not seem
enthused about these proposed treatments.

To find out more about the range of treatments for hepatitis C, read on.
Chapter 4 describes the medical and surgical therapies available to treat
hepatitis C, including interferon therapy and liver transplantation.
Chapter 5 presents information about so-called "alternative" therapies,
while *Chapter 6* describes the role of diet and exercise.

MEDICAL AND SURGICAL TREATMENTS FOR HEPATITIS C

CHAPTER 4

"I have not done interferon, as I did not feel it was the right choice for me."

"I just started on interferon and have no opinion, other than it is not fun."

"I was a partial responder to interferon and a complete responder to interferon and ribavirin."

—Perspectives on interferon medical therapy
from three persons with HCV

Get sick, take a pill. If you're really ill, you may need an operation. That's how most of us are used to dealing with disease and illness. And for many health problems, that's pretty much what happens. However, unlike treatments for many other health problems, medication and surgery currently make up a relatively small part of the treatment for hepatitis. This is true for most forms of the disease, and is especially the case with hepatitis C. In fact, only two medications are approved for use in treating hepatitis C: interferon and ribavirin. These drugs, as well as most other currently being studied, are considered *antivirals*, since they work by directly attacking the virus responsible for the disease, in this case HCV. We'll describe what interferon and ribavirin are, how they work, who benefits from them, and side effects you should know about. Then we'll discuss other medications that are currently being tested for treating hepatitis C as well as other treatments you may want to consider under certain circumstances. Finally, we'll talk about liver transplantation and when it might be needed.

Interferon

Interferon is a protein normally produced by the body's cells during the immune response, but which may be generated in lesser amounts by people infected with HCV. Interferon is actually created by the cells that are infected with the virus. Somehow, interferon "sticks" to healthy cells to protect them from becoming infected. There are three types of interferon—*alpha interferon, beta interferon,* and *gamma interferon.* Synthetic versions of these body proteins are used to combat several types of cancer and diseases thought to be caused by viruses, such as multiple sclerosis, rheumatoid arthritis, and hepatitis C.

Alpha interferon was the first drug approved by the U.S. Food and Drug Administration (FDA) to treat hepatitis C. It is also used to treat hepatitis B, as well as genital warts (an STD), some AIDS-related diseases, and several types of cancer. No one knows exactly how alpha interferon works, but there are three effects it creates:

- It keeps a virus from replicating (duplicating) itself in other cells

- It keeps some tumor cells from growing

- It helps T cells fight the virus more effectively

Three types of alpha interferon are currently approved by the Food and Drug Administration. The first to be approved (and also approved to treat hepatitis B) is interferon alfa-2b (Intron A), manufactured by Schering. Interferon alfa-2a (Roferon-A), manufactured by Roche, is approved for use in hepatitis C only. Interferon alfacon-1 (Infergen) by Amgen is a synthetic consensus interferon. It combines pieces of various natural interferons in hopes that the end product can be more effective with fewer side effects. Other forms of interferon are currently being tested and may also receive approval.

Candidates for Interferon Therapy

Interferon is a powerful drug, but is only effective under certain conditions. This means that only about half of all people diagnosed with HCV are appropriate candidates for therapy with interferon. And of the persons who undergo interferon therapy, a fairly low percent will respond positively. Although treatment criteria are not clear cut, the National Institutes of Health *Consensus Development Statement on the Management of Hepatitis C* recommends the following criteria be used in determining who should try interferon therapy:

- If you are at greatest risk for developing cirrhosis. This includes persons with consistently high ALT levels, a positive PCR test, and a liver biopsy that shows signs of scarring or at least moderate inflammation and cell death.

- If you have acute hepatitis. Interferon treatment at this acute stage often keeps persons from developing chronic hepatitis.

- If you have a condition called essential mixed cryoglobulinemia, which seems to be caused by HCV. Levels of cryoglobulin (a substance involved in the body's immune response) in the blood rise, restricting blood flow, especially to the arms and legs. Symptoms include cold hands and feet, liver inflammation, and fatigue.

- If you also have HIV, but are relatively healthy.

- If you have consistently high ALT levels but little liver damage. If you fall into this category, you could consider interferon therapy now, or wait and in the meanwhile monitor ALT levels, and repeat liver biopsies every 3–5 years.

- Other groups of persons with HCV should consider interferon, but the recommendation is less clear since there isn't much data addressing the use of interferon in people with few symptoms or little liver damage, or in children under 18 years of age and adults over 60. If you have cirrhosis but no serious effects such as jaundice or abdominal swelling, are under age 18, or are over age 60, be sure to discuss interferon use with your doctor.

If you drink excessive amounts of alcohol or use injection drugs, you should not undertake interferon therapy unless alcohol or drug use has been stopped for at least six months. It is also probably not wise to undergo interferon therapy if you are on methadone treatment for overcoming heroin addiction. Others for whom interferon therapy is generally not recommended include persons who have had major depressive illnesses, certain blood problems (low levels of certain types of blood cells), hyperthyroidism, kidney transplant, or another autoimmune disease. If you have one of these conditions and still want to try interferon, it's recommended that you undergo treatment in a clinical trial, which is highly supervised.

Weighing the Disadvantages and Advantages of Interferon

Before electing to try interferon—or any other treatment—you need to consider both the risks and benefits of the therapy. In some cases, the risks are worth it. In other cases, the disadvantages may lead you to choose not to have a particular treatment. For interferon, the disadvantages and advantages are as follows:

Disadvantages/Risks	Advantages/Benefits
Serious side effects	Possible cure
Reactivation of liver disease	Possible remission
Need to self-inject	Possible delay in progression
High cost	of liver disease

Add your own thoughts to this list, discuss these with your doctor and others who have tried interferon therapy, and make a thoughtful decision that is in your best interest.

For all other persons with HCV, whether or not to try interferon therapy is really a personal decision to be made after serious discussion with your physician. Three factors that may make interferon treatment more effective include the following:

- Having genotype 2 or 3 usually requires a shorter treatment course and shows substantially higher rates of success than having genotype 1.

- People who start off with lower HCV levels tend to have lower rates of relapse after interferon therapy.

- Patients with only slight liver damage and no cirrhosis respond better to treatment.

Other factors that may make treatment more successful include:

- Being at your "normal" body weight

- Being female

- A younger age

- Short duration of infection

- Lower iron levels

Also keep in mind that treatment may slow the progression of liver disease no matter what your response to interferon initially may be. These factors make whether to try interferon a decision that merits careful consideration and discussion.

What Happens During Interferon Therapy?

Usually, alpha interferon (2a or 2b) is injected under the skin three times a week. Standard therapy had been for six months, but treatment is usually continued for up to two years. If a person receiving interferon doesn't respond within three months, treatment is usually discontinued. It may be later restarted at a higher dose, a different dosage schedule (such as every day), or with a different type of interferon. Response to interferon is measured by testing ALT and HCV levels in the blood. Other blood tests should also be done periodically to check for side effects and other possible problems.

For most people, interferon therapy will lower ALT levels to normal and reduce HCV levels as long as the treatment continues. When treatment continues for 12 to 24 months, as many as 20 to 30 percent of those treated are potentially cured, that is, their body is rid of HCV. For some people, ALT levels drop for a few weeks, then rise again. In others, HCV disappears from circulation, but some virus still remains in the liver. But even if treatment does not permanently chase the virus away, there is evidence that people whose ALT levels remain high despite interferon therapy may have a slower progression of liver damage as a result of the treatment.

If you try interferon therapy and have no initial positive response, or you have an initial response that dissipates after therapy has ended, retreatment is an option. You may receive different dosages, take interferon for a longer time, have a daily dosing schedule, use a different type of interferon, or receive interferon along with another drug.

Unfortunately, side effects from interferon therapy are common and often severe. Most common are flu-like symptoms, which occur within six to eight hours after injection. These include fever, chills, headaches, muscle and joint pain, fatigue, rapid heart rate, and weakness. Usually these symptoms go away after the first few treatments and can be treated with *acetaminophen* (Tylenol) or a nonsteroidal anti-inflammatory drug. Symptoms can also be lessened by taking interferon at night. Other symptoms that occur as treatment continues include the following:

- Depression
- Apathy, anxiety, drowsiness, confusion, irritability, and cognitive changes
- Suicidal tendencies
- Difficulty sleeping
- Hair loss
- Fatigue, malaise, nausea

Terms You May Hear

Viral load: The amount of HCV RNA detected in blood tested by RT-PCR or bDNA.

Response to treatment: After 12 weeks of treatment, ALT levels are normal or HCV RNA is undetectable.

End-of-treatment response (ETR): Positive response to interferon treatment. By the end of the 12- to 24-month course of treatment, ALT levels are normal and the PCR test detects no HCV RNA.

Sustained response (SR or SR-6): ETR is maintained for at least six months after therapy has ended.

Relapse: After treatment ends, ALT increases and the PCR test detects HCV RNA.

Nonresponse: Despite treatment, ALT levels do not return to normal and the PCR test continues to detect HCV RNA.

- Muscle aches, headache, or other pain
- Thyroid problems
- Seizures
- Diarrhea
- Suppression of bone marrow production

If side effects are severe, the dose can be reduced; however, the treatment then may not be as effective in lowering ALT and HCV RNA levels.

Another potential problem arising from interferon therapy is the development of neutralizing antibodies to the drug. These antibodies develop in response to the interferon and can make the drug less effective. It makes sense when you think about it. The alpha interferon substances created by the pharmaceutical companies are very close to—but not exactly the same as—human alpha interferon. The body may begin to treat these drugs just as if they were any other foreign invader, creating antibodies to the synthetic alpha interferon that help attack and disable it. This makes the drug less and less effective and may cause an increase in side effects. Some companies hope that interferon created from human cells will pose less of a risk of developing neutralizing antibodies.

Despite the low rate of total remission and the potential for side effects, many people have decided that trying interferon therapy is worth it. If interferon therapy is an option for you, weigh the risks and benefits carefully, discuss your concerns with your doctor, talk to others who have undergone the treatment if possible, and then make an informed decision. If you are concerned about the cost of interferon therapy and it is not covered by your health insurance, check with the manufacturer. You may qualify for programs to help pay for the treatment.

Combination Therapies

Besides interferon, no single therapy has been used successfully to treat hepatitis C. Instead, these medications are added to the interferon treatment regimen, resulting in two- or three-drug combinations.

Ribavirin (Rebetrol) is an antiviral drug originally approved for use in viral pneumonia and now also approved for treating hepatitis C. Use of ribavirin alone seems to cause ALT levels to drop during treatment, but they rise again afterward. However, levels of HCV RNA do not change. When ribavirin is used along with interferon, sustained response (normal ALT and negative HCV RNA levels) may be more than two times

What About Drug Costs?

Drugs used to treat hepatitis C can be very expensive—and many patients understandably resent these costs. For example, interferon can run up to $8,000 or more per year. But these high prices are not usually attributable to corporate greed. The drug development and approval process on average takes about 15 years. Since the 22-year patent protection begins at the start of drug testing, this leaves the pharmaceutical company with only seven years to recoup their expensive initial investment before competitors can develop and offer "me too" drugs at much lower costs.

higher than when interferon is used alone. Side effects of ribavirin include anemia, dry mouth, nausea, indigestion, fatigue, mood swings and rashes. Currently, ribavirin is available only in combination with Schering's interferon, Intron A. This combination therapy is called Rebetron. Ribavirin is taken orally every day, while interferon is injected into the skin usually three times a week.

Amantadine and rimantadine are antiviral drugs that are approved to treat certain types of flu (influenza A) and Parkinson's disease. Both help keep viruses from entering the body's cells. Used alone, neither has been shown to reduce ALT levels in a sustained fashion. However, they may help make interferon and interferon/ribavirin therapy more effective, although use of these drugs remain experimental and long-term response is still unknown. Side effects include insomnia, dizziness, dry mouth, confusion, concentration problems, blotchy skin, constipation, cardiovascular problems, and depression.

Experimental Treatments

New drugs to treat hepatitis C are available only if you participate in a *clinical trial*. Clinical trials are tests on humans conducted to determine whether a drug is both safe and effective in treating a particular condition. Clinical trials are usually one of the last stages in drug development before FDA approval. Some of the drugs described below have not yet received FDA approval; some physicians will prescribe an existing drug for you even though it has not been approved specifically to treat hepatitis C. To add new indications for use of existing drugs, the manufacturer must submit appropriate documentation to the FDA. Following are descriptions of some of the drugs—both new and existing (but approved for other uses)—that are currently under investigation for use in treating hepatitis C.

Beta interferon is manufactured by several companies. It is injected under the skin or into muscle tissue. Like alpha interferon, each type of beta interferon comes from a different source (such as certain bacteria, Chinese hamster ovary cells, or human cells). Beta interferon is already approved for use in treating multiple sclerosis. Clinical trials are in progress to determine whether it is useful in treating hepatitis C. Side effects are similar to alpha interferon, including the chance of developing neutralizing antibodies.

Immune globulin is currently used to help prevent hepatitis A. So far, its effectiveness in preventing or treating hepatitis C has not been proven. However, it may help prevent hepatitis C in persons who receive an organ transplant. Note, though, that immune globulin is not intended to eliminate hepatitis C in persons who already have the virus and receive a liver transplant.

Other types of interferon, such as alfa-n1, alfa-n3, leukocyte, or lymphoblastoid interferons, are types of "natural" interferon, created from human cells.

Ketoprofen is a nonsteroidal anti-inflammatory drug (NSAID) that is available over-the-counter as Orudis and Actron. It is thought that ketoprofen may help reduce liver inflammation and ALT levels.

Pegylated (PEG) interferon is a slow-release, long-acting form of interferon alfa-2a or alfa-2b. It is hoped that this form can help reduce the fluctuating effects found in the typical three-times-per-week interferon dosage schedule. PEG interferon is now being tested in humans.

Protease inhibitors block viruses from replicating themselves. The N53 protease has been identified as a key enzyme in HCV replication. If this enzyme could be "deactivated," replication of the virus could not occur. With this theory in mind, several substances are under development that target this protease.

Thymosin alpha-1 is an immunomodulating agent (that is, it affects the body's immune response). It has been used in small trials with humans and seems to be effective in reducing ALT levels to normal in some people when used in combination with interferon. Studies are continuing to assess thymosin alpha-1's potential use in treating hepatitis C.

Continued research in understanding how HCV affects the body yields new ideas for drugs. For example, cytokines are special cells that help control the body's immune response. As researchers learn more about how certain types of cytokines work—or don't—to control HCV, they can then look for new compounds that enhance the action of these

The FDA Drug Development Process

Before they can be used in the U.S., drugs must undergo a rigorous approval process through the FDA. New drugs and existing drugs intended to be used for a new purpose must receive FDA approval before they can be marketed.

Steps in the drug development process include the following:

- Isolation and description of the substance to be tested.

- Analysis of the drug's action and toxicity in animals.

- Application to the FDA to evaluate the drug in humans. In order to have the request approved, the researchers have to submit extensive protocols (exact plans for how the drug will be tested).

- Testing to determine the maximum dose and any toxic effects (phase I trials). Persons enrolled in these early human studies may have already unsuccessfully undergone other therapies. The level of the drug is increased until intolerable side effects are noted.

- Testing to determine if the drug has any therapeutic effects in treating a particular disease (phase II trials). Persons in these studies are often very ill, with no other treatment options available to them.

- Testing to compare the safety and efficacy of the drug to other standard treatments (phase III trials). These tests are done on larger groups of people. They usually include a control group (who receives no treatment or a placebo, a treatment that will not affect them in any way), a group receiving standard treatment, and a group receiving the new treatment.

- FDA approval comes after all test results have been reviewed and a recommendation has been made by a committee of experts in the particular disease.

can then look for new compounds that enhance the action of these cytokines.

In addition, several companies are working toward developing a vaccine to protect against hepatitis C. A vaccine is a preparation manufactured from a weakened or disabled virus that can't infect you but enables your immune system to create antibodies that protect from future infection. No vaccine currently exists for hepatitis C. Chiron Corporation and Ciba-Geigy Corporation are two companies currently involved in developing a vaccine.

If you have hepatitis C and are interested in participating in any of the clinical trials, you should know that trials are usually conducted at university-based medical centers or large urban hospitals. Costs of participating are covered by the sponsoring organization, usually a pharmaceutical company. The trials include extensive testing and close monitoring. Clinical trials can be a great way to be involved in unique therapies—although you must accept that you may fall into the *control group* (the group receiving the placebo) or the group receiving standard therapy. Just as important is the feeling you get from helping to contribute to our knowledge about hepatitis C and its treatment. The best way to become involved in a clinical trial is to ask your doctor about trials in your area, or contact the American Liver Foundation for a list of current trials (see Resources).

Other Treatments for Hepatitis C

Besides the use of interferon and investigational drugs to treat hepatitis C, there are several other treatments that may be appropriate for you in some circumstances. Be sure to talk with your doctor about any of these treatments. Some of these treatments offer more promise than others.

Iron reduction. We've all heard about the importance of having enough iron in the blood. You may even recall unpleasant incidents when your great Aunt Bessie insisted on feeding you calf's liver because she thought you looked "anemic." However, people with hepatitis C are likely to have the opposite problem—too much iron in the blood. You see, not only is iron needed for your cells to remain healthy and continue reproducing, but viruses also rely on iron for the same reason. Normally in people who are fighting off viral infections, one of your the body's responses is to reduce the amount of iron in your blood—an effort to sort of "starve" the virus. But many people with hepatitis don't seem to have this drop in their iron levels. In addition, some researchers have noted that people who respond best to interferon treatment have lower iron levels. Furthermore, reducing iron levels also seems to help lower ALT levels, although it does not appear to lower HCV RNA levels. It may also make interferon therapy more effective.

So if iron reduction is so great, how do you go about doing it? Women may have a natural advantage since they tend to have lower iron levels due to menstruation. Drinking a lot of alcohol can actually raise iron levels, among other dangerous effects on your liver, so avoiding alcohol can help keep iron levels under control. If you are asked to reduce your iron intake, you should work with a dietitian to identify foods free of iron. You can also avoid iron cookware (iron can leach into the food you prepare in it). In severe cases, blood is periodically let out until iron levels become normal, a procedure called phlebotomy.

Anti-inflammatories. Several nonsteroidal anti-inflammatory medications, such as tenoxicam, ketoprofen, and aspirin, as well as herbs with anti-inflammatory properties, may be used to help reduce inflammation by interfering with the body's ability to use prostaglandin, a hormone involved in the anti-inflammatory reaction. They may also relieve other symptoms of hepatitis C, including side effects from interferon therapy. Side effects from anti-inflammatories include gastric ulcers.

Antioxidants. Seems like these days antioxidants are hailed as the latest cure for everything from dry skin to cancerous tumors. And it's no wonder. The more scientists learn about the role of antioxidants, the more potential uses they find for them. Inside your body, antioxidants cause dangerous substances to break apart or become inactivated before they can cause you any great harm. Some of these dangerous substances contribute to the growth of scar tissue (*fibrosis*) in the liver. Studies have shown the antioxidant vitamin E (alpha-tocopherol) re-

---

Summary of Treatments for Hepatitis C

Approved and/or accepted

- Interferon
- Ribavirin and interferon
- Vaccination against hepatitis A and hepatitis B
- Surgical procedures to treat complications
- Liver transplantation

Investigational and/or uncertain

- Amantadine or rimantadine and interferon
- Iron reduction
- Anti-inflammatories
- Antioxidants
- Hydrophilic bile salts
- Immunomodulating agents
- Investigational drugs

---

duces ALT levels and liver inflammation. Researchers don't know yet, though, whether this has any long-term effects on hepatitis C, cirrhosis, or liver cancer.

Hydrophilic bile salts. These medications, such as ursodeoxycholic acids (UDCA), have been used to treat gallstones and cirrhosis. These salts reduce chronic inflammation of the liver and also seem to reduce ALT levels. However, they do not appear to alter HCV RNA levels, even when taken in combination with interferon. Side effects are few, and include abdominal discomfort.

Immunomodulating agents. "Immunomodulating" is simply a big word meaning something that affects the immune system's response. Several of these agents have been used in limited trials to treat hepatitis C. Most substances have met with little positive response. Granulocyte/monocyte colony stimulating factor (GM-CSF) and isoprinosine are two examples. Other substances are still being tested to see if they may be effective against hepatitis C.

Other medications. You may be given other medications if you develop certain liver problems related to hepatitis C. For example, *lactulose* and *neomycin* are prescribed if ammonia levels in the blood get too high as a result of eating more protein than your liver can process, a problem that can occur with cirrhosis.

Surgical procedures. Surgical procedures may be done to help relieve certain complications resulting from hepatitis C. Shunting procedures may reroute blood that would otherwise back up at the liver when the portal vein becomes blocked due to scarring. Excessive buildup of fluid in the abdomen can be drained, usually by the insertion of a catheter.

Vaccinations. If you have hepatitis C, you should get vaccinated for both hepatitis A and hepatitis B. The combination of hepatitis C with either of these other forms of hepatitis can be deadly. Vaccinations have been shown to be safe and effective for people with hepatitis C.

Liver Transplantation

"I got the call at about 2:30 p.m., and I was in surgery in Gainesville by 5 p.m. They whizzed me in there. Even my kids didn't know. [After surgery] I had so much energy lying in that bed. I couldn't wait to get up because I knew I was going to fly. I celebrate my birthday twice a year now." That's how a Florida woman describes her 1993 liver transplant experience. Others who can personally relate to her experience include the singer David Crosby and motorcycle stuntman Evel Kneivel, both of whom have undergone liver transplants because of hepatitis C. Almost 12,000 people are awaiting liver transplants in the U.S. and up to 25 percent of these persons have hepatitis C. About 4,000 liver transplants are performed annually in the U.S.

Thankfully, most people with hepatitis C will never become sick enough to need a liver transplant. However, liver transplants can be one way to regain health when the liver is failing. The decision to have a transplant is not an easy one. First off, there is no guarantee that a liver will be available immediately. The surgery is expensive, and the risks are great. But for many people whose livers have failed, transplants have proven to give them new and active lives.

Transplants are recommended when it becomes clear that a person will not survive without the transplant. However, the transplant is usually done before the person becomes too ill to withstand the stress of surgery and recovery. Once a transplant is suggested, risks of the procedure are discussed with the patient and family. These risks include the following:

- Becoming too ill to have the transplant while waiting for a suitable donor.
- All the risks of any major surgery (such as bleeding, infection, and reaction to the anesthesia).
- Not having any liver function for a short time during surgery.
- The new (donor) liver may not work properly.
- The body may reject the "foreign" donor liver.

In addition, you must take a variety of medications to prevent infection and rejection of the new liver. It requires a lot of effort on the part of the patient and family to make a transplant successful. But if you need a transplant, the risks and effort are worth it. Most people (80 percent to 90 percent) survive the transplant procedure and leave the hospital,

The Great Need for Organ Donations

There are far more people needing liver and other organ transplants than there are available organs. Yet, according to a 1995 Gallup poll, 90 percent of respondents would give permission for donation of a deceased family member's organs if the family member would have discussed the donation previously. Health care professionals are often unlikely to bring up donation at such a painful time.

If you have hepatitis C, you are unable to donate your organs; however, you can certainly encourage your friends and family to consider it. If they wish to donate organs upon their death, they should make their decision known to other family members, as well as carry a written authorization for donation along with their driver's license. In many states, the Department of Motor Vehicles makes it easy to indicate the desire to be a donor right on your driver's license.

after having spent a few days in intensive care and one or two weeks having their progress carefully monitored in a less intensive setting. After that, the medical center may have you stay for a period of time in an apartment or hotel near the hospital if you live far away.

Even after you return home, if problems arise, such as infection or rejection, they can usually be treated with medication. If the new liver doesn't function fully, it may still work well enough for you to maintain a relatively normal lifestyle. Failed transplant livers can also be replaced. But the fact is, people who make it through the first year after a transplant usually survive many years thereafter.

One of the most bothersome aspects of living with a transplanted liver may be side effects from medication. Steroidal drugs similar to cortisone cause fluid retention and may lead to osteoporosis. Cyclosporine and tacrolimus (formerly FK-506; Prograf) are given to help prevent rejection. Cyclosporine may lead to high blood pressure, growth of body hair, and kidney problems. Tacrolimus may cause headaches, tremor, diarrhea, nausea, and kidney problems. Despite such side effects, about 80 percent of those people resume full activities in their lives.

Unfortunately, the new liver is not immune from infection by HCV. In fact, reinfection occurs in virtually all cases. However, as was probably the case when you first contracted HCV, it usually takes many years or decades before the new liver suffers serious problems caused by hepatitis C.

Monitoring Your Treatment Plan

Be sure to review your treatment plan periodically with your doctor. After all, this is one area in which many changes are likely to occur. As knowledge from AIDS drug research is applied to hepatitis C and more is learned about HCV itself, more effective agents are likely to be introduced over the next several years. For example, it is now believed that most people will need more than one drug to stop HCV, so there will be a growing emphasis on combination therapies. You can help by participating in clinical trials and by urging researchers and the FDA to place a higher priority on finding ways to combat this widespread disease. If you are interested in other therapies that may help, turn the page to *Chapter 5.*

"ALTERNATIVE" TREATMENTS FOR HEPATITIS C

CHAPTER 5

"With high worldwide incidence of viral hepatitis, further study of isolated phytochemicals is important in relation to the potential antiviral activity against the different hepatitis viruses."

—M. I. Thabrew and R. D. Hughes in "Phytogenic Agents in the Therapy of Liver Disease." *Phytotherapy Research.* September, 1996.

In other words, plants *are* important to the treatment of HCV. Botanical and other "alternative" treatments may finally be coming into their own, if for no other reason than that so few medical treatments are available for treating hepatitis C. To many people, though, when the term "alternative" is applied to a treatment, it automatically implies last-ditch quackery. In this book, we'll take a different approach. When we refer to "alternative treatments," we mean therapies that may not yet be totally accepted by the traditional Western medical community. This doesn't mean that these therapies have no merit. In fact, whenever you swallow a little pill, chances are great that the medication's origin is plant-related (phytochemical). Furthermore, a growing number of medical doctors recognize the importance of specific herbal or other alternative therapies in the treatment of hepatitis or its symptoms and complications, even if they don't subscribe to all of the underlying philosophy behind the alternative treatment.

Determining Whether a Therapy Will Work

One reason alternative therapies are looked down on by the Western medical community is that these therapies have often not been subjected to the same type of excruciatingly rigorous testing such as that required by the FDA for drug approval. To be considered scientifically valid, a treatment has to go through a series of clinical trials, usually of the double-blind, placebo-controlled, randomized variety, to prove that the therapy is both safe and effective. The goal is to control as many variables as possible to guarantee that any effects that were observed are directly attributable to the substances being studied.

In plain English, this means that researchers usually develop a complex protocol placing patients in one of three treatment groups. The characteristics of the participants in each group must be more or less the same—such as all participants having a similar health status. Participants are assigned to each group at random. Neither they nor the investigators know which treatment they are receiving ("double-blind"). One group, referred to as the control group, receives no treatment at all. To ensure the double-blind aspect of the trial, they receive a substance that looks similar to the substance being tested, but which will have no effect on their health (placebo). The second group receives the standard, already-accepted therapy. The third group receives the investigational substance. Throughout the study, appropriate tests are frequently conducted on each participant.

After the study, the results are analyzed. Researchers determine if the new therapy is better than no therapy at all and how it compares to the existing standard therapy. In addition, they want to identify side effects and other special information about the new therapy, such as whether it works better in certain types of patients than in others.

A Variety of Medical Traditions

Believe it or not, the Western world did not invent the concept of medical care. Several medical traditions have existed for hundreds or in some cases even thousands of years. These include the following:

- **Ayurvedic medicine** is a medical tradition that developed in India. Its philosophy and practices are similar to naturopathy, using diet, herbs, fasting, and yoga as its primary therapies.

- **Chinese medicine** is based on the concept of *qi* or *chi*, energy that flows throughout the universe and through all living organisms, including humans, as *yin* (dark energy) and *yang* (light energy). To maintain health, you need to have *chi* flowing freely, which means you need a balance between *yin* and *yang*. This balance is achieved when all of the organs are in balance, including the liver. When the balance is upset, certain therapies can be prescribed to help restore free-flowing *chi*, including the use of botanicals, acupuncture, massage, diet, and the practice of *chi kung* (*qi gong*), similar to *tai chi*.

- **Homeopathy** treats illness with substances that are similar to the illness itself, such as giving persons with hepatitis C medications that contain very low amounts of HCV. The goal is to stimulate the immune system to fight off the infection and allow the body to heal itself. Note that not only is this approach different from traditional Western medicine, it is *opposite*.

- **Naturopathic medicine** focuses on using natural means of healing, relying primarily on diet, fasting, and techniques such as yoga to promote healing. There are several naturopathic schools in the U.S.

Each tradition has something to offer the person with hepatitis C. But before madly dashing off to visit a practitioner of each, make sure you have a clear understanding of what to expect from the particular type of medicine and how it might work with any traditional medical treatments you may be undergoing.

Alternative therapies have not usually undergone this type of testing, for a couple of different reasons. First off, clinical trials are tedious, time-consuming, and incredibly expensive. Most alternative therapies don't have the backing of large, cash-flush pharmaceutical companies to fund such a venture. In addition, many health care professionals who practice alternative medicine question the necessity and validity of clinical trials. Sure, they prove whether or not a therapy is effective, but at what cost? In the meanwhile, potential help to sick patients is being denied. It may be that our reliance on science to determine the validity of a treatment is merely a Western culture-bound, short-sighted attitude. After all, even medications that have successfully survived clinical trials often rose to the attention of some physician or researcher because of anecdotal evidence of their effectiveness. And anecdotal evidence—individual reports of a therapy's effectiveness—as well as years of established tradition passed from practitioner to apprentice form the basis of acceptance of most alternative therapies.

Some alternatives have such strong anecdotal evidence that researchers are beginning to take a more serious look at them. In addition, respected scholars including plant biologists, pharmacologists, and osteopathic physicians form a sort of bridge between medical and alternative therapies. A lot of research is now being conducted to isolate plant substances that have therapeutic uses and to quantify the effects of such non-plant therapies as acupuncture. Slowly, it seems, the lines between traditional Western and alternative medicine are blurring.

Therapies with Plant Origins

We'll use the term "plant" loosely here and include the fungus family along with the "green stuff." Plants have been used for millennia throughout the world to alleviate symptoms and cure a range of ills. When it comes to treating hepatitis C, botanicals can have a direct effect on the disease or the virus, or they may help indirectly by aiding digestion or making it easier for the liver to do its job. In this context, herbs may be used that have the following effects:

- Reducing fever

- Aiding relaxation

- Killing viruses

- Reducing inflammation

- Increasing appetite

- Removing toxins

- Decreasing fluid retention

Botanicals (substances derived from plant sources) form an important component of naturopathic, Ayurvedic, and Chinese medicine. They are also increasingly being used in traditional Western medicine. Various plant substances slow the destruction of liver cells, normalize liver enzyme levels, restore the function of liver cells, reduce liver inflammation, restore immune system function, and can even destroy the causative virus. Let's take a look at some plants that seem to have a beneficial effect on the hepatitis virus itself, liver function in general, or specific symptoms or complications related to chronic hepatitis. These plants and fungi are listed in alphabetical order. Because there is sometimes conflicting information about using botanicals when you have liver problems, it's best to consult someone such as an herbalist or a physician with knowledge about herbal medicine before using herbs. They should carefully monitor your use. And always let all members of your health care team know about any herbs you may be using.

Aloe vera gel or powder from the plant is eaten to detoxify the body and enhance the immune system.

Alstonia scholaris **R. Br.** has lowered certain liver enzymes and affected liver cell inflammation and death in rats. Note that for this substance and others in which animal testing has occurred, hepatitis is usually induced in animals by administering a high dose of acetaminophen or carbon tetrachloride. This is only an approximation of hepatitis in humans, making animal studies a less than ideal model for understanding the plant's role in human hepatitis. However, it is one of the first steps toward documenting a substance's effectiveness in Western medical research tradition.

Artium lappa (burdock root, lappa, fox's clote, beggars buttons) is from Europe. It cleans the blood and liver and may boost the immune system.

Astralagus membranaceus (*huang chi*) roots may reduce fluid retention, increase energy, and boost the immune system.

Berberis vulgaris (barberry, pipperidge bush) bark may help the immune system destroy the virus.

Bupleurum chinense **DC** (Chinese bupleurum, *chai hu*, thorough wax) root is a Chinese herb that reduces fever and sweating and detoxifies the liver. It is recognized as the standard herbal therapy for hepatitis, to which other botanicals being tested are often compared.

Cascara sagrada (California buckthorn, sacred bark, chittem bark) from North America helps bile flow.

Chelidonium majus (garden celandine) leaves from Europe detoxify the liver and blood.

Cimicufuga racemosa (black cohosh, black snake root, bugbane) is a Native American medicine that may reduce fluid retention.

Citrus aurantum (*zhi ke*, bitter orange) is a Chinese herb that aids digestion and reduces constipation.

Cnicus benedictus (blessed thistle, holy thistle) helps relieve symptoms of acute hepatitis. It originates in southern Europe.

Coptis root (*huang lian*) is an another Chinese herb with antiviral and sedative effects.

"I became a strong believer in alternative therapies when my doctor told me I was terminal and he could not help me."

—Nutritional counselor

So Do You Just Pick the Leaves and Chew?

Definitely not! For one thing, different parts of the same plant can have dramatically different effects on your body, ranging from relieving your symptoms to releasing you from this world forever. Just as some plant substances seem to help hepatitis, others can actually induce hepatitis. The information about botanicals is provided here simply to give you a general sense of the range of possible botanical therapies. Work with a qualified health practitioner to select the treatments that are most appropriate for you, and make sure you purchase any herbs from a reputable source. Rather than being handed a bunch of leaves or roots, you'll probably take the botanical substance in some altered form. Powder, capsule, extract, and tea are four common formulations.

Cynara scolymus (artichoke) leaves, stem, or roots may help rid the body of excess fluid and aid liver cell regrowth.

Desmodium ascendens stems and leaves may protect liver cells. This herb comes from Africa.

Dioscorea paniculata (wild yam, colic root, rheumatism root) is an anti-inflammatory.

Echinacea angustifolia (purple coneflower, snakeroot) may help the immune response and reduces inflammation. This plant was used widely before the discovery of antibiotics.

Echinops grijisii is a Taiwanese folk remedy thought to help protect the liver.

Eclipta prostata (Linn.) is a folk remedy from Taiwan used to treat hepatitis. It has been tested in mice and rats with mixed results, depending on the cause of hepatitis.

Eleutherococcus senticosus (Siberian ginseng, touch-me-not, devil's bush)—NOT Asian ginseng (*Panax ginseng*), which may be toxic to persons with HCV. Siberian ginseng is a general tonic.

Fungus japonicus (kombucha) is a fungus used in China and central Europe to boost the immune system. Kombucha also contains antioxidants that may help protect the liver. It is used along with black or green tea to make a carbonated beverage or is taken in extract form.

Ganoderma lucidum and G. japonicum (reishi mushroom) is an overall energizer and increases the immune system's resistance to stress and disease. No side effects have been noted, except when used for longer than three to six months. Then, dizziness and digestive problems have occurred.

Garlic boosts the immune system and is an antioxidant.

Ginkgo biloba (maidenhair tree) may help relieve problems associated with hepatitis C, including concentration difficulties and circulation problems. It must be taken for several months before effects are noticeable.

Glycyrrhiza glabra (licorice, *gan t'sao'*) may be an effective botanical against flu-like symptoms associated with chronic *viral hepatitis* (hepatitis caused by viruses rather than from drugs).

Grifola frondosa is a mushroom that has been found to normalize liver enzyme levels in rats and has been used in humans as well. Before trying any mushroom-based remedy, be sure that you are working with a qualified practitioner. Many mushrooms are extremely toxic to the liver, quickly causing severe illness and death.

Hydrastis canadensis (goldenseal, puccon root, yellow root) may help with digestive problems associated with hepatitis.

Hypericum perforatum (St. John's wort) may have antiviral effects against HCV. It also reduces fluid retention.

Isatis root (*ban lan gen*) is a Chinese plant used to release toxins from the blood and reduce inflammation.

Larrea tridentata (chaparral) is an antiviral used for many conditions in addition to hepatitis. It may make hepatitis worse, so it's important to work with a qualified health professional when using this herb.

Ledebouriella divaricata (*fang feng*, sileris) is a Chinese herb that works on the immune system, relieving the flu-like symptoms of hepatitis as well as symptoms associated with rheumatoid arthritis.

Questions to Ask About Herbs

Before using any herbal preparation, make sure you know the answers to the following questions. Check with a qualified health professional or the company who manufactures the product.

- How will this herb affect my liver and my health?
- Will it interact with any other medications I'm taking?
- Should I avoid certain foods, drink, or medicines when using this herb?
- What are the side effects associated with this herb?

Lentinus erodus is a mushroom that has been found to normalize liver enzyme levels in rats and has been used in humans as well. Before trying any mushroom-based remedy, be sure that you are working with a qualified professional. Many mushrooms are extremely toxic to the liver, quickly causing severe illness and death.

Mahonia aquifolium (Oregon grape root) relieves symptoms of chronic hepatitis.

Paeonia lactiflora (peony root, *shao yao*) comes from Great Britain and is used to detoxify the liver and blood.

Panax quinquefolium (American ginseng, five fingers)—NOT Asian ginseng (*Panax ginseng*), which may be toxic to persons with HCV. American ginseng is a general tonic.

Peumus boldus (boldo) is native to Chile and used medicinally for a range of digestive and liver conditions. The active substance boldine causes the liver to secrete more bile. However, this herb also contains ascaridote, a toxic substance, so use this herb with care. Although boldo is supposed to help liver problems, some people recommend *not* using it if you have liver problems.

Phyllanthus amarus (euphorbia) comes from Africa, the Middle East, and India. Roots are used for jaundice. It has been used along with milk thistle to treat cirrhosis caused by hepatitis B and hepatitis C infection. In one case, symptoms resolved, liver function tests returned to close to normal, and the patient seemed to become rid of the viruses within five weeks. Because of its potential toxicity, work with a qualified health professional when using this herb.

Picorhiza kurroa (*hu huang lian*) comes from India, Nepal, and Tibet, where it has been used for centuries to treat liver problems, including hepatitis. An extract from this perennial shrub's roots and rhizomes, called picroliv, is undergoing formal human testing in India. Animal studies have shown this herb to protect rats from liver damage and to stimulate liver regrowth. Picroliv appears to be even stronger than silymarin.

Radix angelicae (*pang gui, dong quai*, Angelica root) is a Chinese root that improves circulation.

Radix paeoniae alba (*bai shae yao*, white peony root) is a Chinese root used to relieve night sweats and high blood pressure.

Rhizoma atartylodis (*bai zhu, pai shu*) is a Chinese herb that helps in the production of liver enzymes, helps reduce the buildup of excess fluids, and improves energy.

Rumex crispus (yellow dock, curly dock) reduces liver inflammation, cleanses the blood, and increases bile flow.

Sambucus nigra, S. canadensis (elder flowers) relieve flu-like symptoms associated with hepatitis C.

Plants to Avoid

Some botanicals can be toxic or deadly when you have hepatitis C. Plants to avoid include the following:

- Plants of the *Senecio, Crotalaria*, and *Heliotropium* families
- Jamaican bush tea
- Gordolobo yerba, a Southwest American tea

Sarsaparilla officinalis is more than just a refreshing beverage. It is a mild liver detoxifier.

Schisandra chinensis, S. sphenanthera, and others helps the body adapt to stress and protects the liver, according to many small studies. It may also help improve symptoms of chronic hepatitis. Side effects include stomach upset.

Silybum marianum (milk thistle, St. Mary's thistle, silymarin) is probably the most frequently used herbal remedy for hepatitis C. It is an antioxidant, protecting the liver from toxins. Its seeds are crushed and used. In one documented case, it was used with *Phyllanthus amarus* to treat cirrhosis caused by hepatitis B and hepatitis C infection. Symptoms appeared to be resolved, liver function tests returned to close to normal, and the patient seemed to become rid of the viruses within five weeks. Side effects of milk thistle may include rash.

Swertia mileensis is a Chinese folk medicine used to treat viral hepatitis. Several substances have been isolated from this plant that have beneficial effects on the liver, including chemicals called *secoiridoid glucosides*.

Tabebuia heptaphylla (pau d'arco) is a South American herb that boosts the immune system. A tea is made from the inner bark.

Taraxacum officinale (dandelion) roots and leaves (yes, those very same weeds you are always pulling out of your lawn) may help the liver work more effectively to cleanse the blood.

A Word of Caution

If you are pregnant or trying to become pregnant, make sure your health care provider knows. Many herbs and even traditional medicines such as interferon can damage your unborn child, especially during early stages (the first three months) of pregnancy.

Combinations of herbs may be prescribed to use in teas. Before self-prescribing herbs or herbal teas, be sure to check them out with a qualified health practitioner. Some combinations could do you more harm than good.

Tricholoma lobayense is a mushroom that has been found to normalize liver enzyme levels in rats and has been used in humans as well. Before trying any mushroom-based remedy, be sure that you are working with a qualified practitioner. Many mushrooms are extremely toxic to the liver, quickly causing severe illness and death.

Other plants besides the ones listed here have shown promise in fighting hepatitis B. These include extracts from *Rheum palmatum* rhizomes, *Poligonum cuspidatum* roots, *Panax japonicum* roots, and *Terminalia arjuna* bark. This may be good news if you have both B and C. But if you have only hepatitis C, don't try a botanical simply because it worked for another type of hepatitis. Even though the names are similar and they all cause liver inflammation, each hepatitis virus is very different. What works for one hepatitis virus may not work for another.

Other Therapies

In Chinese medicine, massage and acupuncture are two techniques to help *chi* flow freely through the body, restoring health. In addition, other massage and stress-reduction techniques may provide relief, ranging from restoring some liver function, to resolving symptoms associated with hepatitis C, to helping you deal with the stress and frustration of living with a chronic illness.

Massage can have a range of therapeutic effects, depending on the practitioner's philosophy and technique. Chinese massage (*an mar*) and its Japanese counterpart *shiatsu*, for example, strive to restore balance to the body, restoring the free flow of *chi* and, thence, your health. Other types of massage work off similar theories. In addition, massage has the effect of relaxing you, which not only has the psychological payoff of helping you feel better, but also allows your immune system to function better.

Professional masseuses, physical therapists, chiropractors, naturopaths, and other health practitioners may offer massage services. But massage doesn't have to be performed by a professional for you to benefit from it. Recruit a concerned friend or relative. And even self-massage

A Quick Mental Trip Provides Relief

It's no substitute for a regular relaxation program, but a short mental trip can still provide relief from stress. Find a quiet location where you won't be bothered for a few minutes. Even a stall in a restroom will do in a pinch. Get comfortable, and follow these steps:

1. Close you eyes. Breathe slowly in through your nose and out through your mouth for a minute or so.

2. As you begin to calm yourself, imagine a peaceful place you would like to visit. Perhaps it's an isolated mountain top; a sunny, warm beach; or a babbling brook in the forest.

3. Picture yourself in this location. Imagine the breeze. The sun. The water. The clouds floating through the sky. The sounds of birds. The smell of the trees.

4. After a few minutes in your paradise, return mentally to your restroom stall, office, or wherever you happen to be, hanging on to the serenity you acquired.

can make a significant difference in how you feel. At the very least, buy one of those little wooden massage critters at the store, roll a tennis ball against the soles of your bare feet, gently massage your scalp with a hairbrush, or try rolling a cool can of soda on the back of your neck. Doesn't it feel good just thinking about it?

Acupuncture can have more precise effects than massage. By insertion of small needles into specific locations, acupuncture removes blockages to *chi* and manipulates warm (*yang*) and cool (*yin*) energy in the body to achieve the desired effects. For persons with hepatitis C, acupuncture may help maintain liver function, boost the immune system, and relieve insomnia. Make sure you use a qualified practitioner, and be sure the needles provided are sterile or used only for you.

Other stress reduction techniques include meditation, yoga, guided imagery, prayer, a ten-minute cat nap, or just about any other practice in which you can reach a calm, quiet state. Reducing stress in any of these ways can keep you healthier by helping your immune system function more effectively. Look for classes on relaxation techniques through the adult education program of your school district, the YMCA or YWCA, or a local hospital. For a quick stress reducer, try finding a quiet spot, sitting comfortably with your eyes closed, and slowly breathing in through your nose and out through your mouth for about ten minutes. Focus on your breathing, and soon you'll notice how much calmer you feel.

Thymic therapy is a novel but unproven approach to treating hepatitis B and hepatitis C developed by the late Carson Bergstiner, MD, a specialist in obstetrics and gynecology. Bergstiner developed hepatitis B while operating on an infected patient, and had the disease for seven years before he came up with an idea that made him well for many years.

He posited that the *thymus*, a small gland located in the chest that manufactures immature white blood cells critical to the body's immune system, is crucial for our health, even though it shrinks and is nonfunctional by our early 20s. Like diabetes or menopause, supplemental hormones should be given to replace the enzymes normally released by the thymus, thereby helping the immune system fight off viral infections like hepatitis.

He prepared a combination of thymic enzymes and a vitamin–mineral supplement containing B complex vitamins, vitamin C, vitamin E, selenium, zinc, and beta carotene (a form of vitamin A). Within six weeks, he was free of the hepatitis B virus.

Some results of his small, informal studies were positive, including disappearance of symptoms in people with hepatitis B, hepatitis C, rheumatoid arthritis, lupus, multiple sclerosis, psoriasis, and squamous cell skin cancer, all conditions considered to be immune system disorders.

Bergstiner stressed that his results were purely anecdotal. The FDA would probably never support a study of his regimen, since it contains too many variable factors.

Expanded Possibilities for Treating Hepatitis C

For many people with hepatitis C, alternative therapies have proven to be a viable option, giving them both hope and health. If you are interested in any of the therapies described here, be sure to seek the advice of a qualified health professional. Talk to other people with hepatitis C who have tried the same therapy you are considering. Keep your medical doctor informed of any treatment you undertake. And look for updated information, as many of these treatments are starting to undergo the rigors of formalized clinical trials to document their safety and efficacy.

THE ROLE OF DIET AND EXERCISE

CHAPTER 6

"Be sensible. Be moderate. Let Solon, the 7th-century Greek philosopher, be your guide: 'Nothing to excess.'"

—Dominic Nompleggi, MD, and Herbert Bonkovsky, M.D.
Diet and Chronic Liver Disease: An Updated Research Report
American Liver Foundation, 1997

Of course, the problem is that one person's sense of moderation is likely to be perceived as excess by another. But Solon's advice is still sound and worth keeping in mind as we take a look at the role of diet and exercise in hepatitis C. For, after all, this aspect of your life should play a part in your overall plan to manage hepatitis C. Diet and exercise probably won't cure you of the disease, but they can certainly make a difference in the health of your liver as well as your overall health and well-being. Even more, what you eat and how you exercise are two areas of your management plan in which you have a lot of control.

"Great," you may say. "But what should I be eating? How can diet help me with hepatitis C? What about exercise?" These are fair questions

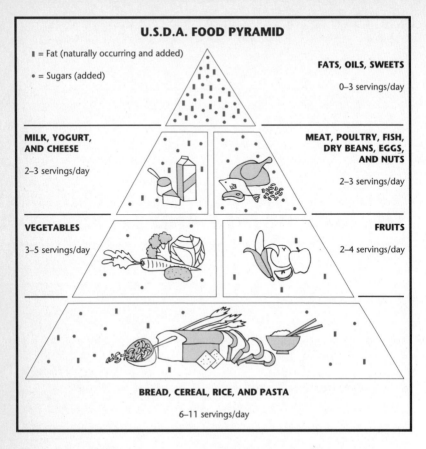

U.S.D.A. FOOD PYRAMID

▮ = Fat (naturally occurring and added)

• = Sugars (added)

FATS, OILS, SWEETS

0–3 servings/day

MILK, YOGURT, AND CHEESE

2–3 servings/day

MEAT, POULTRY, FISH, DRY BEANS, EGGS, AND NUTS

2–3 servings/day

VEGETABLES

3–5 servings/day

FRUITS

2–4 servings/day

BREAD, CEREAL, RICE, AND PASTA

6–11 servings/day

to be asking. After all, your doctor may not have said much about diet or exercise, unless you are experiencing serious symptoms of liver problems. To answer your concerns, first we'll take a look at general dietary guidelines as well as some suggestions for modifying your diet in specific circumstances. Then we'll review the role of supplements—vitamins, minerals, and other nutrients. Finally, we'll discuss how exercise may help.

Eating from the Pyramid

That odd-looking U.S.D.A. (United States Department of Agriculture) food pyramid you may have noticed on the packaging of much of the food you purchase deserves a closer look. Even though it is intended for use by the general, healthy public, this pyramid still forms the basis for a liver-healthy diet.

Starting from the base of the pyramid, let's take a look at each of the blocks of this structure and see how they might apply to your eating habits.

Bread, cereal, rice, and pasta—in other words, foods containing *carbohydrates*. Most of the calories you consume each day come from this group. Carbohydrates form the foundation for the rest of your diet. But just what are they? Basically, sugars—the fuel every cell in your body needs for generating energy. After carbohydrates break down during digestion, they are stored in the liver as *glycogen*. The liver releases glycogen into the blood as needed, helping you maintain a

---

Make the Most of Your Carbs

Not only is it important to get enough servings of carbohydrates each day, you can also benefit from the type of carbohydrates you choose. Here are two ways to help out your health—especially your digestion—even more:

- **Choose more complex carbohydrates.** Sugar and alcohol are carbohydrates, too. But since they are very simple forms of carbohydrates, they fly through your digestive system with the greatest of ease, overloading your liver and raising your blood glucose level to unhealthy heights. Stick to foods that have less sugar and more substantive carbohydrates, such as grains, rice, and pasta.

- **Load up on fiber.** When given a choice between white and wheat breads, go for the wheat. Try brown rice rather than white rice, which contains almost no fiber at all. What's the big deal about fiber? Fiber prevents constipation and other digestive problems that many people with chronic hepatitis experience. Fiber also lowers your cholesterol level, and reduces your risk of several types of cancers.

---

more or less constant level of energy throughout the day. That's why you need 6–11 servings of carbohydrates each day. Does that sound like a lot? No, you won't need to stuff yourself with a bag full of rice morning, noon, and night. The use of the term "serving" is a little misleading. Perhaps some examples would help. A single serving of carbohydrates includes:

- 1 slice of bread (A sandwich gives you two servings right off the bat!)

- 1 ounce of ready-to-eat cereal (You probably eat 5 or 6 ounces in a regular bowl of cereal.)

- ½ cup of cooked cereal, rice, or pasta (How many ½-cup servings would your big plate of spaghetti fill?)

So it probably won't take too much effort to meet this carbohydrate requirement each day.

Vegetables and fruits form a vital part of your diet, supplying critical fiber, vitamins, and minerals. Try to have 3–5 servings of vegetables and 2–4 servings of fruit every day. If this seems like a lot, it probably is. Most people don't come anywhere near these goals, resulting in vitamin deficiencies, a situation you cannot afford to be in these days. Don't ignore those "Eat 5" ads on the produce bags in the grocery store (if you add it up, you'll notice that 5 is the minimum number of combined daily servings of fruits and vegetables). Do something about your vegetable deficit. Make sure you have a serving or two of vegetables and fruits at every meal. Use veggies and fruits for snacks instead of chips and candy bars. To help you assess what you need to shoot toward, here are examples of servings of vegetables and fruits:

- 1 cup of raw leafy vegetables

- ½ cup of cooked vegetables

- ½ cup of chopped raw vegetables or fruit

- ¾ cup of vegetable or fruit juice

- 1 medium apple, banana, or orange

Expand Your Vegetable Horizons

Did you grow up eating peas and carrots until they were coming out of your ears? Do you still hear your mother's voice chiding you to eat all your vegetables before you can have dessert? Maybe it's time to shake some old habits and discover exciting new fruits and vegetables. Not only may your taste buds appreciate the change of pace, but your body may, too. One of the goals of healthy eating is to have a variety of foods. That's one way to ensure that you get not only those necessary vitamins and minerals, but also all those undiscovered substances that may be beneficial to your health. Look at your daily intake of fruits and vegetables as a sort of informal botanical therapy.

Milk, yogurt, and cheese—dairy products—should form an important part of your diet. Not only do dairy products provide you with vital carbohydrates, vitamins, and minerals, they also are a valuable source of protein for people with liver disorders. It is thought that the proteins contained in milk may be easier for your liver to process than meat proteins. That's why you should do all you can to get the 2–3 servings a day. Some people find yogurt, hard cheese, or lactose-free milk easiest to digest. But just what constitutes a serving of dairy products? Here are some examples:

- 1 cup of milk or yogurt
- 1 ½ ounces of natural cheese
- 2 ounces of processed cheese

Meat, poultry, fish, dry beans, eggs, and nuts are all good sources of protein. Unless your doctor tells you otherwise, try for 2–3 servings each day. Some people with hepatitis may want to reduce their protein intake, especially if their liver shows signs of having difficulty in processing the protein (high levels of certain types of protein or ammonia in the blood may indicate problems). You may also need to reduce the protein in your diet if you have encephalopathy (a condition caused by cirrhosis). However, you should talk with your doctor before taking any steps to reduce protein in your diet. It's easy for people with liver problems to become malnourished, and there's probably not a lot of sense in cutting back on protein unless there's a good reason to do so.

Some health professionals suggest that if you have hepatitis, you may be doing your liver a favor if you choose your proteins from vegetable and dairy sources rather than from meat. That's because the protein in nonmeat sources is made up of different *amino acids* (the substances that form the building blocks of protein) than the protein in meat. Nonmeat sources of protein may be easier for your liver to process.

Fats, oils, and **sweets** sit atop the pyramid. You'll also see them as the little circles and triangles scattered throughout the pyramid. That's because you'll find these as ingredients in many of the foods you eat. Besides the obvious sources of these foods—butter, oils, margarine, lard, shortening, sugar, honey, corn syrup, and molasses—you're likely to also find them in salad dressing, soft drinks, candy, fried foods, and sweet desserts. Use fats, oils, and sweets sparingly. They add on calories quickly, while providing little nutrition. Fats should make up no more than 30 percent of the total calories you eat. This is especial-

What About Amino Acids?

Proteins are made up of a variety of amino acids, usually a combination of 25–30 of these acids per type of protein. Over 50 amino acids have been identified in the world around us. You need to eat eight of them (*essential amino acids*) on a regular basis to survive as a living, breathing human being. Why only eight? Your body can find a way to create all the others. The essentials are methionine, leucine, isoleucine, valine, lysine, threonine, tryptophan, and phenylalanine. Amino acids also serve other purposes in the body, such as directly providing cells with energy and aiding the work of certain vitamins. In addition to eating certain types of protein, your doctor may also recommend amino acid therapy as part of your treatment plan (see the section on supplements coming up in a few pages).

ly important for your liver, which must produce bile to help digest fats. If you have bile backing up in the liver (*cholestatis*), you may need to use fat substitutes such as medium chain triglycerides (MCT) oil and safflower oil in cooking and baking, because bile isn't available to digest the fat you eat. Instead, it passes out of the body in stool. Severe weight loss can result. This condition is called steatorrhea.

Beyond the Pyramid

The food pyramid gives you a pretty good idea about what to eat. If you follow the principles embodied in the food pyramid, you're likely to get balanced levels of carbohydrates, protein, fiber, vitamins, and minerals. But for people with hepatitis C, there's more to a well-balanced, liver-healthy diet than taking that cute little triangle to heart. Talk to your doctor about dietary goals. Often, people with liver problems need to eat more calories, possibly between 2,000 and 3,000 calories each day. And there are other dietary principles you may want to implement as well:

Reduce the amount of sodium in your diet. Sodium is most frequently found in salt, and is added to many foods as a seasoning and a preservative. You probably already have heard that people with high blood pressure should avoid salt. What you may not know is that people with liver conditions should probably avoid salt as well, especially if you have abdominal swelling (ascites) or swelling in your feet (edema). Salt helps the body retain fluids. But your body may already be retaining too much fluid as it is, especially if circulation of blood and fluids through your liver is impaired by cirrhosis or inflammation. Where is sodium likely to be hiding out? Obviously in your salt shaker. Other sources of sodium include the following:

- Canned foods such as peas, refried beans, soups, or chili

- Condiments such as mayonnaise and ketchup

- Cured meats such as ham, bacon, and lunchmeat

- Boxed foods such as macaroni and cheese

- Dairy products such as cheese and sour cream

- Snacks such as potato chips and peanuts

- Fast food such as burgers and fries

Take a look at your cupboards. You're likely to find at least some of these items residing there. But don't panic. You can purchase low-salt alternatives for practically all high-sodium foods. In addition, try some of these tips when shopping, cooking, or eating out.

• **Read labels**. Look for ingredients such as salt, sodium nitrate, and monosodium glutamate (MSG), all of which can cause fluid retention.

• **Look for "Nutrition Facts."** Most packaged food in the U.S. now provides this information about sodium and other nutrients right on the label.

• **Ask your doctor for a specific sodium goal**. The recommended amount for the general public is less than 2,400 mg (milligrams) of sodium a day. That's right around 1 teaspoon. Compare that with the 4,000–7,000 mg of sodium a day the average adult in the U.S. eats!

• **Buy fresh**, whenever possible. Generally speaking, the less processing, the less sodium there is likely to be—and another benefit, fresh food items usually contain more vitamins, minerals, and fiber, too.

• **Cook salt-free**. Don't add salt when preparing food. It may take awhile to get used to the new taste, but over time your taste buds will begin to notice flavors that were covered up by the salt. Use other herbs and spices to flavor your foods. Try lemon, garlic (not garlic salt!), basil, oregano, ginger, chili powder, sage, and more. If you're not sure where to start, read the label on the spice jar. Often they list suggestions for use. Or buy spice combinations that don't contain salt, such as Italian seasonings or poultry spices.

• **Choose restaurant food wisely**. Not only is restaurant food often loaded with salt, it may be high in fat, too. But you can make choices that are healthier for your liver. Ask to have foods grilled or baked without added salt or butter. Ask for sauces on the side. Order turkey or roast beef sandwiches at the deli. Choose Asian dishes that have no

Let the Label Be Your Guide

The Nutrition Facts label on most packaged foods can help you make wise choices about sodium content and nutrients. This label for potato chips shows high levels of sodium and fat, low fiber, relatively little carbohydrate and protein, and few vitamins and minerals—except for iron, which you may not want anyway. Probably okay for an occasional treat, but overall not a very liver-friendly food!

Nutrition Facts

Serving Size 1 package
Servings Per Container 1

Amount Per Serving

Calories 230   Calories from Fat 140

	% Daily Value*
Total Fat 15g	**24%**
Saturated Fat 4g	**21%**
Cholesterol 0mg	**0%**
Sodium 270mg	**11%**
Total Carbohydrate 22g	**7%**
Dietary Fiber 1g	**6%**
Sugars 0g	
Protein 3g	

Vitamin A 0%	●	Vitamin C 15%
Calcium 0%	●	Iron 2%

* Percent Daily Values are based on a 2,000 calorie diet. Your daily values may be higher or lower depending on your calorie needs:

	Calories:	2,000	2,500
Total Fat	Less than	65g	80g
Sat Fat	Less than	20g	25g
Cholesterol	Less than	300mg	300mg
Sodium	Less than	2,400mg	2,400mg
Total Carbohydrate		300mg	375mg
Dietary Fiber		25g	30g

Calories per gram:
Fat 9   ●   Carbohydrate 4   ●   Protein 4

added MSG—and watch the soy sauce! Order side salads rather than French fries.

Avoid alcohol. Alcohol is just plain bad for your liver. Even moderate use of alcohol can lead to cirrhosis in some people. And if you have hepatitis C, you need to be even more careful. If you're a woman, you should be beyond careful. Alcohol seems to cause liver damage more readily in women. This may be due to the higher level of body fat in women, causing the body to digest alcohol differently than in men. Here are some other reasons to avoid alcohol:

- Persons with HCV who drink alcohol tend to develop cirrhosis and hepatocellular carcinoma (liver cell cancer) more quickly.

- Persons with HCV who drink are at more than eight times greater risk of developing liver cancer than people with HCV who do not drink.

- Alcohol may cause HCV to replicate more readily. This may be due to higher levels of iron generated by alcohol. The virus needs iron to duplicate itself.

- Alcohol makes hepatitis more active.

- Alcohol makes interferon therapy less effective. Studies show that people who drink are less likely to clear the virus from their bodies.

Need any more reasons to avoid alcohol? You ought to question whether even a drink once in a while is worth the risk. But stopping drinking can be easier said than done, even when you understand the need to abstain. If you find that you can't stop drinking—even if it's only a few drinks a day—it's time for some outside help. Contact the local AA group or ask your doctor for a referral to an alcohol treatment program. Your liver and your health are worth it!

Avoid certain drugs. Remember that your liver is primarily responsible for processing any drugs you take. If your liver's function is impaired, it may make it more difficult to process any drugs, legal or otherwise. First off, avoid any illicit drugs. These drugs are generally hard on your liver and many suppress the immune system, something you don't need right now. Plus, you probably don't want to share a needle and risk passing HCV to others—or risk acquiring another virus such as HIV.

Even many "legal" medications should be used cautiously. Acetaminophen, for example, can be toxic to the liver, even in moderate doses and especially when combined with alcohol. Some medications used to treat side effects of hepatitis C or interferon therapy should be used cautiously. Talk with your doctor about these medications, and weigh the risks and benefits carefully. For example, using an antidepressant for a short while to help you cope with depression may certainly be worth the extra temporary stress on your liver. Realistically, your doctor may not be aware of each drug's interaction with your illness and with your other medications. That's where the advice of your pharmacist can be invaluable. Your pharmacist can't change a prescription for you, but they can discuss potential side effects and may even notify your doctor if they suspect the prescription may cause problems.

Avoid smoking. By now, you've probably heard all the arguments to quit. Besides all the effects you're aware of, smoking can be a contributing factor in the development of liver cancer. It can make some conditions associated with hepatitis C worse, such as circulation problems. And smoking depletes your supply of immune system-enhancing substances such as vitamin C.

Avoid excess iron. If you have any liver damage, you may have too much iron in your blood. And high levels of iron may also make treatment less effective. Make sure you monitor your iron intake. Don't take extra iron in supplements (most vitamin and mineral supplements contain iron). Don't use iron cookware. Ask your doctor about foods to avoid.

Avoid food additives. Doctors may tell you that you shouldn't worry about preservatives, additives, fertilizers, and pesticides used in growing and processing the food you eventually eat. Other "alternative" practitioners may tell you just the opposite. It may be the additives themselves that wreak some damage to the liver. Although there is no evidence to point either way, it does make sense to avoid added chemicals whenever possible. After all, the liver has to deal with it, and one of your management goals is to make life as easy on the liver as possible. Select food products containing no additives such as preservatives. Buy "organic" whenever possible—organic products have not been sprayed with chemical pesticides. Consider using bottled water, since many local water supplies contain levels of chemicals and organisms that may be unhealthy for persons with weak immune systems.

What About Supplements?

Controversy continues to rage concerning the role of supplements in treating hepatitis C. Even practitioners within the Western medical community debate whether supplements are helpful or harmful. This is one area in which you'll need to make your own decision based on what you think is best for you. One thing that everyone agrees on, however, is that persons with hepatitis C should not take megadoses of nutritional supplements. These substances, like all other nutrients, need to be processed by the liver. Megadoses can be toxic when the liver is unable to function fully.

Theoretically, you should get most of the nutrients you need if you follow the dietary principles described earlier. However, persons with hepatitis C may have some nutritional deficiencies related to the disease, may have deficiencies due to diet restrictions, and may have an increased need for certain supplements to fight off HCV and preserve liver health. Talk with your doctor before trying any of these supplements.

Vitamins help the body use energy more effectively. Vitamins fall into two classes: water-soluble and fat-soluble. Since persons with hepatitis C and cirrhosis may have problems digesting fat, they may be deficient in fat-soluble vitamins; however, megadoses of fat-soluble vitamins can be dangerous. Fat-soluble vitamins include A, D, E, and K. Vitamins A and D are especially toxic, and can cause death if an overdose is taken. The other fat-soluble vitamins should be taken only under the guidance of your doctor. A form of vitamin A, beta carotene,

Getting Nutritional Advice

It's likely your doctor doesn't know a whole lot about the role of nutrition in hepatitis C. You may need to seek out some extra advice. Make sure whoever you talk with is qualified to discuss nutritional matters. Here are some people who may be able to help:

- **Dietitians** have usually gone through a bachelor's degree program or more and should be certified as an RD (registered dietitian). Most dietitians work out of hospitals or other health care practices. They usually have a traditional Western medical view of the role of diet in health, but many dietitians are learning more about the role of herbs and nutritional supplements in maintaining health.

- **Nutritionists or certified nutrition counselors** have usually completed a master's degree or higher in nutrition. They may also be registered dietitians. They often have a broader view of the role of diet in health.

- **Practitioners of other medical traditions** often provide advice about diet and liver health, since diet is seen by them as an important therapeutic tool. Look for qualified, credentialed practitioners of naturopathy, Chinese medicine, or homeopathy.

---

and vitamin E are taken with several other vitamins when undergoing thymic therapy (see Chapter 5). Vitamin E (tocopherol) is an antioxidant that helps immune system function, can help combat fatigue, and may even help prevent cirrhosis from developing or getting worse. Vitamin K aids in blood clotting. A good source of vitamin K is yogurt containing "live" cultures.

Water-soluble vitamins, such as the B vitamins, are not only more easily absorbed by people with hepatitis C, but also have some potentially beneficial effects. In general, the B vitamins help break down carbohydrates, proteins, and fats so that your body can use the resulting sugar as energy. Because of this central role, the B vitamins affect everything from your moods to the health of your heart. In addition,

B complex vitamins are not only part of thymic therapy, but also support the immune system and help the liver detoxify. Despite the value of the Bs, most people are deficient in B vitamins, leading many health experts to recommend B supplements, even in healthy people. B complex vitamins include the following:

- **B$_1$ (thiamin)** breaks down carbohydrates and assists in maintaining your body's network of nerves. It may, along with vitamins B$_2$ and B$_6$, reduce depression and related symptoms such as memory loss in older people. B$_1$ may also be helpful to the spleen. People with hepatitis are often deficient in this vitamin.

- **B$_2$ (riboflavin)** aids in the breakdown of fats. It also helps cells use oxygen. And it makes your urine look more yellow (just so you're not too surprised if you take this vitamin). It may also help lessen signs of depression in older people. It works with vitamin A to prevent cataracts and eye fatigue.

- **B$_3$ (niacin)** has a range of benefits. It opens up your blood vessels. This might be one of the reasons it has been linked to relieving symptoms of arthritis: increased blood flow to affected joints may speed healing. Your cholesterol levels are regulated in part by B$_3$. Niacin and nicotinic acid—both names for vitamin B$_3$—are often prescribed for people with high cholesterol levels. B$_3$ is also involved in maintaining the health of your nervous system and in creating hormones.

- **B$_5$ (pantothenic acid)** is involved in almost every process your body undertakes. It may help relieve symptoms associated with rheumatoid arthritis and fatigue.

- **B$_6$ (pyridoxine)** helps you digest and use proteins and fats. It also regulates the amount of sodium and potassium in the body in order to maintain correct fluid levels. Related to this benefit is B$_6$'s association with lower risk of artery disease. Along with vitamins B$_1$ and B$_2$, vitamin B$_6$ may also relieve symptoms of depression. Vitamin B$_6$ is crucial for maintaining a strong immune system. It helps you develop the white blood cells you need to fight off HCV and other infections. This vitamin may also play a role in maintaining healthy skin. Some physicians prescribe high doses of B_6 to relieve symptoms of carpal tunnel syndrome, which can cause tingling in the wrists and arms. However, too much B_6 can cause these very same symptoms. With all the potential benefits from an adequate intake of vitamin B_6, it's unfortunate that most people only get about half of the daily requirement of this critical vitamin.

- **B_{12}** helps keep the nervous system strong. It's often recommended for people experiencing fatigue. Inadequate levels of B_{12} are also linked with increased levels of artery disease, heart attacks, and strokes. Not only can vitamin B_{12} reduce the level of the artery-clogging amino acid homocystein, it actually changes this amino acid into methionine, an amino acid that helps prevent cancer. Vitamin B_{12} (along with folic acid) has also been shown to reduce symptoms of depression, dementia, memory loss, and confusion. It seems to enable people to think more clearly, even when they don't have a serious mental health disorder such as depression. The problem with vitamin B_{12} is, as you get older, it's more difficult for your body to absorb it, so you may need to increase your intake.

- **Biotin** is a B vitamin without a number. It helps break down fats. It may also aid in the reduction of gray hair and hair loss. That's probably why you'll sometimes see biotin as an ingredient in hair shampoos and conditioners. Biotin also helps T cells do their work, an important benefit to people with hepatitis C, who need to keep their immune systems as strong as possible.

- **Folic acid** (also called folate or folacin) is another numberless B vitamin that is now coming into its own. As recently as 1989, folic acid was not considered to be very useful, causing the National Academy of Sciences to cut the requirement in half. Even at this lower level, the average intake of folic acid is just over half the recommended level. But recommendations about folic acid are changing as researchers discover more about its role. You may already know that folic acid's primary function is to help your body use iron more effectively. This is essential for producing red blood cells and for keeping your iron levels under control. In fact, many people would never need iron supplements if they just consumed enough folic acid. Folic acid has a range of other benefits, as well. Birth defects are reduced when expectant mothers have adequate folic acid intake. Women who are considering pregnancy are now being advised to take extra folic acid. Folic acid is crucial for maintaining the health of your arteries, and preventing heart attacks and strokes. Like vitamin B_{12}, it also converts artery-damaging homocysteine into cancer-preventing methionine. Some studies have shown folic acid to help prevent changes in the colon, cervix, and lungs that could eventually lead to cancer. Getting enough of this vitamin can help reverse dementia, reduce symptoms of depression, enhance concentration, improve memory, and even simply help you think more clearly. The amount of folic acid needed by your body may increase as you age. Even if you're younger, the role of folic acid is now considered to be so important that there is discussion about raising the daily amount of folic acid recommended by the USDA. The USDA is also beginning to require food manufacturers to add folic acid to breads, flours, and other grain-based food products.

- **Lecithin (phosphatidylcholine or PC)** is a fatlike, phosphorus-containing substance found in many plants and animals. If you look very closely (with a microscope), you'll find lecithin in your very own cells and in the coverings of your nerves. When you eat lecithin, your body breaks it down into several components: choline, phosphate, glycerol, and some fatty acids. Once in the liver, these components are reformed into lecithin. The lecithin is distributed throughout the body, where it protects nerves and helps get rid of fat. Lecithin has been used to help relieve symptoms of liver problems, such as lack of appetite and liver pressure or pain. There is also some initial evidence that lecithin may help alleviate symptoms of Alzheimer's disease. And due to its qualities as a polyunsaturated fat, theoretically lecithin should help lower cholesterol, although this benefit has never been proven. Using more than 20 grams of lecithin a day can cause digestive problems and sweating.

Vitamin C is another water-soluble vitamin and an immune system supporter. Like the eight essential amino acids, vitamin C is a substance that your body can't manufacture itself. But even though it's readily available in fruits and vegetables (one orange a day would do it), about half of all Americans don't get the daily minimum intake of vitamin C. People with hepatitis C should probably be getting even more, although megadoses can be harmful to people with high iron levels, since vitamin C helps the body take in more iron. Smokers deplete their vitamin C supplies rapidly. And it appears that men, as they get older, need to increase the amount of vitamin C they eat. All this adds up to some basic advice: Don't forget to eat your fruits and veggies.

Vitamin C has been shown to lessen symptoms related to the common cold, allergies, and respiratory infections. It prevents scurvy. It aids in the manufacture of collagen, a protein that helps provide structure to your bones, muscles, blood vessels, skin, and cartilage, and some kidney tissue, which may be damaged in some people with hepatitis C. Vitamin C also keeps your teeth strong and helps prevent and cure periodontal (gum) disease.

There is substantial evidence that vitamin C boosts your immune system and helps lower your risk of cancer. Vitamin C relieves symptoms associated with rheumatoid arthritis and diabetes, both immune system diseases not unlike hepatitis C. Vitamin C may also relieve cancer symptoms, allowing people with terminal cancer to experience a higher quality—and longer—life. It has been used to help alleviate symptoms of some types of potent cancer-fighting drugs, such as adri-amycin and interleukin-2. Some people think vitamin C should even be used as an anticancer drug itself, although the evidence is still unclear. And vitamin C may also protect against cancer-causing food additives such as nitrates and nitrites, which are found in processed meats such as bacon, bologna, ham, and sausage.

How can vitamin C be so all-around beneficial? One reason is that it's an "antioxidant," a sort of natural preservative. You've probably heard about vitamin E and beta carotene as antioxidants—they've gotten most of the press up until recently. But vitamin C fits into this category as well—and, in fact, may be the most potent antioxidant of them all. That's why you'll see vitamin C or ascorbic acid in the list of ingredients of so many foods and drinks. As a preservative, it's cheap, it's effective, and it's even good for you.

Minerals aid the body in effectively using other nutrients. Again, with a balanced, varied diet, you should be receiving at least a good

The Role of Antioxidants

Inside your body, antioxidants cause dangerous substances called "free radicals" to break apart or become inactivated before they can cause you any great harm. These free radicals are created in your body as a byproduct of burning energy. You're also exposed to free radicals from outside sources, especially from air pollutants such as nitrogen dioxide, ozone, radiation, and cigarette smoke. Free radicals include individual atoms or small molecules of oxygen, iron, and copper, among many other substances. They differ from regular, nonradical substances in that they have the wrong amount of "ions," that is, their electrical charge is different than what the substance normally prefers. That's why free radicals are so unstable. They're simply looking for a way to get back to their "normal" charge. But they aren't all bad. Your body needs a few of these unstable free radicals, some of which are used to help disable invading microorganisms. However, too many free radicals roaming through your body can create real trouble. Antioxidants disable free radicals and carry them away to be processed and disposed of through your liver.

baseline level of a range of minerals. Some minerals that are important to people with liver disease include the following:

- **Calcium, cobalt,** and **manganese** aid white blood cell function and phagocytosis (the ingestion of the virus by certain white blood cells), critical for the immune response to HCV.

- **Iodine** may help persons with HCV who have thyroid problems.

- **Potassium** and **sodium** help regulate the body's fluid balance. You probably get more than enough sodium already in your diet. If you take a diuretic (medication that helps the body excrete excess water), you may need extra potassium.

- **Selenium** may help prevent tumors and aids immune system function.

- **Zinc** is often deficient in people with hepatitis C. It helps regulate the immune system.

Amino acids are found in the protein you eat. However, persons with hepatitis C may be deficient in some amino acids. Normally, as long as you eat enough of the eight essential amino acids, your liver should be able to synthesize the rest. However, in some cases you may need supplementation. Amino acid therapy is controversial, so be sure to talk this over with your doctor carefully. Some amino acids to be aware of include the following:

- **Acetylcysteine** breaks down into glutathione, a nonessential amino acid. Glutathione itself breaks down into cysteine, glutamic acid, and glycine. It helps detoxify the liver and aids in energy production in the cells. Acetylcysteine is the antidote to acetaminophen overdose.

- **Lysine** is an essential amino acid that may help control replication of HCV.

- **Methionine** (an essential amino acid) and **glycine** detoxify the liver. They help rid the body of heavy metals, free radicals, and byproducts of alcohol.

- **Proline** may help reduce inflammation of joints associated with rheumatoid arthritis.

- **Taurine** may help the body digest fats.

- **Tryptophan** is an essential amino acid that may relieve liver inflammation and depression.

Superoxide dismutase (SOD) is an enzyme used by the body to deactivate superoxide radicals produced by inflammation. SOD has been used to treat cirrhosis. Taken orally, it likely has little or no effect, since the digestive acids probably destroy the enzymes. However, an injectable form (orgotein) has been effective in treating cirrhosis and other inflammatory problems in horses and in some humans.

What About Exercise?

Can you exercise HCV away? So far, nobody advocates that approach. In fact, there is evidence that overly strenuous exercise may hurt your immune system. And if you are in an acute stage of hepatitis, you shouldn't exercise at all. However, moderate exercise can have several beneficial effects for most people with chronic hepatitis C:

- Moderate exercise boosts your immune system.

- Exercise can help relieve symptoms of fatigue and depression.

- Exercise can relieve stress, which depresses the immune system.

- Exercise improves the action of your heart and your general circulation, which can be especially important if you have circulation problems along with hepatitis C.

- Sweating during exercise is one way to help your body rid itself of some toxins.

Before beginning an exercise program, check with your doctor. Start slowly and gradually increase the time and intensity of your exercise. Aim for at least a half-hour of aerobic activity three times a week. Aerobic exercise gets your heart beating faster and your lungs work-

Examples of Aerobic Exercise

Aerobic exercise includes any activity that gets your major muscles working in a continuous and rhythmic fashion for more than 12 minutes and that forces you to breathe deeply. Examples include:

- Walking briskly

- Bicycling

- Inline or ice skating

- Swimming

- Water exercises

- Stationary machines such as exercise bicycles, rowing machines, stair climbers, treadmills, cross-country ski simulators

- Aerobic exercise videotapes

ing harder, resulting in a healthier cardiovascular system. This increases your endurance and improves muscle tone.

Choose a variety of activities you enjoy—walking, riding a bike, swimming, inline skating, and dancing are just a few examples. Exercise with a friend or with your kids. And be sure to wear supportive shoes and other gear as needed to protect yourself from injuries. After all, exercise is supposed to do you some good, not leave you worse off than before you started!

Now It's Up to You

The food pyramid, other principles for good eating, moderate exercise. These are weapons you can use in your fight against HCV. You don't need a special prescription. All you need is the determination to get started. Pick one area to begin with—such as eating enough fruits and vegetables each day for a week. When you complete that goal, pick another—such as walking the dog after dinner—and add it to your routine. Soon you'll be on your way to healthier eating, regular exercise, and best of all, a healthier, happier you.

PART III
OTHER STEPS TO TAKE

"Take responsibility for your own treatment. Learn as much as possible about the disease, and find a doctor who will act as a partner/coach in the healing process. Be holistic in your approach: Don't just take drugs or herbs, but change your diet, exercise, meditation, etc. Don't get angry, get well. Convince yourself that you are not alone."

—44-year-old man with hepatitis C

Your hepatitis C treatment plan—including diet, medications, exercise, and alternative therapies—can help you take responsibility for your health. The following chapters describe other steps you can take as well. These steps may not restore your immune system to its pre-HCV state. But they will help you in other ways that may be just as important at this point in your life.

Reaching out for support can help turn feelings of isolation and discouragement into a sense of togetherness and hope. By reaching out, you will find that you are not alone in your struggle to deal with hepatitis C. You may be surprised to find out how similar your experience is to thousands of others. And you may be pleased to learn that you probably have some words of advice that can help others, too.

Taking steps to halt the spread of HCV gives you a greater purpose— to help others stay healthy and free from HCV. Personally, you can make sure you don't spread the hepatitis C virus to anyone else. And you can help fight hepatitis C by advocating for more education and research.

As we've said before, pursuing more information about HCV has several benefits. It helps you make sure you're getting the best possible treatments for hepatitis C. And it puts you in touch with a group of people throughout the world who understand what you're going through.

SEEK OUT SUPPORT

CHAPTER 7

"What has been the most positive thing that has happened as a result of having HCV? Discovering new abilities as a result of becoming very active in our local support group."

—50-year-old woman who was probably infected
with HCV from a blood transfusion in 1970

Living with hepatitis C isn't easy, despite what many doctors may tell you. Even if you don't have dramatic symptoms, the fatigue and other problems associated with hepatitis C can be frustrating, even more so when doctors, family, or friends don't understand why you may not feel well. When asking people who have hepatitis C to give advice to those who have just been diagnosed with the disease, two messages are repeated by almost everyone:

1) Learn everything you can about the disease

2) Find support

These folks ought to know. Many of them have been struggling for years with unexplained symptoms that were supposedly "all in their head." Even after diagnosis, many were told that they shouldn't be having any physical problems associated with HCV and perhaps what they really needed was to see a psychiatrist. It's not unusual to hear cases where people lost jobs, homes, and spouses before realizing what was making them sick and that there were others out there with the same symptoms. If you have hepatitis C, benefit from their advice and experience now. If you know someone with hepatitis C, understand that their disease is both real and frustrating. Don't give up on them.

This book can help get you started with the first piece of advice, and it may be a relief to finally learn something about hepatitis C. But no book can provide real emotional support. We can point you in some directions, but you'll have to take it from there.

Why Support Is Critical

Remember that just a few years ago, HCV wasn't even identified. Since its discovery in 1989, knowledge about the virus and the problems it causes has grown. But there's still a long ways to go. The support of others can make understanding and living with hepatitis C much more bearable, whether or not a "cure" is found soon. Finding support from others can help you

- Stay up-to-date as new information and treatments for hepatitis C become available

- Understand that you're not alone in dealing with this confusing, often-frustrating condition

- Find insights that help you deal with issues such as employment, disability claims, life insurance, and the managed health care system

Where to Look for Support

It's surprising where you may find support—and perhaps just as astonishing to learn where you may find less support than you anticipated. Let's take a look at some groups you can look to for support.

Your doctor is certainly a good place to start. First off, the advice to work with a doctor who will act as a partner/coach is wise, indeed. If your doctor takes this attitude toward your relationship, then you are likely to see your doctor as a source of solid support. You will be more confident in treatment recommendations. And you will feel like you are really an integral part of your health care team. Unfortunately, many doctors know little about hepatitis C, and may even discourage you from seeking treatment or having routine testing as long as your symptoms are "mild." If you have run into this situation, realize that it's not unusual. Depending on how you feel about your relationship with your doctor, you can respond in a number of ways:

- **Find another primary care doctor** who is better informed and more flexible in dealing with hepatitis C. Don't be afraid to set up a short interview with one or more doctors before making a switch. Usually there is no charge for an initial 10- to 15-minute meeting. Prepare a list of questions to guide you through the interview.

- **Encourage your doctor to learn more** about hepatitis C. Knowledge is changing so rapidly, even if your doctor read a good summary article or attended a seminar about the disease last year, the information is probably out of date.

- **Help educate your doctor** about hepatitis C. Many persons with this disease arm themselves with the latest research before each doctor's appointment. They find their doctors asking them questions about hepatitis C, rather than the other way around. Then doctor and patient jointly research how they can best manage the disease.

- **Ask for a referral to a specialist**. But don't be surprised if you run into the same problem again. Even some gastroenterologists and, to a lesser extent, hepatologists are surprisingly uninformed about hepatitis C and its ramifications.

- **Learn how to "work" your health care plan** to your benefit. If you seek referrals to specialists or want to try interferon therapy, make sure your health care plan covers it. You may have to use their list of approved participating providers. Or you may need special permission or documentation to get approval. Otherwise, you may end up paying for all or part of the cost. It's always a good idea to call your insurance company first before scheduling an appointment to see a specialist.

Family and friends can be great supporters, but you may need to "prep" them on how to effectively assist you. They themselves may be feeling frustrated about your illness and their inability to help you get better. Try some of these ideas:

- **Help them understand HCV** and related problems. Give them a copy of this book or one of the American Liver Foundation brochures to read. Ask them to talk to someone else who has been living with a diagnosis of HCV for awhile.

- **Make them part of your health care team**. Ask a concerned family member to go with you to your doctor appointments, especially if your doctor is knowledgeable about hepatitis C and recognizes the potential seriousness of any symptoms you might have.

- **Give specific suggestions** for how you'd like friends and relatives to deal with your condition. For example, if comments such as "But you look just fine" bother you, gently remind them that most people with hepatitis C look normal, but may still be experiencing symptoms that are hard to deal with.

- **Get them involved in groups** focusing on the concerns of friends and family members of persons with chronic illness. Of course it's difficult dealing with a loved one who has an illness such as hepatitis C. But you're probably not the best one to help them cope—you may be having a hard enough time dealing with the disease and your own reactions to it. Ask your doctor if there are any local groups for your family and friends. Check with area hospitals. Call the American Liver Foundation or the Hepatitis C Foundation to see if there are such groups in your area. Check out resources on the Internet. For example, there's a weekly discussion group on America Online for spouses of persons with hepatitis C (Hepmates) on Wednesday evenings, 10 p.m. to 11 p.m. EST in the PEN (Personal Empowerment Network) conference room.

Interviewing a Doctor

As awkward as it may feel, you have every right to interview any doctor you are considering using. When you call his or her office, let the person scheduling the appointment know that you want to set up an interview to meet the doctor. There should be no charge for this service (you may have to remind them of this after your appointment when you are checking out). Write down questions ahead of time. Here are some suggested questions to keep in mind:

- What is your experience in dealing with patients who have hepatitis C? With other chronic illnesses such as diabetes or multiple sclerosis?

- What is your understanding of hepatitis C and its treatment? What do you perceive to be the current "standard of care"?

- What is your opinion of alternative treatments such as herbs or acupuncture?

- What resources do you have available to help with issues such as diet and exercise?

- As a primary care physician, how do you see your role in working with a specialist such as a gastroenterologist or hepatologist in managing my condition?

Your employer and coworkers may be a source of support, but you'll need to deal with this issue cautiously. First, decide whether or not to tell anyone about having hepatitis C. Why would you tell your employer? It might make sense for the following reasons:

- Under the Americans with Disabilities Act, employers must make reasonable accommodations to anyone with a disability. Chronic illnesses, including conditions such as multiple sclerosis, rheumatoid arthritis, diabetes, and chronic hepatitis, are considered disabilities for the purposes of the act. Your employer can only accommodate your needs if he or she knows about them. Accommodations could include a range of things depending on your job and your health condition: perhaps more flexible work hours, allowing you to do some work at home, or reassignment to less taxing duties.

- Telling your employer may help you retain your job. If you think your employer is upset because you miss a lot of work or are unable to perform duties such as heavy travel, then it might make sense to tell your employer of your condition rather than simply allow yourself to be fired.

- It could help you get along with coworkers who may be feeling like you're not pulling your "fair share." If they understand that you have a chronic illness, they may be more supportive than if they believe you are simply shirking your duties for some unknown reason.

On the other hand, you may feel it is none of your employer's business to know about your health problems. Or you may be concerned that you'll be shunned by coworkers or passed up for promotions if your condition becomes known. All these concerns are valid, which is why a decision to tell your employer that you have hepatitis C is one to think through carefully.

As an alternative, many people with chronic symptoms of hepatitis C have found that self-employment is a good option. This lets them tailor their work to their energy level. Sales, computer consulting, writing, graphic design, and almost any type of service job are good examples of self-employment that provide flexibility.

Organizations devoted to the needs of people with hepatitis C, both national and international, can provide information and support. Here are groups to contact right away:

- **The American Liver Foundation** is a voluntary health organization in the United States. Its goal is to prevent, treat, and cure a variety of conditions related to the liver and gallbladder, including hepatitis C. It sponsors research and educational initiatives. It also has support groups, some of which are specifically for persons with hepatitis C and others that are for persons with any chronic liver condition. It has several chapters throughout the U.S.:

  Main office: American Liver Foundation
  1425 Pompton Avenue, Cedar Grove, NJ 07009-1000
  (201) 256-2550
  fax (201) 256-3214
  Toll-free hotlines: (800) GO-LIVER (465-4837)
  and (888) 4HEP-ABC (443-7222)
  web site: www.liverfoundation.org

- **American Digestive Health Foundation** is a volunteer organization that focuses on research and education for a variety of digestive disorders, including hepatitis C.

  American Digestive Health Foundation
  7910 Woodmont Ave, 7th floor
  Bethesda, MD 20814
  (301) 654-2635
  fax (301) 654-1140
  Toll-free hotline: (800) 668-5237
  web site: www.adhf.org

- **Hepatitis C Support Project** primarily provides support for persons with hepatitis C. They publish a newsletter as well.

  Hepatitis C Support Project
  P.O. Box 427037
  San Francisco, CA 94142-7037
  (415) 834-4100
  Bay Area support groups: (415) 676-4888

"Learn all you can about your disease. The level of ignorance in the medical establishment regarding HCV, and its symptoms, is mind boggling. Treat it early, even if discouraged to do so by your physician. Join a support group (e.g., the Hepatitis C Foundation or the Internet-based HEPV-L Discussion List)."

—46-year-old man who received HCV
from a blood transfusion 14 years ago

Support groups can be a lifesaver for people with hepatitis C. If you have hepatitis C and feel like nobody can possibly understand what you're going through, a support group can do you a world of good. Usually these groups are fairly informal. They may or may not be led by a health care professional. The focus of the group may vary, but usually includes providing emotional support and information about hepatitis C to the participants. Even the location and format of the groups vary. Most groups meet monthly. There are literally hundreds of small support groups throughout the U.S. Check these sources for more information about local support groups:

- One of the national foundations, such as the American Liver Foundation. Most national groups have local chapters that sponsor support groups.

- Your local hospital.

- Your local Alcoholics Anonymous or Narcotics Anonymous groups. Many people rely on alcohol or drugs to help them through the day. But alcohol and drugs can be dangerous for people with hepatitis C, both because of the damage they do to the liver and because of the association of alcohol with quicker replication of the hepatitis C virus. Furthermore, many doctors may not provide treatment such as interferon therapy to active users of alcohol or drugs. If you find you need help stopping alcohol or drug use, check your phone book White Pages for the numbers of your local AA or NA groups.

Computer on-line support is a less traditional but highly accessible resource for people with hepatitis C. If you don't own a computer that is able to get you onto the Internet, you ought to seriously consider purchasing one. You may also find access to the Internet through computers at your local library. If you're new to the Internet, take a course or two on how to access and use the Internet. Short classes are offered by computer stores, community colleges, and community education programs. Many people with hepatitis C have found the Internet to be the single best way to access information and support. Believe it or not, this particular section of cyberspace is friendly, supportive, and extremely human. All you need to do is learn how to get there. Resources for hepatitis C are available in a variety of ways via the Internet, including web sites and discussion groups. Besides learning a lot about hepatitis C, you'll also meet people who have similar experiences to yours. And you'll even get an introduction to the quirky humor that people with hepatitis C have developed to help them cope with such a frustrating, chronic condition. Here are a few places to look up:

- **America Online** sponsors a hepatitis C support group "chat" every Wednesday night from 8 to 9 p.m. EST. You must subscribe to America Online in order to access this chat group. They often have guest speakers who are experts in some aspect of hepatitis C. Other America Online chat groups related to hepatitis C include Hepterminal and HCV (a private chat room). All these take place in the PEN (Personal Empowerment Network) conference room. If you subscribe to another service, such as CompuServe or Prodigy, check out their sections on chronic illness or alternative/ natural medicine to find resources and discussion groups related to hepatitis C.

- **Focus: Hepatitis C International Web Site** provides lots of information and first-person accounts about various aspects of hepatitis C. The internet address is pages.prodigy.com/ hepc/index.htm.

- **Ask Emaliss** is a monthly on-line magazine devoted to hepatitis C information and support. It feels lots more personal than a printed magazine, since you can leave messages for Emaliss and jump from the magazine site to other relevant sites and then back again. Plus, the site is filled with the personality of its creator (who has hepatitis C), making your visit an enjoyable as well as an educational and supportive experience. The address is soli.inav.net/~webbsite.

- **Yahoo** provides easy access to several "clubs" you can join to discuss concerns about hepatitis C. Reach these clubs at clubs.yahoo.com.

- **Hepatitis Web Ring** is a web site that provides access to just about every other web site that deals with hepatitis, including sites by persons with hepatitis, sites by health practitioners who treat hepatitis C, information sites, and support and discussion group sites. The Hepatitis Web Ring address is www.hepring.org.

Professional counselors are also a critical area of support. Although you may disagree if your doctor suggests that your symptoms from hepatitis C are "all in your head," there is still merit in seeking the services of a therapist. After all, you are likely to be going through some stressful times, and since hepatitis C is chronic, you need to prepare yourself for dealing with all the issues associated with chronic illness. The type of counselor isn't so important. It could be a psychiatrist (a medical doctor who has special training in psychiatric problems and can prescribe medication), psychologist (a person with an advanced degree in clinical psychology), counselor, social worker, minister, priest, or rabbi (all these counselors usually have at least a master's degree in their field). What is important is that you feel comfortable talking with the counselor and that he or she has some experience in dealing with persons who have chronic illness. Just like choosing a doctor, don't be afraid to set up an informational interview with a counselor to assess his or her philosophy toward and experience in dealing with chronic illness, as well as checking to make sure the type of therapy fits comfortably with your own philosophy and beliefs.

The Benefits of Reaching Out

At first, looking for the support of people who understand what you're going through may seem unnecessary. After all, finding support will not cure you of the disease. However, just by taking any of these steps to get support, you're likely to find yourself feeling a bit better and more in control of your health. The payoffs can go even further, providing you with invaluable insight and information, and removing you from the isolation that so many people with hepatitis C encounter. One woman with hepatitis C sums up how getting—and giving—support can make a difference: "Every time I pick up the phone and hear someone say they have just been diagnosed with hepatitis C, my heart goes out to them, as I know the long road ahead is not a pretty one. I feel I MUST help them. If I did not, it would be like leaving the scene of an accident. Those people need someone who can relate to their situation, give them moral support, and help them deal with this virus in every way possible. So, basically, it has given me a purpose in life—to devote myself to helping others, to get as much education as possible to enable me to do this. I have thus far received my certification in nutrition and am currently working on my Ph.D. in natural healing."

STOP THE SPREAD OF HCV

CHAPTER 8

"First, we need to intensify efforts to educate primary care physicians and patients.

- *Physicians must be armed with state-of-the-art information about diagnostic testing and optimal care.*

- *Physicians and patients must be empowered to make informed decisions about treatment.*

- *We must educate and motivate people at highest risk to prevent new infections."*

—American Liver Foundation Statement on Hepatitis C

Remember those statistics from Chapter 1? Almost 4 million people are infected with HCV in the U.S. and up to 400 million people worldwide. The problem is, most of these people may not yet have discovered that they have hepatitis C. They may be unwittingly passing the virus, infecting millions and millions more. With such a widespread problem, is there any hope of stopping HCV?

Luckily, the answer is "yes." But stopping HCV requires that everyone who knows about this virus—whether you have it or not—take personal responsibility to halt its spread. This comes down to four steps:

1. Protecting others from acquiring HCV from you if you are a carrier of the virus.

2. Protecting yourself from acquiring HCV if you are not a carrier of the virus.

3. Supporting efforts to educate others about the dangers posed by HCV.

4. Advocating for more research into treatments and vaccines.

Let's take a look at each of these four steps to see how you can implement them in your own crusade to stop the spread of HCV and hepatitis C.

You Can Protect Others from HCV

It's bad enough to learn that you have a virus as dangerous as HCV. You may feel even more frustrated to know that you may have passed it on to others. Now that you know more about HCV and how it spreads, you can take measures to protect those you love. Follow these precautions:

- Tell all your health care providers that you have hepatitis C so they can protect themselves when caring for you. This includes telling your doctors, dentist, and any other health care professionals you work with. If you encounter an emergency, make sure you or someone with you informs any emergency personnel.

- Don't share needles used for injection drugs, tattoos, or body piercing. Remember, bleach won't kill HCV.

- Do not donate blood or agree to be an organ donor.

- Cover all cuts, scrapes, or other skin wounds or sores with bandages. Treat these wounds yourself whenever possible.

- Don't share personal care items such as razors and tooth-brushes with anyone else.

- Decide along with any partners whether you should use a condom or not when having sex. Chances of spreading HCV through sex are low (about 2–5 percent), especially in a mutually monogamous relationship, but it is still possi-ble.

- If you're a woman, decide whether you want to take the risk of spreading HCV to an unborn child. Again, HCV rarely spreads from mother to child during childbirth, but it does occur about 5 percent of the time.

Taking these steps will help protect others from HCV. But just because you have to be careful in some areas doesn't mean you have to cut yourself off from all human contact. There is no evidence that HCV spreads through casual contact such as hugging a friend or using the family dinnerware.

Protect Yourself from HCV

If you don't have HCV, your goal is to stay clear of it. Take these steps to protect yourself:

- Don't share personal care items such as razors or tooth-brushes with anyone else.

- Don't share needles used for injection drugs, tattooing, or body piercing. Bleach will not kill HCV.

- Make sure any needles you use for acupuncture are steril-ized or used only for you.

- If you work with patients where the potential for exposure to blood exists, always follow all universal precaution pro-cedures. Wear protective gloves and other clothing as need-ed. Use and dispose of needles properly. Never try to recap a needle. Always discard needles and other blood- contam-inated items in appropriate biohazard containers. If a tube breaks or you must clean up a blood spill, wear protective clothing and follow the procedures indicated by your employer.

- If a partner has HCV, decide together whether you should use a condom or not when having sex. Chances of spreading HCV through sex are low, especially in a mutually monogamous relationship, but it is still possible.

- If you're at risk for developing HCV, consider testing to see if you have the virus. This won't prevent you from getting HCV, but if you do have the virus, you can take steps to be treated and to prevent its spread to others.

Taking these precautions helps protect you from HCV. But don't overreact and isolate yourself from the rest of the world. There is no evidence that HCV spreads through casual contact. Even if you know a person is infected with HCV, it's still okay to touch them. Sharing household items such as plates and silverware will not spread HCV, either.

Advocate for Education

Just like the educational efforts that have been made to heighten our awareness about HIV and AIDS, so should everyone be informed about HCV and hepatitis C. Knowledge about the danger posed by HCV is the first step toward changing our behaviors. Now that you know more about HCV, don't let that knowledge just sit in the back of your brain. Do more than simply nod your head and agree that educating people about HCV is important. Take some concrete steps to make sure that education occurs. Here are some suggestions:

- Join the American Liver Foundation or the Hepatitis C Foundation. Your contributions help support their educational efforts.

- Contact governmental agencies at all levels: local, county, state, and federal. Find out what information they have

Research Funding for HCV/Hepatitis C and Other Diseases

Dramatic differences in funding for research exist for HCV, HIV/AIDS, and rheumatoid arthritis. Take a look at these numbers from the Hepatitis C Foundation for average yearly research funding for each disease from 1991 to 1995:

Disease Funding

HCV $4.5 million/year

Rheumatoid arthritis $169 million/year

HIV/AIDS $1.15 billion/year

about hepatitis C and encourage them to increase their educational outreach programs.

- Become involved in local issues that affect the spread of HCV. For example, one way HCV spreads is through sharing needles used to inject drugs. Reducing drug use would certainly go a long way toward reducing the spread of HCV. Also, needle exchange for injection drug users is a proven way to prevent the spread of deadly viruses such as HCV and HIV. Yet needle-exchange programs are illegal in most areas.

Advocate for Research

Ideally, one day there will be a vaccination to prevent the spread of HCV and a treatment to cure people who have the disease. However, research in these areas is very time-consuming and expensive. Government funding for HCV is incredibly low, and not likely to increase dramatically unless you and others concerned about hepatitis C join your voices to insist on more funding. Both the American Liver Foundation and the Hepatitis C Foundation are actively encouraging more support for research. The American Liver Foundation even attempts to fund some studies itself. By joining one of these organizations, you'll be more likely to hear regularly about research funding needs. You can also write to your congressional representatives to encourage them to address the issues surrounding the research funding for HCV.

You Can Make a Difference

Whether it's protecting others from HCV, protecting yourself, or encouraging educational and research efforts, you can make a difference in preventing the spread of HCV. Don't assume that some large government bureau of something or other will take up the slack. It's only due to the efforts of individuals like yourself that changes get made. That's what made the difference in funding for research, education, treatment, and support for HIV/AIDS. And your efforts can do the same for HCV.

GLOSSARY

Acetaminophen: A nonaspirin pain reliever (Tylenol is one common brand). Called paracetamol in the United Kingdom.

Acquired immunodeficiency syndrome (AIDS): A disease caused by the human immunodeficiency virus (HIV). When you have AIDS, your body's defenses are weakened, leaving you open to attack from a range of other diseases. AIDS was considered to be fatal until recently. With powerful new drugs, the virus seems to be suppressed or possibly eliminated in many people with HIV/AIDS.

Acute hepatitis: A stage of liver inflammation which occurs suddenly. Persons with hepatitis C are less likely to have acute hepatitis than persons with hepatitis caused by other viruses.

AIDS: See Acquired immunodeficiency syndrome.

Alanine aminotransferase: See ALT.

Albumin: A protein synthesized in the liver. If the liver is damaged, it cannot produce enough albumin. Therefore, lower levels of albumin in the blood are a sign of liver damage.

Alkaline phosphatase: An enzyme that in high levels in the blood may indicate some sort of blockage in the common bile duct or within the smaller bile ducts inside the liver itself. Alkaline phosphatase is also found in bones, the placenta, and the intestines; therefore, another enzyme (GGT) is measured at the same time to confirm results.

Alpha interferon: Currently the only substance approved to treat hepatitis C. Three types of alpha interferon are approved for treating hepatitis C. Some forms of alpha interferon are also used to treat hepatitis B, as well as genital warts (an STD), some AIDS-related diseases (such as Kaposi's sarcoma), and several forms of cancer (some types of leukemias and lymphomas, multiple myeloma, melanoma, renal cell cancer, ovarian cancer, and bladder cancer). No one knows exactly how interferon works, but it keeps the virus from replicating (duplicating) itself in other cells, it keeps some tumor cells from growing, and it helps other cells fight the virus more effectively.

ALT (alanine aminotransferase) levels: An enzyme found in liver cells. When the liver is damaged, ALT escapes out into the blood. Therefore, ALT levels in the blood indicate some sort of possible liver damage. ALT levels are often measured in routine blood testing. This test used to be called the SGPT. Very high levels suggest hepatitis or another liver disease that has killed many liver cells. Moderately high levels may be a sign of conditions such as chronic hepatitis, gallbladder disease, or mononucleosis. Slightly elevated levels may indicate cirrhosis or a heart attack. Many medications (such as aspirin, barbiturates, narcotics, and some immunosuppressant drugs can also affect ALT levels. Previously, physicians relied on ALT levels exclusively to guide decisions on when and how to treat chronic hepatitis and liver damage. However, since it is known that persons with HCV can suffer liver damage and still have normal ALT levels, your doctor should be using other indicators in addition to ALT to monitor your progress.

Amantadine: An antiviral drug that is approved for use in preventing and treating certain types of flu and Parkinson's disease. It may reduce levels of HCV in some people, especially if used in conjunction with interferon or interferon and ribavirin.

Amino acids: Chemicals that form the "building blocks" of proteins. Over 50 amino acids have been identified; the human body uses almost 30 of them. Your body is able to create most of the amino acids you need. However, eight must be eaten in order to maintain an adequate supply. These eight are called essential amino acids.

Anecdotal evidence: Evidence for the effectiveness of a given substance based on accounts of individuals who responded positively to the substance. Collecting anecdotal evidence is often the first step in determining whether a given therapy is effective. Anecdotal evidence for the effectiveness of many alternative therapies exists. Alternative health practitioners usually consider anecdotal evidence sufficient for prescribing an herbal or other "nonmedical" therapy. Most medical doctors, however, are skeptical about such treatments unless the therapy has undergone more rigorous, controlled study.

Anemia: A condition in which there are too few red blood cells in the blood.

Antibody: A substance created during the immune system response that helps disable foreign substances. Antibody "sticks" to antigen, the marked foreign substance. Antibody helps disable the foreign substance and signals to certain white blood cells to ingest the substance to help complete the immune response.

Antigen: A foreign invader in the body that is marked so that white blood cells and other substances can find and disable it.

Anti-HCV: The antibody for the hepatitis C virus.

Anti-inflammatories: Substances that reduce inflammation throughout the body in a variety of ways. Several anti-inflammatories seem to help reduce liver inflammation as well as ALT levels.

Antiviral drugs: Medications that work by killing the virus responsible for a given disease. Antivirals are relatively new. Several have recently been developed for treating HIV/AIDS. The knowledge gained from creating these drugs is now being put to use in research for antivirals that will combat hepatitis C. One antiviral drug is currently approved for treating hepatitis C: alpha interferon. Ribavirin and other antivirals are currently in clinical trials (human testing) to determine whether they are effective in treating hepatitis C.

Ascites: Fluid accumulation and swelling of the abdomen caused by blocked blood flow through the liver. This condition is associated with chronic hepatitis and other liver problems such as cirrhosis. Treatment includes reducing salt intake and taking diuretics. Sometimes fluid can be drained by a catheter.

Aspartate aminotransferase: See AST.

AST (aspartate aminotransferase) levels: An enzyme often measured in routine blood testing. This test used to be called the SGOT. Like ALT, AST can escape out into the blood when the liver is damaged. But it can also leak out from muscle tissue, including the heart. This means that a high AST level in and of itself does not necessarily indicate a liver problem.

Ayurvedic medicine: The medical tradition that developed in India. There are Ayurvedic-based treatments for hepatitis that attempt to slow the destruction of liver cells, normalize liver enzyme levels, restore the function of liver cells, reduce liver inflammation, restore immune system function, and destroy the causative virus.

B cells: Cells produced by the lymph system. During the body's immune response, B cells produce antibodies to combat the specific antigen that has invaded the body.

dBNA (branched DNA) assay: A test to detect HCV directly. It is easy to perform and can be replicated. But it is not as sensitive as the RT-PCR test. This means you may get a negative (no HCV present) result even though you may be a carrier of HCV.

Beta interferon: One type of interferon made by the body to protect cells from invading viruses. Beta interferon can be made synthetically, such as from bacteria or animal cells or cloned from human interferon. It is currently being used to treat multiple sclerosis and some researchers believe it may prove to be somewhat useful in treating hepatitis C.

Bile: A digestive juice made by the liver, containing bilirubin, accounting for its greenish yellow color. Bile travels from the liver through the common bile duct, which empties into the duodenum and into the small intestine. Excess bile is stored in the gallbladder, near the duodenum, where it can be released as needed to aid digestion.

Bilirubin: A bile pigment that causes yellowing of the skin and eyes (jaundice). It is created when red blood cells break down. The liver processes these cells, then secretes the bilirubin into the bile. There is normally a little bilirubin circulating in blood. However, if the liver is unable to process bilirubin, it accumulates at higher levels in the blood.

Carrier: A person whose body harbor a virus such as HCV, but who may not necessarily show signs of having the disease associated with the virus. Whether or not the carrier has symptoms of the disease, the carrier can still pass on the virus to others.

Cell-mediated response: Part of the immune system response to a foreign invader. T cells become activated and differentiate into several forms, each of which has a role in the immune response. Some T cells help disable the invading substance and ingest it.

Chemotherapy: The use of toxic substances to destroy cancerous tumors. Chemotherapy is often used to fight hepatocellular carcinoma, a type of liver cancer that can occur as a result of hepatitis C.

Chinese medicine: The tradition of medical practice that developed in China and is now fairly popular in the U.S. There are Chinese medicine-based treatments for hepatitis that attempt to slow the destruction of liver cells, normalize liver enzyme levels, restore the function of liver cells, reduce liver inflammation, restore immune system function, and destroy the causative virus.

Chronic hepatitis: Liver inflammation that does not go away. Many people have chronic hepatitis and don't realize it. Over time, chronic hepatitis can lead to severe liver damage.

Cirrhosis: A liver condition in which normal liver cells that become damaged are replaced by scar tissue. This new tissue is unable to perform the various functions carried out by normal liver cells. Scar tissue also blocks blood from flowing through the liver. As scar tissue builds, the liver gradually performs fewer and fewer of its vital functions. Fluid can accumulate in the abdomen (ascites) and back up into the veins near the esophagus. These veins can burst, causing the person with cirrhosis to vomit up blood. Because the liver cannot remove toxic substances, they build up in the skin (leading to jaundice and itching).

Clinical trials: Tests on humans conducted to determine whether a drug is both safe and effective in treating a particular condition. Clinical trials are usually one of the last stages in drug development before FDA approval.

Clotting factors: Chemicals manufactured by the liver that enable blood to clot when needed, such as when skin is damaged by a cut. These clotting factors are absent in people with hemophilia, requiring them to use clotting factor from donated blood. Before HCV was isolated, using clotting factor placed hemophiliacs at great risk for acquiring hepatitis C. Now, blood is screened for HCV.

Cognitive dysfunction: A condition that can occur as a result of severe liver problems. As toxins build up throughout the body and the brain, thinking is less clear. A person may become confused and disoriented.

Consensus interferon: A type of synthesized alpha interferon that includes amino acids from several different types of natural alpha interferons. It is one of the three types of interferon licensed by the FDA under the name interferon alfacon-1 (Infergen), manufactured by Amgen.

Control group: The group participating in a clinical trial that receives no treatment at all.

Cryoglobulinemia: See essential mixed cryoglubulinemia.

Delta hepatitis: Another name for hepatitis D.

Drug-induced hepatitis: Liver inflammation caused by long-term use of certain medications.

Edema: Swelling of the hands and feet due to fluid retention. A symptom of chronic hepatitis.

EIA-2 and -3 (second- and third-generation enzyme immunoassay) blood tests: Tests for anti-HCV, the antibody to the hepatitis C virus. If detected, an initial diagnosis of hepatitis C is made, but follow up testing to confirm the actual presence of the virus should be done, since the EIA is not able to detect the virus itself.

Encephalopathy: A condition resulting from cirrhosis in which the person becomes confused. Left untreated, coma results. Treatment includes medication, reducing protein—especially animal protein—in the diet, and controlling intestinal bleeding.

Enteric non-A, non-B hepatitis: Another name for hepatitis E.

Enzyme: A substance that helps cells generate energy without being used up itself. Many enzymes are found in the liver, each with a different function. When the liver enzymes alanine aminotransferase (ALT) or aspartate aminotransferase (AST) are found in the blood, liver damage is suspected.

Epidemic non-A, non-B hepatitis: Another name for hepatitis E.

Essential amino acids: The eight amino acids that cannot be created by the human body; therefore, some of these acids must be eaten on a regular basis. The eight essential amino acids are methionine, leucine, isoleucine, valine, lysine, threonine, tryptophan, and phenyl-alanine.

Essential mixed cryoglobulinemia: A condition that is thought to be caused by HCV. Levels of cryoglobulin (a substance involved in the body's immune response) in the blood rise, restricting blood flow, especially to the extremities. Symptoms include cold hands and feet, muscle and joint pain, dermatitis, nerve problems, liver inflammation, and fatigue.

FDA: See Food and Drug Administration.

Fibrosis: One of the effects of hepatitis C on the liver. Fibrosis occurs as old tissue is destroyed and replaced by new, nonfunctional tissue. Over time, the liver begins to function less and blood becomes backed up in the main vein and surrounding channels in the liver.

Floaters: A condition that some people with chronic hepatitis C complain of. Floaters are wispy cobweb-like substances that float inside the eye, interfering with the visual field. Usually floaters are not harmful, and most people see some as they grow older.

Food and Drug Administration (FDA): An agency within the Department of Health and Human Services of the U.S. government. The FDA is responsible for regulating and approving all drugs (prescription and over-the-counter) in the U.S.

Gamma globulin: A substance that helps initiate the body's immune response. Gamma globulin can be given before or sometimes right after exposure to protect against some types of hepatitis, but not to protect against hepatitis C.

Gamma-glutamyltranspeptidase: See GGT.

Gamma interferon: One type of interferon made by the body to protect cells from invading viruses. It is thought to be involved in the development of rheumatoid arthritis.

Gastroenterologist: A medical doctor (MD) or doctor of osteopathy (DO) who has received additional training in the diagnosis and treatment of stomach and other digestive system problems. Many gastroenterologists have a special interest and expertise in treating liver problems, since the liver is considered part of the body's digestive system. Gastroenterologists may perform certain diagnostic procedures, but are not trained to do surgery.

Genotypes: The various forms that a virus may take. HCV comes in many genotypes, making it harder to diagnose and treat than other types of hepatitis. Known genotypes of HCV and their predominant locations are type 1, type 2 and type 3 (worldwide); type 4 (Middle East and Africa); type 5 (South Africa); and type 6 (Asia). Type 1 is the predominant genotype in the U.S.

GGT (gamma-glutamyltranspeptidase or GGTP): An enzyme that in high levels in the blood may indicate some sort of blockage in the common bile duct or within the smaller bile ducts inside the liver itself. High levels may also indicate liver cancer. Alcohol use can dramatically affect results. GGT is usually measured along with another similar enzyme, alanine phosphatase.

GGTP: See GGT.

Glomerulonephritis: Inflamed kidneys caused by an immune system reaction and sometimes seen in persons with HCV. Symptoms include weakness, aching near the kidneys, high blood pressure, anemia, and the presence of high levels of certain waste products (urea, creatinine, and protein) in the blood and urine. Over time, hemodialysis may be needed to help the kidneys function.

Glycogen: The form in which sugar is stored in the liver.

HCV: Hepatitis C virus, the virus that causes the disease called hepatitis C. HCV is classified as a RNA virus.

Hemophilia: A condition that occurs when the body is unable to manufacture a factor that helps the blood clot. Many people with hemophilia have hepatitis C, due to using clotting factors created from infected donated blood.

Hepatectomy: Surgical removal of all or part of the liver. Usually used to treat hepatocellular carcinoma (HCC), a form of liver cancer that affects 6 percent to 8 percent of persons with HCV.

Hepatitis: Inflammation of the liver. Can be caused by viruses, drugs, or alcohol.

Hepatitis A: Formerly called **infectious hepatitis** because its virus spreads through contaminated water and food. It is more common in developing countries, but is also found in the U.S. There is a vaccine to prevent hepatitis A. Gamma globulin can also be taken to help protect against exposure for a shorter period of time.

Hepatitis B: Formerly called **serum hepatitis** because its virus, HBV, spreads through blood and other body fluids. It is often considered the most serious form of hepatitis. Hepatitis B can be transmitted from a pregnant woman to her baby. Most people recover from hepatitis B, but some may retain chronic infection. There is a vaccine to prevent hepatitis B. A special gamma globulin can also be taken to protect against exposure.

Hepatitis C: Formerly called **non-A, non-B (NANB) hepatitis**. HCV spreads through blood and is the most common form of hepatitis. The initial illness is often so slight that most people don't even notice it, yet few people recover completely. Most people with HCV go on to develop chronic hepatitis infection. Currently, there is no vaccine to prevent hepatitis C. Gamma globulin does not seem to protect against hepatitis C.

Hepatitis D: Formerly called **delta hepatitis**. It is only found along with hepatitis B and is rare in the U.S.

Hepatitis E: Formerly called **enteric** or **epidemic non-A, non-B hepatitis**. It is similar to hepatitis A. It is rare in the U.S. and is most common in areas around the Indian Ocean.

Hepatitis G: has only recently been discovered. The HGV virus (there are at least three subtypes of this virus) spreads through blood and is often found along with HBV, HCV, and HIV (the virus that leads to AIDS). In otherwise healthy people, HGV seems to cause no problems. It is thought that HGV may simply be a sort of marker for other, yet-undiscovered hepatitis viruses.

Hepatocellular carcinoma (HCC): A type of cancer of the liver that is associated with hepatitis C.

Hepatologist: A medical doctor (MD) or doctor of osteopathy (DO) who has received additional training in the diagnosis and treatment of liver problems, including surgery. There are not many practicing hepatologists. Most are located in large university research centers or large urban medical centers.

Herpes virus: A group of viruses, including the virus that causes chickenpox, that can sometimes lead to hepatitis.

HIV: See Human immunodeficiency virus.

Homeopathy: A medical system that treats illness with substances that are similar to the illness itself, such as giving persons with hepatitis C medications that contain very low amounts of HCV. The goal is to stimulate the immune system to fight off the infection and allow the body to heal itself. Note that not only is this approach different than traditional Western medicine, it is *opposite*.

Human immunodeficiency virus (HIV): The virus that causes AIDS (acquired immunodeficiency syndrome), in which the body's defenses are weakened, leaving you open to attack from various diseases.

Humoral response: Part of the immune system response that includes the creation of antibodies by B cells in response to antigen. Antibodies then attach to antigen, help disable the foreign substance, and signal to phagocytes to ingest the cell.

Hydrophilic bile salts: Substances that reduce chronic inflammation of the liver. Hydrophilic bile salts also seem to reduce ALT levels.

Immune system: The body's mechanism for dealing with foreign invading substances.

Infectious hepatitis: Another name for hepatitis A.

Inflammation: One of the results of the immune response to a foreign invader. As fluid, cells, and other substances accumulate at the site of the invasion, swelling occurs.

Interferon: A protein produced by the body's cells during the immune response. It is actually produced by the cells that are infected by the virus or other invader, and protects other cells from infection. There are three types of interferon—called alpha interferon, beta interferon, and gamma interferon—which are used to combat several types of cancer and diseases thought to be caused by viruses, such as multiple sclerosis, rheumatoid arthritis, and hepatitis C.

Interferon alfa-2a: One of two types of alpha interferon treatments approved for hepatitis C. Interferon alfa-2a (Roferon-A) is manufactured by Roche. See Alpha interferon.

Interferon alfa-2b: The first of two types of alpha interferon treatments approved for hepatitis C. Interferon alfa-2b (Intron A) is manufactured by Schering. See Alpha interferon.

Interferon alfacon-1: A synthetic alpha interferon (Infergen) that includes amino acids from several different types of natural alpha interferons. See Consensus interferon.

Irritable bowel syndrome (IBS): A condition sometimes associated with chronic hepatitis. IBS may come and go, making eating very difficult.

Jaundice: A yellowing of the eyes and skin that occurs as bilirubin builds up in the tissues. Normally, bilirubin is broken down and removed by the liver. Jaundice is a sign of liver problems.

Lactulose: A medication used to help rid the blood of excess ammonia. Ammonia is a byproduct of the digestion and use of protein. When a person has cirrhosis, the liver may be less able to process proteins properly, leading to a rise in the ammonia level in the blood.

Lichen planus: Small, itchy, purple bumps that form on the insides of the wrists or in the mouth. An immune system condition that is often seen in people with hepatitis C.

Liver: An organ in the abdomen that is responsible for processing all food that passes out of the digestive tract, storing and distributing nutrients, and breaking down toxic substances in the body.

Liver function tests (LFTs): Blood tests that measure a range of substances normally found in the liver, including ALT, AST, alkaline phosphatase, GGT, bilirubin, serum albumin, prothrombin time, and other substances related to more rare liver conditions.

Lymph: Body fluids created by the lymph glands that assist with the immune system.

Lymphoblastoid-alfa N1 interferon: See natural interferon.

Multiple sclerosis (MS): A condition in which the body's immune system attacks the lining (myelin) of the nerves. This results in problems such as pain, spasm, an inability to move, and other central nervous system symptoms. Like people with hepatitis C, people with MS often feel fatigued and combat depression. Another type of interferon (beta interferon) is used to treat MS.

Mutations: Variations that occur in viruses and cells as they replicate. Mutations make it difficult to create effective treatments and vaccines for the hepatitis C virus.

N-acetylcysteine: An anti-inflammatory that may help reduce ALT levels and liver inflammation in persons with hepatitis C. Note that N-acetylcysteine is not approved by the FDA for this use, however.

Natural (lymphoblastoid-alfa n1 and alfa n3) interferon: A type of alpha interferon currently being tested for treating hepatitis C; this drug is not yet approved for use in persons with hepatitis C. Interferon alfa-n1 and alfa-n3 are actually produced from human cells, whereas other alpha interferons are generally created from *e. coli* bacteria. Sustained response in persons treated with alfa-n1 or alfa-n3 appear to be higher than for other alpha interferons. Further studies are underway to continue to assess this drug's safety and effectiveness.

Naturopathic medicine: A medical tradition that focuses on using natural means of healing, including botanicals. There are naturopathic-based treatments for hepatitis that attempt to slow the destruction of liver cells, normalize liver enzyme levels, restore the function of liver cells, reduce liver inflammation, restore immune system function, and destroy the causative virus. Several schools of naturopathy exist in the U.S. A naturopath should have completed a program at one of these schools and is certified to practice.

Neomycin: A medication used to help rid the blood of excess ammonia. Ammonia is a byproduct of the digestion and use of protein. When a person has cirrhosis, the liver may be less able to process proteins properly, leading to a rise in the ammonia level in the blood.

Non-A non-B (NANB) hepatitis: Another name for hepatitis C.

Nonspecific: The term used by doctors to describe symptoms that are general in nature and could be associated with a number of different medical conditions. Examples of nonspecific symptoms include flu-like symptoms, fatigue, and sleep problems. Many nonspecific symptoms are associated with hepatitis C.

PCR (polymerase chain reaction): See RT-PCR.

Phagocyte: A white blood cell that ingests and destroys invading substances.

Phagocytosis: The process by which certain white blood cells ingest and destroy invading substances.

Portal hypertension: A condition that occurs as a result of cirrhosis. As blood is less able to flow through the liver, it backs up into the vein that connects the intestines and liver (portal vein). As blood continues to back up into surrounding veins, smaller vessels can burst, leading to life-threatening bleeding. Blood may be vomited up.

Prothrombin time (Protime or PT): A test to determine how long it takes for your blood to clot. The liver makes the proteins used for blood clotting. If the liver is damaged, it takes longer for blood to clot. The result is often expressed as the International Normalized Ratio or INR.

Protime: See Prothrombin time.

PT: See Prothrombin time.

Recombinant immunoblot assay: See RIBA-2 and -3.

Referred pain: Pressure on nerves in the liver and abdomen caused by swelling can also cause sensations of pain around the right shoulder. This may occur most frequently after liver biopsy.

Remission: A state in which the virus and symptoms seem to disappear. Interferon therapy and possibly some alternative therapies cause remission for some people with hepatitis C. If therapy is discontinued, however, the virus may reappear.

Rheumatoid arthritis (RA): A condition caused when the body's immune system attacks the lining (synovia) of the joints. Symptoms include joint pain, swelling, and loss of function of joints. Like hepatitis C, people with RA often feel extreme fatigue, depression, and other symptoms associated with immune system disorders.

RIBA-2 and -3 (second- and third-generation recombinant immunoblot assay): Blood tests that, like EIA-2 and EIA-3, detect antibodies to HCV, but do not detect the virus itself.

Ribavirin: An antiviral drug that by itself is not very effective against HCV but seems to make interferon therapy more effective.

Rimantadine: An antiviral drug similar to amantadine that is approved for use in preventing and treating certain types of flu and Parkinson's disease. It may reduce levels of HCV in some people, especially if used in conjunction with interferon or interferon and ribavirin.

RT-PCR (qualitative reserve transcription polymerase chain reaction): Tests the blood for the presence of the hepatitis C virus itself. Used to confirm HCV infection.

Seasonal affective disorder (SAD): A condition in which a person's mood changes in relation to the amount of light. During the winter, people with SAD can become extremely depressed. Treatment includes phototherapy, that is, receiving adequate exposure to certain types of bright light.

Secoiridoid glucosides: Substances thought to be helpful to liver function. They are found in many plants, including *Swertia mileensis*.

Serotype: The various forms of a virus, as measured indirectly by looking at its antibodies. HCV serotypes roughly correlate with HCV genotypes, although the serotype process does not always provide definitive results.

Serum hepatitis: Another name for hepatitis B.

Sexually transmitted disease (STD): Any of a number of diseases that are spread through sexual intercourse. STDs include HIV/AIDS, genital herpes, vaginitis, chlamydia, gonorrhea, syphilis, condyloma, and many other diseases. It is thought that HCV may in some cases be transmitted through sexual intercourse; however, incidence of acquiring HCV is extremely low in persons involved in a mutually monogamous relationship with a partner who has HCV. As a result, many physicians do *not* generally recommend that a person with HCV use barrier protection (condoms) when in a monogamous relationship.

T cells: White blood cells that enable the immune response. T cells are primarily responsible for cell-mediated immunity, where they disable and digest invading substances. They also play a role in humoral immunity, where certain T cells trigger B cells to create antibody.

Thymosin alpha-1: An immunomodulating agent (that is, it affects the body's immune response. It has been used in small trials with humans and seems to be effective in reducing ALT levels in some people to normal when used in combination with interferon. Studies are continuing to assess thymosin alpha-1's potential use in treating hepatitis C.

Thymus: A gland located in the chest, just under the neck. The thymus is responsible for manufacturing T cells, white blood cells that aid the body's immune response. By the time most people reach 20 years old, the thymus has shrunken and no longer produces these cells. It may be that replacing enzymes normally created by the thymus may help the body's immune response against viruses such as those that cause hepatitis B and hepatitis C.

Transfusion: Giving blood from a donor to a patient who has experienced blood loss. Transfusion was one of the major ways of transmitting HCV until a test was devised in 1991 to test donated blood for the virus.

Viral hepatitis: Hepatitis caused by a virus (such as hepatitis A and hepatitis C). Hepatitis can also be caused by some medications.

Virus: An extremely small organism, invisible to the eye and even to all but the strongest microscopes. There are two classes of viruses: DNA (deoxyribonucleic acid) and RNA (ribonucleic acid). HCV is considered an RNA virus.

RESOURCES

Resources for information and support concerning hepatitis C abound. You just have to know where to start looking. Here are a few sources that seem to be the most useful. They will lead you to others.

General Information About Hepatitis C

The American Liver Foundation, a voluntary health organization in the United States. Its goal is to prevent, treat, and cure a variety of conditions related to the liver and gallbladder, including hepatitis C. It sponsors research and educational initiatives and publishes a series of brochures on liver disease. The ALF also has several regional chapters and support groups.

> 1425 Pompton Avenue, Cedar Grove, NJ 07009-1000
> (201) 256-2550
> fax: (201) 256-3214
> Toll-free hotlines: (800) GO-LIVER (465-4837)
> and (888) 4HEP-ABC (443-7222)
> web site: www.liverfoundation.org

The American Digestive Health Foundation, a health organization that focuses on research and education for a variety of digestive disorders, including hepatitis C.

7910 Woodmont Ave., 7th floor
Bethesda MD 20814
(301) 654-2635
fax: (301) 654-1140
Toll-free number: (800) 668-5237
web site: www.gastro.org

Digestive Health Initiative Viral Hepatitis Education Campaign is sponsored by the American Digestive Health Foundation and the American Liver Foundation. Among other public information services, the campaign also publishes a quarterly newsletter. For information, call either sponsoring organization.

Ask Emaliss, a monthly on-line magazine devoted to hepatitis C information and support. Provides a wealth of information about HCV, a personal approach to what it's like to live with HCV, and links to many other HCV-related sites.

The Internet address is: soli.inav.net/~webbsite

Contact the **Hepatitis Foundation International** at (201) 239-4139.

Support Groups

The American Liver Foundation has chapters and support groups throughout the U.S., as well as hotlines. For how to contact, see the listing under "General Information" on the previous page.

The Hepatitis C Foundation is a nonprofit advocacy and education group for persons with hepatitis C. The foundation has a more "activist" approach than the American Liver Foundation. It provides a support hotline as well as support groups throughout the country. The Hepatitis C Foundation also strongly advocates for more federal funding in the U.S. for hepatitis C research and education. It also provides some information about alternative treatments for hepatitis C.

Hepatitis C Foundation
1502 Russett Drive
Warminster, PA 18974-1176

(215) 672-2606
fax (215) 672-1518
Support line: (800) 324-7305
web site: www.hepcfoundation.org

The Hepatitis C Support Project primarily provides support for persons with hepatitis C. They publish a newsletter, as well.

Hepatitis C Support Project
P.O. Box 427037
San Francisco, CA 94142-7037
(415) 834-4100
Bay Area support groups: (415) 676-4888

America Online sponsors a hepatitis C support group "chat" every Wednesday night from 8 to 9 p.m. EST. You must subscribe to America Online in order to access this chat group. They often have guest speakers who are experts in some aspect of hepatitis C. Other America Online chat groups related to hepatitis C include Hepterminal and HCV (a private chat room). All these take place in the PEN (Personal Empowerment Network) conference room. If you subscribe to another service, such as CompuServe or Prodigy, check out their sections on chronic illness or alternative/natural medicine to find resources and discussion groups related to hepatitis C.

Yahoo sponsors or provides access to clubs for a variety of interests, including several support groups dealing with hepatitis C.

web site: clubs.yahoo.com

Alternative Therapies

The Hepatitis C Foundation provides some information about alternative treatments for hepatitis C. See listing under "Support Groups."

Nature's Response is an Oklahoma-based company that provides vitamins, herbs, other nutritional supplements, and homeopathic remedies. Its owner is a certified nutritional counselor who provides consultations. To request a catalog, call (800) 216-5195 or fax (888) 842-8168. For nutritional counseling, call (405) 878-6778.

Preventative Therapeutics provides information and products for thymic therapy. Contact them at P.O. Box 956248, Duluth, GA 30136, 770-409-0900, fax 770-409-0110.

If you subscribe to an on-line service (America Online, CompuServe, or Prodigy), check in the Natural Medicine or Alternative Medicine forums.

Drug Therapy

The American Liver Foundation tries to maintain a current database of drugs undergoing clinical trials. To contact them, see the listing under "General Information About Hepatitis C" on page 132. Their web site also has some "hot links" connecting directly to web sites of some of the drug manufacturers.

Interferon information can be received by any of the three manufacturers of alpha interferon:

Amgen: 1-888-508-8088

Roche: 1-888-300-7284

Schering: 1-888-437-2608

REFERENCES

Alcohol and the Liver. American Liver Foundation. 1997.

Alter, Harvey J., MD. *Blood Donors with Hepatitis C.* NIH Consensus Development Conference on Management of Hepatitis C. March, 1997.

Alter, Harvey J.; Nakatsuji, Yoshiyuki; Melpolder, Jacqueline; Wages, John; Wesley, Robert; Shih, J. Wai-Kuo; Kim, Jungsuh P. "The Incidence of Transfusion-Associated Hepatitis G Virus Infection and Its Relation to Liver Disease." *New England Journal of Medicine.* March 13, 1997. 336(11): 747-754.

Alter, Miriam J., MD. *Epidemiology of Hepatitis C.* NIH Consensus Development Conference on Management of Hepatitis C. March, 1997.

Amantadine (Systemic). *USP DI-Volume II Advice for the Patient: Drug Information in Lay Language.* 1996. Edition 16: 167.

Anstett, Patricia. "Naomi Judd Spreads Hope Fighting Hepatitis C." *San Jose Mercury News.* Wednesday, June 24, 1998.

Batchelder, H.; Hudson, T.; Sodhi, V.; Ergil, K.; Dharmananda, S.; Scalzo, R. "Therapeutic Approaches to Viral Hepatitis." *Protocol Journal of Botanical Medicine.* Autumn, 1995. Vol. 1, no. 2: 129-72.

Bonkovsky, Herbert L., MD. *Other Options for Treatment of Hepatitis C.* NIH Consensus Development Conference on Management of Hepatitis C. March, 1997.

Cancer of the Liver. American Liver Foundation. 1997.

Carithers, Robert L. Jr., MD. *Therapy of Hepatitis C: Interferon Alfa-2b.* NIH Consensus Development Conference on Management of Hepatitis C. March, 1997.

Cheung, Ramsey C., MD, Keeffe, Emmet B, MD, and Greenberg, Harry B, MD. "Hepatitis G Virus: Is It a Hepatitis Virus?" *Western Journal of Medicine.* July, 1997. Vol. 167: 23-33.

Chronic Hepatitis. American Liver Foundation. 1997.

Cirrhosis: Many Causes. American Liver Foundation. 1997.

Complications: Portal Hypertension. *Focus: On Hepatitis C International Newsletter.* December 1994.

Davis, Gary L., MD. *Hepatitis C: Therapy.* American Liver Foundation. 1997.

Davis, Gary L., MD. *Predictive Factors for a Beneficial Response.* NIH Consensus Development Conference on Management of Hepatitis C. March, 1997.

Davis, Gary L., MD, Esteban-Muir, Rafael, MD, Rustgi, Viunod, MD, et al. "Interferon Alfa-2b Alone or in Combination with Ribavirin for the Treatment of Relapse of Chronic Hepatitis C." *New England Journal of Medicine.* Vol. 339, no. 21: 1493.

Davis, Gary L., MD, Esteban-Muir, Rafael, MD, Rustgi, Viunod, MD, et al. "Interferon Alfa-2b Alone or in Combination with Ribavirin as Initial Treatment for Hepatitis C." *New England Journal of Medicine.* Vol: 339, no: 21: 1493.

DiBisceglie, Adrian M., MD. *Hepatitis C and Hepatocellular Carcinoma.* NIH Consensus Development Conference on Management of Hepatitis C. March, 1997.

DiBisceglie, Adrian M., MD, editor. *Treatment Advances in Chronic Hepatitis C.* Thieme Medical Publishers, New York. 1999. Vol. 19, supplement 1.

Dienstag, Jules L., MD. *Sexual and Perinatal Spread of Hepatitis C Virus Infection.* NIH Consensus Development Conference on Management of Hepatitis C. March, 1997.

Diet and Your Liver. American Liver Foundation. 1997.

Disease Burden from Viral Hepatitis A, B, and C in the United States. Centers for Disease Control and Prevention, Hepatitis Branch. February, 1996.

Dolan, Matthew. *The Hepatitis C Handbook.* Catalyst Press, London. 1996.

Drugs for Liver Disease Currently in Clinical Trials or Development. American Liver Foundation. 1997.

Dusheiko, Geoffrey, MD. *Side Effects of Interferon Alpha in Viral Hepatitis.* NIH Consensus Development Conference on Management of Hepatitis C. March, 1997.

EASL International Consensus Conference on Hepatitis C: Consensus Statement. *Journal of Hepatology.* 1999. Vol. 30: 956-961.

English, Richard and Foster, Graham. *Living with Hepatitis C.* Robinson Publishing Ltd., London. 1997.

Farrell, Geoffrey C., MD. *Interferon Alfa-n 1 Trials.* NIH Consensus Development Conference on Management of Hepatitis C. March, 1997.

Focus: On the Liver & Cirrhosis. *Focus: On Hepatitis C International.* September/October/November 1994.

The Food Guide Pyramid. United States Department of Agriculture. 1992.

Getting Hip to Hep: What You Should Know About Hepatitis A, B, & C. American Liver Foundation. 1996.

Gish, Robert G., MD. Alternatives in the Treatment of Chronic Hepatitis C Infection. *Liver Lifeline.* Summer, 1998.

Gish, Robert G., MD. FDA Approves Rebatron Combination Therapy for Chronic Hepatitis C. *Liver Lifeline.* Summer, 1998.

Hepatitis C. American Liver Foundation. 1997.

Hepatitis C: Diagnostic Techniques and Monitoring Strategies. Amgen, Inc. 1997.

Hepatitis C: Predictors of Therapeutic Response to Disease Progression. Amgen, Inc., 1997.

Hepatitis C Fact Sheet. Centers for Disease Control, Hepatitis Branch. March 6, 1997.

"Hepatitis/Liver Pain?" *Focus: On Hepatitis C International Newsletter.* November, 1994.

Hepatitis Surveillance: Issues and Answers:. Report 56. Centers for Disease Control and Prevention. April, 1996.

Hoofnagle, Jay H., MD. *Hepatitis C: The Clinical Spectrum of Disease.* NIH Consensus Development Conference on Management of Hepatitis C. March, 1997.

Hubner, John. Insidious Disease on the Upswing. *San Jose Mercury New.* March 7, 1999.

Interferon Treatments for Hepatitis B and C. American Liver Foundation. 1997.

Keeffe, Emmet B., MD. "Treatment of Chronic Hepatitis C." Personal paper and slides, 1998.

Keeffe, Emmet B., MD and Hollinger, F. Blaine, MD. *Consensus Interferon Trials. Hepatology.* 1997. Vol. 26, no. 3, supplement 1: 1015.

Keeffe, Emmet B., Iwarson, Sten, McMahon, Brian J., et al. "Safety and Immunogenicity of Hepatitis A Vaccination in Patients with Chronic Liver Disease." *Hepatology.* 1998. Vol. 27: 881-886.

Kikuzaki, H.; Kawasaki, Y.; Kitamura, S.; Nakatani, N. Secoiridoid Glucosides from *Swertia mileensis. Planta Medica.* February, 1996. Vol. 62, no. 1: 35-38.

Koff, Raymond S., MD. *Cost-Effectiveness Analysis*. NIH Consensus Development Conference on Management of Hepatitis C. March, 1997.

Laboratory Blood Tests. Focus: Hepatitis C International Web Site. 1997.

Lee, William M., MD. *Therapy of Hepatitis C with Interferon Alfa-2a*. NIH Consensus Development Conference on Management of Hepatitis C. March, 1997.

Lin, C. C.; Lin, C. H. "Pharmacological and Pathological Studies on Taiwan Folk Medicine: The Hepatoprotective Effect of the Methanolic Extract from *Echinops grijisii*." *American Journal of Chinese Medicine*. 1993. Vol. 21, no. 1: 33-44.

Lin, S. C.; Lin, C. C.; Lin, Y. H.; Supriyatna, S.; Pan, S. L. "The Protective Effect of *Alstonia scholaris R. Br.* on Hepatotoxin-induced acute liver damage." *American Journal of Chinese Medicine*. 1996. Vol. 24, no. 2: 153-164.

Lin, S.; Yao, C.; Lin, C.; Lin, Y. "Hepatoprotective Activity of Taiwan Folk Medicine: *Eclipta prostrata (Linn.)* against Various Hepatotoxins induced acute hepatotoxicity." *Phytotherapy Research*. September, 1996. Vol. 10, no. 6: 483-490.

Lindsay, Karen L., MD. *Therapy of Hepatitis C: Overview*. NIH Consensus Development Conference on Management of Hepatitis C. March, 1997.

Liver Biopsy. American Liver Foundation. 1997.

The Liver Biopsy Guide. Focus: Hepatitis C International Web Site. 1997.

Liver Disease in the United States—A Fact Sheet. American Liver Foundation. 1997.

Liver Function Tests. American Liver Foundation. 1997.

Loftus, Mary J. "Transplant Allows Woman to Live—Not Just to Be Alive." *Lakeland [Florida] Ledger*. June 1, 1997.

Lok, Anna, MD and Gunaratnam, Naresh T., MD. *Diagnosis of Hepatitis C*. NIH Consensus Development Conference on Management of Hepatitis C. March, 1997.

Low Sodium Eating: Tips for Kicking the Salt Habit. Krames Communications. 1996.

Management of Hepatitis C. National Institutes of Health Consensus Development Statement. Revised draft, March 27, 1997.

Marcellin, Patrick, MD. *Treatment of Patients with Normal ALT Levels.* NIH Consensus Development Conference on Management of Hepatitis C. March, 1997.

McPartland, J. M. "Viral Hepatitis Treated with *Phyllantus amarus* and Milk Thistle (*Silybum marianum*): A Case Report." *Complementary Medicine International.* March/April, 1996. Vol. 3, no. 2: 40-42.

McQuillan, G. M., Alter M. J., Moyer, L. A., et al. "A Population Based Serologic Study of Hepatitis C Virus Infection in the United States." *Viral Hepatitis and Liver Disease: Proceedings of IX Triennial International Symposium on Viral Hepatitis and Liver Disease.* Edizioni Minerva Medica, Turin, Italy. 1997.

Miyakawa, Yuzo and Mayumi, Makoto. "Hepatitis G Virus—A True Hepatitis Virus or an Accidental Tourist?" *New England Journal of Medicine.* March 13, 1997. 336(11): 795-796.

Most Common Symptoms. Emaliss On-Line Newsletter. 1997.

Nompleggi, Dominic J., MD, and Bonkovsky, Herbert L., MD. *Diet and Chronic Liver Disease: An Updated Research Report.* American Liver Foundation. 1997.

Ooi, V. E. Hepatoprotective Effect of Some Edible Mushrooms. *Phytotherapy Research.* September, 1996. Vol. 10, no. 6: 536-538.

Perrillo, Robert P., MD. *Role of Liver Biopsy.* NIH Consensus Development Conference on Management of Hepatitis C. March, 1997.

Petro, Beth Ann. *The Book of Kombucha: Unlocking the Secrets of the 2000-Year-Old Chinese "Tea Mushroom."* Ulysses Press, Berkeley, CA. 1996.

Pierce, Andrea. *The American Pharmaceutical Association Practical Guide to Natural Medicines.* William Morrow Co., New York. 1999.

Purcell, Robert H., MD. *Hepatitis C Virus: An Introduction.* NIH Consensus Development Conference on Management of Hepatitis C. March, 1997.

Reichard, Elle, MD, and Weiland, Ola, MD. *Ribavirin Treatment Alone or in Combination with Interferon*. NIH Consensus Development Conference on Management of Hepatitis C. March, 1997.

Rosenfeld, Isadore, MD. "Do You Have Hepatitis C? Are You Sure?" *Parade*. January 29, 1999.

Schalm, Solko W., MD. *Treatment of Patients with Cirrhosis*. NIH Consensus Development Conference on Management of Hepatitis C. March, 1997.

Schiff, Eugene R., MD. *Hepatitis C and Alcohol*. NIH Consensus Development Conference on Management of Hepatitis C. March, 1997.

Seeff, Leonard B., MD. *Natural History of Hepatitis C*. NIH Consensus Development Conference on Management of Hepatitis C. March, 1997.

So, Samuel and Keeffe, Emmet B., MD. "Liver Transplantation for Hepatitis B and C." *Medical Progress*. December, 1998. Page 63.

Thabrew, M. I. and Hughes, R. D. "Phytogenic Agents in the Therapy of Liver Disease." *Phytotherapy Research*. September, 1996. Vol. 10, no. 6: 461-467.

Tuller, David. "Deadlier Form of Hepatitis C Has No Cure: List of 'C' Victims Grows—But Research Funding Doesn't." *San Francisco Chronicle*. May 31, 1997.

Viral Hepatitis: An Epidemic in the Making. New Approaches to the Prevention, Diagnosis and Treatment of Viral Hepatitis. American Digestive Health Foundation and American Liver Foundation. 1996.

Who Is at Risk for Hepatitis and Other Liver Diseases? American Liver Foundation. 1997.

Yasko, Joyce M.; Kearney, Brian; and Conrad, Kathryn. *Biotherapy in Cancer: Continuing Education for Oncology Nurses*. Berlex Laboratories. 1996.

Your Liver: A Vital Organ. American Liver Foundation. 1997.

INDEX

ULYSSES PRESS HEALTH BOOKS

A Natural Approach Books

Written in a friendly, nontechnical style, *A Natural Approach* books address specific health issues and show you how to take an active part in your own treatment. Believing that disease is more than a combination of symptoms, these books offer integrated mind/body programs that take a positive, preventative approach.

ANXIETY & DEPRESSION
ISBN 1-56975-118-8, 144 pp, $9.95

CANDIDA
ISBN 1-56975-153-6, 208 pp, $11.95

ENDOMETRIOSIS
ISBN 1-56975-088-2, 184 pp, $9.95

FREE YOURSELF FROM TRANQUILIZERS & SLEEPING PILLS
ISBN 1-56975-074-2, 192 pp, $9.95

IRRITABLE BLADDER & INCONTINENCE
ISBN 1-56975-089-0, 112 pp, $8.95

IRRITABLE BOWEL SYNDROME
2nd edition, ISBN 1-56975-188-9, 256 pp, $13.95

MIGRAINES
ISBN 1-56975-140-4, 240 pp, $10.95

PANIC ATTACKS
2nd edition, ISBN 1-56975-187-0, 144 pp, $9.95

Other Health Titles

THE ANCIENT AND HEALING ART OF AROMATHERAPY
ISBN 1-56975-094-7, 96 pp, $14.95
Discusses the benefits and history of aromatherapy.

THE ANCIENT AND HEALING ART OF CHINESE HERBALISM
ISBN 1-56975-139-0, 96 pp, $14.95
Offers a beautifully illustrated history and demonstrates the uses of Chinese herbalism.

THE BOOK OF KOMBUCHA
ISBN 1-56975-049-1, 160 pp, $11.95
Explains the benefits of and addresses concerns about Kombucha, the widely used Chinese "tea mushroom."

CIDER VINEGAR: THE NATURAL REMEDY
ISBN 1-56975-141-2, 144 pp, $8.95
Gives detailed information—not just hype—about the safe use of cider vinegar.

PRAISE FOR
Three Wishes

"I adored *Three Wishes* by Liane Moriarty. . . . It's fresh, very, very funny, accessible, and entertaining. But it's also intelligent and unsentimental about family dynamics. Moriarty doesn't pull any punches, and I appreciated how she didn't produce any last-minute sugar-coating out of the hat. I really did believe in the strength of the characters to pull through. In fact, it made me believe in the resilience of the human race!"

—Marian Keyes, author of
Sushi for Beginners and *Under the Duvet*

"Liane Moriarty is a wonderfully perceptive observer of women. More than accomplished, this is a stunning debut. Bright, funny, smart, and warm. A winner. A joyful, bighearted valentine to sisters. Full of charm and cleverness. Perceptive, right-on. A rich, enticing birthday cake of a book."

—Patricia Gaffney, author of *The Saving Graces*

"Why it's a beach read: because three funny heroines are three times the fun." —*Dallas Morning News*

"An entertaining exploration of an offbeat, yet surprisingly ordinary, family. You'll long to make friends with these delightful young women." —*Woman's Day*

"Moriarty's first novel, written with wisdom, humor, and sincerity, is an honest look at sisters who have a bond stronger than anything life throws their way." —*Booklist*

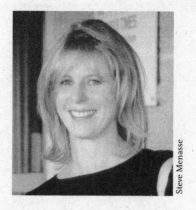

Steve Menasse

About the Author

The eldest of six children, LIANE MORIARTY grew up in Sydney and was one of those annoying little girls whose friends had to hide their books when she came to play. She grew up to be an advertising copywriter and has written everything from Web sites and catalogs to television commercials and cereal box copy. She is writing her second novel.

Three Wishes

Three Wishes

A NOVEL

Liane Moriarty

HARPER PERENNIAL

NEW YORK • LONDON • TORONTO • SYDNEY • NEW DELHI • AUCKLAND

HARPER PERENNIAL

A hardcover edition of this book was published in 2004 by HarperCollins Publishers.

HarperCollins books may be purchased for educational, business, or sales
promotional use. For information, please e-mail the Special Markets Department
at SPsales@harpercollins.com.

First Perennial edition published 2005.

Reissued in Harper Perennial in 2014.

Designed by C. Linda Dingler

The Library of Congress has catalogued the hardcover edition as follows:

Moriarty, Liane.
  Three wishes : a novel / Liane Moriarty.—1st ed.
    p. cm
  ISBN 0-06-058612-5 (alk. paper)
   1. Adult children of divorced parents—Fiction. 2. Birthday parties—
Fiction. 3. Australia—Fiction. 4. Triplets—Fiction. 5. Sisters—Fiction.
I. Title.

PR9619.4.M67T47 2004
823'.92—dc22   2003056992

ISBN 978-0-06-058613-3 (reissue)

19 20 21 LSC 40 39

For my four little sisters and brother:
Jaci, Kati, Fiona, Sean, and Nicola

ACKNOWLEDGMENTS

I am so grateful to the following long-suffering friends and family members for reading drafts, making suggestions, and encouraging me to keep writing: Vanessa Proctor, Jaci Moriarty, Colin McAdam, Petronella McGovern, Marisa Medina, and Diane Moriarty. A special thank-you to my U.S. agent Faye Bender for her wonderful support of the book and everyone at HarperCollins, especially my lovely editor, Alison Callahan.

The book *Twins: Genes, Environment and the Mystery of Identity* (1997) by Lawrence Wright was very helpful to me in understanding the special relationships between triplets.

Three Wishes

PROLOGUE

It happens sometimes that you accidentally star in a little public performance of your very own comedy, tragedy, or melodrama.

You're running for your morning bus, briefcase swinging jauntily, when you trip and tumble playground-style to the footpath. You're trapped in the heavy-breathing silence of a crowded elevator when your lover says something infuriating (*What* did you just say?), or your child asks a rather delicate question, or your mother calls on your mobile to shriek dire warnings. You're shuffling past a row of knees in the cinema, caught in the spotlight of the previews, when you tip your popcorn into a stranger's lap. You're having one of those days of accumulating misery when you argue violently with someone in a position of power: a bank teller, a dry cleaner, a three-year-old.

You either ignore your silently grinning spectators, glower at them, or shrug humorously. If you're a flamboyant type, you might even give a little bow! It doesn't really matter much what you do, because you have no control over your role in the amusing little anecdotes they're already busy composing; if it suits them, they will rob you of even more dignity.

It happened to three women one cold June night in Sydney.

(Actually, it had been happening to them all their lives, but this time their performance was especially spectacular.)

The setting was a busy seafood restaurant endorsed as "full of surprises" by Sydney's *Good Food Guide,* and their audience excluded only those suffering from excessive good manners. Everyone else witnessed the entire show with complete, bug-eyed enjoyment.

Within hours this little incident was being described and reenacted for the pleasure of baby-sitters, roommates, and partners waiting at home. By early the next day at least a dozen versions of the story were doing the rounds of office cubicles and coffee shops, pubs and preschools. Some were funny, others disapproving; many were censored, a few were spiced up.

Of course, no two were the same.

The Birthday Brawl

Last night? Eventful.

No mate, not that sort of eventful. The blind date was a disaster.

It wasn't too soon after Sarah, I told you, I'm ready to get back out there. The problem was her voice. It's like trying to hear someone on a bad line.

I'm not being picky, I can't hear the woman! There's a limit to how many times you can ask someone to repeat themselves before it gets bloody awkward. All night I was leaning halfway across the table, squinting my ears, making wild guesses at what she was whispering. At one point, I chuckled appreciatively at what I thought was a punch line and the poor girl looked horrified.

She could be really nice. She just needs someone with better ears. Preferably bionic ones.

But forget about the date. I'm sure she has. Actually, I'm sure she hasn't because as I say, it was . . . eventful.

The restaurant was jam-packed and we had a table right next to

three women. At first I didn't even register them because I was busy per-
fecting my lip-reading skills. The first time I even looked over was when
one girl got her handbag strap tangled around her chair.

Yep. Nice-looking. Although, I did have a preference for—but I'm
getting ahead of myself.

So, at first these three girls were having a great time, roaring with
laughter, getting louder and louder. Each time they laughed, my date and
I smiled sadly at each other.

About eleven o'clock, we cheered up because the end was in sight. We
got the dessert menu and she used sign language to suggest we share the
blueberry cheesecake. Obviously I didn't completely ruin her night by
mentioning my missing sweet tooth. What is it with women and sharing
desserts? It makes them so happy.

But we never got to order because that's when the action started.
The lights in the restaurant went off and three waitresses appeared, each
of them lugging these three huge bloody . . .

. . . birthday cakes if you don't mind!

And I said to Thomas, Well for heaven's sakes! *Three* cakes! One for
each girl! All ablaze with those noisy sparklers, which I personally think are
a fire hazard. So then they sang "Happy Birthday"—three times! Thomas
thought it was ridiculous. Each "Happy Birthday" got louder and more
boisterous and by the end of it everyone in the restaurant was singing.

Except for Thomas of course. He'd been upset about the noise from
the three girls all night. He even complained to the waitress! They
seemed like nice, high-spirited young people to me. Well, they did in the
beginning, anyway. The pregnant one smiled very nicely at me when she
went to the Ladies.

They all had very generous portions of their cake! Not dieting, obviously! And they all helped themselves to spoonfuls of each other's. That
was nice, I thought.

Well, I kept a little eye on them. They had me intrigued for some reason. I noticed that after their cake they each took a turn reading something out loud. They looked like letters to me. Well, I don't know what in

the world those letters were about, but it was only a few seconds later that the yelling started!

Goodness me! What a terrible tiff! Everyone was staring. Thomas was appalled.

One girl scraped back her chair and stood right up and I've never seen anyone so angry! Her face was all blotchy bright red and she was shaking a fork and screaming, yes, screaming.

Well, I don't know if I can say this part.

Well, all right. Come close and I'll whisper it to you.

She was screaming, "You have both . . .

. . . fucking ruined my life!"

And I think to myself what the fuck is going on here?

I'd just been telling Sam that I was going to score a massive tip from Table Six because they were all having such a good time and they were all pretty drunk.

Even the pregnant girl had a glass of champagne, which is pretty bad, isn't it? Don't you have an alcoholic baby or something if you drink while you're pregnant?

The thing I can't believe is how she could do that to her own sister. I mean I get pretty mad with my sister but this—wow! Her own triplet even!

Did I tell you they were triplets?

They were all out together celebrating their thirty-fourth birthdays. I never met triplets before and they were pretty friendly, so I was asking them questions about what it was like. The two blond ones were identical. It freaked me out! I kept staring at them once I knew. It was like Spot the Difference. Weird.

One of them said it was fantastic being a triplet. She just loved it! The other one said it was terrible! It made her feel like a mutant or something. And the third one said it was just nothing, no big deal, no different from being in any other family.

And then they all started arguing about what it was like to be a triplet. But in a friendly, funny way.

That's why I couldn't believe it when I heard them start fighting. Like really fighting, as if they absolutely despised each other. It was sort of embarrassing, you know? Like they were doing something really private in public.

Sam told me to distract them with their coffees. So I was trying to keep my face normal, walking up to their table, and that's when it happened.

I tell you. It gave me such a shock the coffees were wobbling in my hands.

You know those two old fossils that come every second Thursday? You know, the fat woman always has the crème brûlée? She's got the skinny husband with something right up his arse. Anyway, my hand was shaking so much I sent cappuccino froth flying over the guy's bald head!

O.K., O.K.! Gimme a break, I'm trying to set the scene for you!

One of the girls stood up at the table and she's yelling at her sisters, right? And all the time she's yelling she's sort of poking at the air with her fondue fork.

They shared the special fondue for their entrée, you see. Actually, now I think about it, it was my fault the fondue fork was still sitting there on the table.

Wow. I hope they can't sue me or anything. Ha.

So this girl, she's got the fork and she's yelling like a complete maniac. And then she throws the fondue fork at her. Can you believe it?

And the fork gets stuck in the pregnant one's stomach!

She's just sitting there looking down at her big belly and there's this fork sticking right out of her. It looked just completely bizarre.

The girl who threw it is standing there with her hand sort of held out, frozen, in midair. Like she was trying to stop a glass from falling or something and then realized it was too late.

And then—get this—she faints.

No—not the pregnant one. The one who threw the fork.

She just sort of crumples and falls—really heavy—onto the floor and on the way down she bangs her chin, like bang, really hard, on the edge of the table.

So she's lying on the floor, completely out of it.

The pregnant one, she's just sitting there looking at the fork sticking out of her stomach and she's not making a sound. She's just staring at it in this sort of dreamy way and then she touches her stomach with her finger and holds it up and it's covered in blood! Totally gross!

The restaurant is silent, like so silent, it's loud. Everybody is just sitting there looking at them.

So the third sister. She sort of sighs and shakes her head as if it's no big deal and leans down under the table and picks up her handbag and pulls out . . .

. . . her mobile and rang for an ambulance for the two of them.

Then she rang me on the way to the hospital. I mean really. What a complete debacle.

They're over thirty now, for heaven's sakes, and they're behaving like children. Throwing things at each other in public places! It's disgraceful. And on their birthday of all days!

I think they all need to see a really sensible psychiatrist. I really do.

Remember that restaurant in the city, when they were little? Remember? The manager asked us to leave after Lyn threw her glass of lemonade at Catriona. What a fiasco! I've never been so humiliated in my life. Not to mention the perfectly good bottle of Shiraz we left behind. Cat needed four stitches that day.

I blame you, Frank.

No. It makes perfect sense.

Well, if you like, you can share the blame equally with Christine.

Christine, Frank, was the name of the woman who broke up our marriage. Now that is a perfect indication of how much your mind was involved in that sordid little incident.

I have not strayed from the point, Frank! Our broken marriage clearly damaged our daughters. Today's incident is not normal! Even for multiples!

I was seeing the accountant when I got the call. I was speechless!

I could hardly say, oh, please excuse me, Nigel, my daughter just *broke her jaw after fainting from the shock of throwing a fondue fork at her pregnant sister!*

You should have seen them when I arrived here at the hospital. They were giggling! Treating the whole thing as a hilarious joke. They make me so cross.

I just don't understand them at all.

Don't pretend you understand them any better than me, Frank. You don't talk to them. You flirt with them.

They all smelled unpleasantly of garlic, too. They had some sort of seafood fondue for their entrée apparently. I mean, really, what a strange choice! It doesn't sound edible.

I think they have a drinking problem too.

I fail to see the humor in this, Frank. The baby could have been hurt. It could have died.

Our daughter could have murdered our grandchild!

Dear God, we could have been on the front page of the Daily Telegraph.

No, I do not think I'm being the slightest bit dramatic.

Well yes, obviously, that's what I'd like to know too. It was the very first thing I said to them when I got here:

"What in the world started it?"

CHAPTER 1

You could argue that it started thirty-four years ago when twenty-year-old Frank Kettle, a tall, fair, hyperactive ex–altar boy, fell madly in lust with Maxine Leonard, a long-legged languid redhead just a few days short of her nineteenth birthday.

He was pumping with fresh testosterone. She knew better but did it anyway. In the backseat of Frank's dad's Holden. Twice. The first time involved a lot of head-bumping and grunting and breathless shifts of position, while Johnny O'Keefe bellowed at them from the car radio. The second time was slower and gentler and rather nice. Elvis soothingly suggested they love him tender. In each case, however, the terrible result was the same. One of Frank's exuberant little sperm cells slammed head-on with one of Maxine's rather less thrilled eggs, interrupting what should have been an uneventful journey to nonexistence.

Over the following days, while Maxine was chastely dating more suitable boys and Frank was pursuing a curvy brunette, two freshly fertilized eggs were busily bumping their way along Maxine's fallopian tubes toward the haven of her horrified young uterus.

At the exact moment Maxine allowed the very suitable Charlie Edwards to hold back her long red hair while she puffed out her cheeks and blew out nineteen candles, one egg fizzed with so much friction it split right in two. The other single egg burrowed its way comfortably in between the two new identical eggs.

Guests at Maxine's birthday party thought they'd never seen her look so beautiful—slender, glowing, almost incandescent! Who could have guessed she'd been impregnated with some Catholic boy's triplets?

Frank and Maxine were married, of course. In their wedding photos, they both have the blank-eyed, sedated look of recent trauma victims.

Seven months later, their triplet daughters came kicking and howling into the world. Maxine, who had never even held a baby before, was presented with three; it was the most despair-filled moment of her young life.

Well, that would be Gemma's preference for how it started. Cat would argue that if she was going to begin with their conception, then why not go back through their entire family tree? Why not go back to the apes? Why not start with the Big Bang? I guess I did really, Gemma would chortle, Mum and Dad's big bang. Oh funn-y, Cat would say. Let's look at it logically, Lyn would interrupt. Quite clearly, it started the night of the spaghetti.

And Lyn, quite naturally, would be right.

It was a Wednesday night six weeks before Christmas. A nothing sort of night. An unassuming midweek night that should have vanished from their memories by Friday. *"What did we do Wednesday?" "I don't know. Watch TV?"*

That's what they were doing. They were eating spaghetti and drinking red wine in front of the television. Cat was sitting cross-legged on the floor, with her back up against the sofa, her plate on her lap. Her husband, Dan, was sitting on the edge of the sofa, hunched over his dinner on the coffee table. It was the way they always ate dinner.

Dan had cooked the spaghetti, so it was hearty and bland. Cat was the more accomplished cook. Dan's approach to cooking was somehow too functional. He stirred his ingredients like concrete mix, one arm wrapped around the bowl, the other stirring the gluggy mix so vigorously you could see his biceps working. "So what? Gets the job done."

That Wednesday night Cat was feeling no specific emotion; not especially happy, not especially sad. It was strange afterward, remembering how she sat there, shoveling Dan's pasta into her mouth, so foolishly trusting of her life. She wanted to yell back at herself through time, *Concentrate!*

They were watching a show called *Med School.* It was a soap about a group of very beautiful young medical students with shiny white teeth and complex love lives. Each episode featured a lot of blood and sex and anguish.

Cat and Dan shared a mild addiction to *Med School.* Whenever the plot took a new twist, they responded with loud enthusiasm, yelling at the television like children watching a pantomime: "Bastard!" "Dump him!" "It's the *wrong medication!"*

This week Ellie (blond, cutesy, cropped T-shirt) was in a state. She didn't know whether to tell her boyfriend, Pete (dark, brooding, abnormal abs), about her drunken infidelity with a guest-starring troublemaker.

"Tell him, Ellie!" said Cat to the television. "Pete will forgive you. He'll understand!"

The ad break came on, and a manic man in a yellow jacket bounced around a department store pointing an incredulous finger at the Christmas specials.

"I booked that health and beauty thing today," said Cat, using Dan's knee as a lever to help her reach over him for the pepper. "The woman had one of those gooey, spiritual voices. I felt like I was getting a massage just making a booking."

For Christmas, she was giving her sisters (and herself) a weekend away at a health retreat in the Blue Mountains. The three of them would share an "exquisite experience" of "indulgent pampering." They would be wrapped in seaweed, dunked in mud, and slathered in vitamin-enriched creams. It would be extremely amusing.

She was pleased with herself for thinking of it. "What a clever idea!" everyone would say on Christmas Day. Lyn definitely needed the stress relief. Gemma didn't need it but she'd be right into pretending that she did. Cat herself wasn't especially stressed either, but perhaps she was, because she wasn't pregnant and she'd been off the Pill now for nearly a year. "Don't get stressed about it," everybody said wisely, as if they were the first to pass on that hot little tip. Apparently, the moment your ovaries noticed you were worried about becoming pregnant, they refused to cooperate. *Oh well, if you're going to get all huffy about it, we'll just close down.*

A health insurance ad came on. Dan winced. "I hate this ad."

"It's effective. You watch it more closely than any other ad on television."

He closed his eyes and averted his head. "O.K. I'm not looking, I'm not looking. Oh God. I can still hear that woman's grating voice."

Cat picked up the remote and turned up the volume.

"Aaaagh!" He opened his eyes and grabbed the remote from her.

He was behaving perfectly normally. She remembered that afterward and it made it worse, somehow. Every moment he behaved normally was part of the betrayal.

"Shh. It's back on."

Ellie's betrayed boyfriend, Pete, appeared on the screen, flexing his freakish abs. Ellie gave the TV audience guilty looks.

"Tell him," Cat told her. "I'd want to know. I couldn't stand not to know the truth. Better to tell him, Ellie."

"You think so?" said Dan.

"Yeah. Don't you?"

"I don't know."

There were no bells jangling a warning in Cat's head. Not a single chime.

She had put down her wineglass on the coffee table and was feeling a pimple that had just that very moment appeared on her chin, undoubtedly a malevolent herald of her forthcoming period. Each month it appeared like an official stamp on her chin. There will be no baby for this woman this month. Nope. Sorry, try again! Cat had begun to cackle bitterly, throwing back her head witch-like, as soon as the first treacherous spots of blood appeared. It was such a joke, such a crushing anticlimax, after all those years of anxiously ensuring she *didn't* have a baby, after all those months of "Are we ready to make this momentous change in our lives? I think we are, don't you? Ooh, maybe we should have *one* more month of freedom!"

Don't think about it, she told herself. Don't think about it.

"Cat," said Dan.

"What?"

"I have to tell you something."

She snorted at his ponderous tone, pleased to be distracted from her pimple. She thought he was sending up the show. "Oh my God!" she said and hummed the *Med School* sound track that helpfully warned viewers when something dramatic and awful was about to happen. "What? Have you done an Ellie? Have you been unfaithful to me?"

"Well. Yes."

He looked like he was going to be sick and he wasn't that great an actor.

Cat put down her fork. "This is a joke, right? You're saying you've slept with someone else?"

"Yes." Now his mouth was doing something strange. He looked like a guilty little boy caught doing something disgusting.

She picked up the remote and turned off the television. Her heart was thumping with fear but also a strangely urgent desire, a desire to *know*. It was the sick feeling of excited resistance at the very top of the roller coaster—I don't want to go hurtling over that precipice but I do, I do!

"When?" She still didn't really believe it. She was half laughing. "Years ago, do you mean? When we first started going out? You don't mean recently?"

"About a month ago."

"What?"

"It didn't mean anything." He looked down at his plate and picked up a mushroom with his fingers. Halfway to his mouth, he dropped it and wiped the back of his hand across his mouth.

"Would you just start from the beginning, please? When?"

"One night."

"What night? Where was I?" She fumbled through her mind for events over the last few weeks. *"What night?"*

It seemed that on a Tuesday night, three weeks before, at drinks after squash he met a girl. She came on to *him,* and he was flattered because she was, well, quite good-looking. He was a bit drunk, and so he went back to her place and one thing led to another. It didn't mean anything, obviously. He didn't know why he had made such a stupid, stupid mistake. Maybe all the stress lately with work, and, you know, the baby thing. Obviously it would never happen again and he was very, very, *very* sorry and he loved her so much and God, it was such a relief to have this out in the open!

It was almost like something interesting and unusual had happened to him and he'd forgotten to tell Cat about it until now. She asked him questions and he answered them. "Where did she live? How did you get home?"

He finished his story and Cat stared stupidly at him, waiting for it to hurt. All her muscles were tensed tight in anticipation of pain. It was like giving blood and waiting for the smiling doctor to find her vein.

"What was her name?" she said.

His eyes slid away. "Angela."

Finally. An exquisite twist of her heart because this girl actually had a *name* and Dan *knew* her name.

She gazed at her dinner congealing on her plate, and she could see every snakelike strand of spaghetti in nauseating definition. The lens of a telescope had been clicked, and her previously blurry world was now in sharp-edged focus.

She stared with new eyes at their living room. Casually angled cushions on the sofa, bright wacky rug on polished floorboards. The bookshelf, lined with photos, each one carefully selected and framed as evidence of their happy, active lives. Look! We're so loving and cosmopolitan, so fit and humorous! Here we are smiling and hugging in our ski gear! Here we are having a laugh before we go scuba diving! We party with our friends! We pull ironic faces at the camera!

She looked back at Dan. He was quite a good-looking man, her husband. It used to worry her in a pleasurable, not-really-worried way.

He's been unfaithful to me, she thought, trying it out. It was bizarre. Surreal. Part of her wanted to switch the television back on and pretend it had never happened. I have to iron my skirt for tomorrow, she thought. I should do my Christmas list.

"It was nothing," he said. "It was just a stupid one-night stand."

"Don't call it that!"

"O.K."

"This is all so *tacky.*"

He looked at her beseechingly. A speck of tomato sauce quivered beneath his nose.

"You've got food on your face," she said savagely. His guilt was inflating her, making her powerful with righteousness. He was the criminal and she was the cop. The bad cop. The one that grabbed the criminal's shirtfront and slammed him up against the wall.

She said, "Why are you telling me this now? Is it just to make you feel better?"

"I don't know. I kept changing my mind. And then you said you'd want to know the truth."

"I was talking to *Ellie*! I was watching television! I was eating dinner!"

"So you didn't mean it?"

"For God's sake. It's too late now."

They sat in silence for a few seconds, and suddenly she wanted to weep like a five-year-old in the playground because Dan was meant to be her *friend,* her special friend.

"But, why?" Her voice cracked. "Why did you do it? I don't understand why you would do that."

"It didn't mean anything. It really didn't mean anything." Had his friends told him to say that? "Tell her it didn't mean anything, mate. That's all they want to hear."

If she were on *Med School,* one single tear would have been trickling so slowly, so heartbreakingly down her cheek. Instead, she was making strange, wheezy sounds as if she'd been running.

"Please don't be upset. Cat. Babe."

"Don't be *upset!*"

Dan placed his palm tentatively against her arm. She pushed it violently away. "Don't you touch me!"

They looked at each other in horror. Dan's face was pasty-white. Cat was trembling with the sudden chasm-opening revelation that he must have touched this woman she'd never seen. Properly touched her. He must have kissed her. All the tiny, trivial details of sex.

"Did you take her bra off?"

"Cat!"

"I mean obviously her bra came *off.* I just want to know if she took it off, or you? Did you reach your hand up her back, while you were kissing and undo it? Have any difficulty? Was it a tricky one? Those tricky ones are bad, aren't they? Been a while since you've had to worry about that. How'd you do? Breathe a sigh of relief once you got it undone?"

"Please stop it."

"I will *not* stop it."

"I took her bra off, O.K.! But it was nothing. I was drunk. It was nothing like with us. It didn't—"

"It didn't mean anything. Yes, I know. What meaningless position did you choose?"

"Please, Cat."

"Did she have an orgasm?"

"Please don't."

"Oh, darling. Don't worry. I'm sure she did. Those little techniques of yours are so *reliable.* I'm sure she was very appreciative."

"Cat, I'm begging you to stop." There was a tremor in his voice.

She wiped sweat from her forehead. It was too hot.

She felt ugly. In fact she was ugly. She put her hand to her chin and felt the pimple. Makeup! She needed makeup. She needed makeup, wardrobe, a hair stylist, and an air-conditioned set. Then she'd feel clean, beautiful waves of grief like the stars of *Med School.*

She got to her feet and picked up both their plates.

The back of her throat itched unbearably. Hay fever. Right now, of all times. She put the plates back down on the coffee table and sneezed four times. Each time she closed her eyes to sneeze, an image of a sliding bra strap exploded in her mind.

Dan went into the kitchen and came back with the box of tissues.

"Don't look at me," she said.

"What?" He held out the tissues.

"Just don't look at me."

That was when she picked up one of the plates of spaghetti and threw it straight against the wall.

To: Lyn; Cat
From: Gemma
Subject: Cat

LYN! WARNING, WARNING! DANGER, DANGER! I just spoke to Cat and she is in a VERY, VERY bad mood. I would not recommend ringing her about minding Maddie for another twenty-four hours at least.

Love, Gemma

To: Gemma
From: Cat
Subject: ME
Warning, warning, if you're going to send e-mails about my bad
mood at least make sure I don't get them. That could really put
me in a bad mood.

To: Gemma
From: Lyn
Subject: Cat
G. Need to be careful about hitting "reply all" instead of "reply to
author" on old e-mails. Set up address book!! No doubt Cat v.
impressed. Kara minding Maddie so no problem. L.

To: Lyn; Cat
From: Gemma
Subject: Kara
Dear Lyn,
I don't know how to set up an address book but thank you for
the thought. I don't mean to alarm you but have you heard of
SHAKING BABY SYNDROME? I think leaving Maddie with Kara
could be very dangerous. Once I saw her shaking a box of corn-
flakes FURIOUSLY. She is a teenager and teenagers have problems
with their hormones that cause them to be just a little insane.
Can't you ask Cat, once she has finished her bad mood? Or else I
could cancel my date with the luscious locksmith. I am prepared
to do that to save Maddie's life. Let me know. Love, Gemma

Cat wondered if her face looked different. It felt different, as if it
were bruised and swollen. Both her eyes as if like they'd been
punched. In fact, her whole body seemed strangely fragile. She'd
been holding herself stiffly all day, as if she were sunburned.

It was surprising really, how much this hurt and how *consistently* it hurt. All day at work she kept thinking that she ought to

get a painkiller and then remembering that she wasn't actually in physical pain.

She hadn't slept much the night before.

"I'll sleep on the sofa bed," Dan had announced, looking heroic and pale.

"No, you won't," said Cat, refusing to give him the satisfaction.

But when they got into bed and she lay there looking at the ceiling and listened to Dan's breathing starting to slow—he was actually going to *sleep*—she had snapped back on the light and said, "Get out."

He went, clutching his pillow sleepily to his stomach. Cat lay in bed and imagined her husband having sex with another woman. She was right there, under the covers with them, watching his hands, her hands, his mouth, her mouth.

She couldn't stop. She didn't want to stop. It was necessary to imagine every excruciating second-by-second detail.

In the middle of the night she woke Dan up to ask him what color underwear the girl was wearing.

"I don't remember," he said blearily.

"You do! You do!" She kept insisting until finally he said he thought it might have been black, at which point she burst into tears.

Now Cat looked at the people in the 4:30 P.M. Operations Meeting and wondered if this *thing*, this vile thing, had ever happened to them.

Sales Director Rob Spencer was in his favorite position by the whiteboard, enthusiastically scribbling flamboyant arrows and boxes. "Folks! I think this makes my point very clear!"

Rob Spencer. Well, that was a joke. For the last five years or so Rob Spencer had been having an affair with gorgeous Johanna from accounts. It was the company's favorite secret. Telling new staff the Rob/Johanna legend was part of the induction procedure at Hollingdale Chocolates. The only people who didn't know, presumably, were Rob's wife and Johanna's husband. Everyone stared with enjoyable pity at the two unfortunate spouses when they made their appearance each year at the annual Christmas party.

It occurred to Cat that she now had something in common with Rob Spencer's pathetic wife. She was the faceless wife in *Angela's* amusing story of a one-night stand with a married man. *Well I feel sorry for the wife . . . the wife isn't Angela's responsibility . . . who cares about the wife, just give us the gory details, Ange!*

She swallowed hard and looked down at Rob's analysis for a quick way to humiliate him.

Colorful graphs. Nifty little spreadsheet. All done by his minions, of course.

Aha.

"Rob," she said.

Ten heads turned in relieved unison to face her.

"Catriona!" Rob spun from the whiteboard, teeth flashing against solarium-yellow tan. "Always value your feedback!"

"I just wondered where those figures came from?" she said.

"I do believe the marvelous Margie did the number crunching for me." Rob tapped his figures seductively, as if Margie had given him a rather marvelous blow job at the same time.

"Yes, but what figures did you give Margie to crunch?" asked Cat.

"Ah, let's see," Rob began shuffling vaguely through his paperwork.

She savored the moment before moving in for the kill.

"Looking at the marketing budget here, it seems you've given her last financial year's figures. So your analysis, while fascinating, is also, hmmm, how can I put it best . . . irrelevant?"

Too bitchy. Male egos were so tender, just like their balls. She would pay for that one.

"Crash and burn, Rob, mate!" Hank from production thumped his fist on the table.

Rob held up both hands in boyish surrender. "Team! It seems the Cat has caught me out again with her razor-sharp eye for errors!"

He looked at his watch. "It's nearly five on a Friday afternoon! People, what are we still doing here? Who wants to join me in drowning my humiliation at Albert's? Catriona? Can I shout my nemesis a drink?"

His eyes were opaque little marbles.

Cat smiled tightly. "I'll hold you to it another time."

She bundled up her files and left the room, feeling quite ill with inappropriate-for-the-workplace hatred for Rob Spencer.

To: Cat
From: Gemma
Subject: Drink
Would you like to have a drink?
We can talk about the bad mood you're not in.
Love, Gemma
P.S. Essential that you back me up on Kara issue!
P.P.S. Do you owe me any money by any chance? I don't seem to have any.

Cat sat in a dimly lit corner of the pub with three beers in front of her and waited for her sisters.

She wasn't going to tell them. She and Dan needed time to work it out for themselves. It wasn't necessary to share every single detail of her marriage. It was weird and triplet-dependent. "You tell those two *everything*!" Dan always said, and he didn't know the half of it.

If she told them, Gemma would hug her and rush off to buy supplies of ice cream and champagne. Lyn would be on her mobile ringing friends for referrals for good marriage counselors. They would inundate her with advice. They would argue passionately with each other over what she should and shouldn't do.

They would care too much and that would make it real.

She took a gulp of her beer and bared her teeth at a man who was making hopeful gestures at the two stools she had saved.

"Just checking!" he said, hands up, looking hurt.

She definitely wasn't telling her sisters. Look what happened when she went off the Pill. Her cycle became public property; every month, they'd call to cheerily ask if her period had arrived yet.

They had both stopped calling now but only after she'd said to Gemma that yes, it had come, and yes, she probably was infertile, and now was she satisfied? Gemma had cried, of course. Then Cat had felt sick with guilt as well as period pain.

"Are these seats?"

"Yes, they are seats, but no, they are not free."

"What's *her* problem?"

"Ignore her. Bitch."

Two girls in matching Barbie-doll business suits tottered off disapprovingly on their high heels, while Cat examined her knuckles and imagined jumping up and punching their lipsticked mouths.

She wondered what that girl looked like.

Angela.

She was probably short and curvy like those girls who had now stopped to giggle and gurgle up at a group of, no doubt married, men.

Cat hated curvaceous little women. Feminine, doll-like women who tilted up their sweet faces to Cat like she was some sort of towering, lumbering giant.

Her sisters understood. Tall women understood.

But she didn't want the humiliation of their understanding. In fact, for some reason the thought of their intensely sympathetic faces made her furious. It was *their* fault.

She searched her mind for a rational reason for blaming them.

Of course: it was their fault she'd ever met Dan in the first place.

Melbourne Cup Day over ten years ago. Twenty-one and delightfully drunk on champagne, back when you were still allowed to call cheap sparkling wine "champagne." Betting spectacular amounts of money on every race. Laughing like drains, as their grandmother said. Making a complete spectacle of themselves, as their mother said.

They accosted every boy who walked by their table.

Gemma: "We're triplets! Can you tell? Can you believe it? They're identical but I'm not. I'm a single egg! They're just half of the one egg. Half-eggs. Would you like to buy us a drink? We quite like champagne."

Lyn: "Got any good tips? Personally, I like Lone Ranger in Race Five. We're drinking the $9.99 bottle of champagne if you were thinking of buying us a drink. We've already got glasses, so that's O.K."

Cat: "You seem to have an unusually large head. It's blocking the television and I'm about to win a lot of money. Could you go away? Unless you'd like to buy us a drink."

The boy with the large head sat down in the booth next to Cat. He was very tall, and they all had to squash together to give him enough room.

He had evil green eyes and stubble.

He was gorgeous.

"So," he said. "You're all ex–womb mates."

Gemma thought this was hilarious and dissolved into tears of laughter. Cat sat back, sipping her drink, waiting for the gorgeous boy to fall in love with Gemma. Men generally fell in love with Gemma when she laughed. They couldn't hide their sheepish grins of pride. It became their life mission to make her laugh again.

But this boy seemed more interested in Cat. He put his hand on her knee. She removed it and put it back on the table.

"Did you just put your hand on Cat's knee!?" shouted Lyn, whose voice tended to rise several decibels when she was drunk. *"Gemma!* That boy just put his hand on Cat's knee!"

"Do you like her?" said Gemma. "Do you want to kiss her? She's a good kisser. She says she is anyway. After you've kissed her could you buy us some more champagne please?"

"I don't want to kiss him!" said Cat. "His head is abnormally large. And he looks like a truck driver."

She wanted to kiss him quite a lot.

"If I pick a winner in this race, will you kiss me?" said the boy.

They looked at him with interest. They were all gamblers. It was a rogue gene they'd inherited from their grandfather.

Lyn leaned forward. "WHAT IF IT LOSES?"

"Bottle of champagne," said the boy.

"Deal!" Gemma knocked over Cat's champagne as she reached across to shake his hand.

"What are you two, my pimps?" asked Cat.

He picked a horse called Dancing Girl.

"NO CHANCE!" cried Lyn. "She's fifty to one for God's sake. Why didn't you pick a favorite?"

Gemma and Lyn were screaming on their feet for the whole race.

Cat stayed sitting next to the boy. She kept her eyes fixed on the television. Dancing Girl ran in the middle of the pack until the last few seconds when she broke free and began surging forward. The race caller's voice rose in rapid surprise. Gemma and Lyn wailed.

Cat felt the boy's hand at the back of her head. As Dancing Girl was thundering toward the finish line, the boy was pulling her to him and Cat's eyelids were closing as if she were sinking into a deep, delicious sleep. He smelled of Dunhill cigarettes and Palmolive soap and tasted of Colgate toothpaste and Tooheys beer, and she had never wanted anything so bad as she wanted that boy.

The boy turned out to be Dan and Dan turned out to be her husband and her husband turned out to be a cheat.

Cat drained her beer and started on one of the other two.

Gemma and Lyn had adored Dan from the moment Dancing Girl had come in second and they turned around to claim their champagne, to find him claiming the kiss he hadn't won. He managed to extricate his wallet from his back jeans pocket and hand it to Lyn while keeping his tongue firmly entwined with Cat's. So cool! So sexy! So *dexterous*!

How could she admit the adorable Dan wasn't so adorable after all?

She wasn't going to tell them.

She slammed the beer down on the table, reached for the third, and looked up to see her sisters walking through the pub toward her.

Gemma was dressed, as always, like an oddly beautiful bag lady. She was wearing a faded flowery dress and peculiar holey cardigan that didn't match the dress and was too big for her. Her glinty red-gold hair was all over the place, a tangled mess that fell past her shoulders. Split ends. Cat watched a guy at the door turn to look at her. A lot of men didn't notice Gemma, but the ones who did, *really* did. They were the sort of men who wanted to brush her hair out of her eyes, roll up her cardigan sleeves, and tell her to zip up her bag before her purse got stolen.

Lyn had come from teaching aerobics at the gym. Her straight, blond hair was in a smoothly coiled knot at the back of her head. Her cheeks were pink and healthy. She was wearing jeans and a white T-shirt that looked suspiciously like it might have been ironed. A fair, lanky, sporty-looking girl. Her nose was too pointy, in Cat's opinion, but she was attractive enough. (Although, maybe not?) When Cat saw Lyn she saw herself in three dimensions. Three very vigorous, Lyn-like dimensions.

Cat felt that sense of pleasure and pride that she always felt when she saw her sisters in public. "Look at them!" she wanted to say to people. "My sisters. Aren't they great? Aren't they annoying?"

They saw Cat and sat down on the waiting stools without saying hello.

It was one of their rituals, never saying hello or acknowledging one another. People found it strange, which they found enjoyable.

"So I've been going to this new deli for my lunch," said Gemma. "Whatever I order, *whatever,* it seems to shock the woman behind the counter. I say, I'll have the fruit salad, and her eyes widen and she says, The *fruit salad*! It's the funniest thing."

"I thought you hated fruit salad," said Lyn.

"I do. That's just an example," said Gemma.

"Well, but why not give an example of something that you actually ordered?"

Cat looked at her sisters and felt her limbs becoming weak with relief.

She ran her finger around the rim of her empty beer glass and said, "I've got something to tell you."

The Cabbage-Leaf Trick

Do you know, I can never see a cabbage without thinking of breast milk.

I wonder if they still do that? The cabbage-leaf trick. I can tell you when I first saw it. It would be over thirty years ago now. My first week as a nurse's aide. Everyone at the hospital was in a tizz because a young girl had given birth to triplets. Everyone wanted to see them. They even had reporters from the papers!

I happened to be making beds in the maternity ward when the three babies were wheeled in for their feeds. Sister Mulvaney, the cruelest woman you could ever hope to meet, was directing the whole event. My eyes popped as the nurses undid the mother's bra and peeled off soggy green leaves! Your breasts sometimes become very hard and swollen when you start nursing, you see, and for some reason chilled cabbage leaves soothe them.

Gosh, but that poor young mother was in pain. You could tell. Her face was all set and white. Her three little babies were sound asleep but in those days they were sticklers for routine. You fed them every four hours on the dot. The first little baby did not want to be woken. They tried everything. Undressing her. Moving her around. Eventually, Sister Mulvaney sprinkled some water on her little face. That certainly woke her up. But the moment she started crying, the other two were off. All three screaming!

They got two of the babies and showed the mother how to tuck them back under her arms, one on each breast. But she couldn't get the babies to latch on. Sister Mulvaney was barking out instructions and the mother was doing her best to follow them. By this stage, the babies had worked themselves up into a fine rage. What a racket! The whole ward was watching.

Eventually, they gave up and got a breast pump to try and get her milk started. They were dreadful, clunky old contraptions in those days. You could tell that poor mother was upset, with her babies holler-

ing, Sister Mulvaney tut-tutting, and everyone pretending not to stare. All of a sudden she just burst into tears. My supervising nurse said, very know-it-all, "Ah the three-day blues, all new mothers cry on the third day." And I remember thinking, But my goodness, who wouldn't cry?

CHAPTER 2

"Die, you little motherfucker." Lyn squatted down on the kitchen floor and aimed the cockroach spray like a machine gun.

"Language, young lady!" Lyn looked up to see her stepdaughter, Kara, sucking in her cheeks in a parody of a horrified parent.

"I thought you were gone," said Lyn, feeling a bit silly to be caught doing her private Hollywood gangster act. She didn't normally say things like "motherfucker." In fact, she generally swore only in situations involving cockroaches or her sisters.

"It's escaping!" said Kara helpfully.

Lyn looked back down to see the cockroach scuttling across the tiles to a microscopic tunnel under the sink. No doubt it would now live a long, happy life and give birth to many thousands of sweet little cockroach babies.

Lyn stood up and looked at her watch. It was just on nine o'clock. "Aren't you very late?"

Kara heaved an exhausted sigh to indicate she could not be expected to cope with yet another imbecilic question.

"Well, aren't you?" asked Lyn, because she couldn't help herself.

"Lyn, Lyn, Lyn." Kara shook her head sadly. "What am I going to do with you?"

Kara was six when Lyn first met her, a girly little girl, with butterfly clips in her curly black hair and skinny arms that jangled with sparkly pink bangles. Her most treasured possession was an extra-large pencil case that she called her "Crafty Case"; it had special things in it like glitter, glue, and chunky plastic scissors. Lyn was allowed Crafty Case privileges, and they spent whole Sunday afternoons together, making cardboard and Paddle Pop–stick creations. When Kara eventually began to find other interests, Lyn kept clinging on, making hopeful suggestions for new projects. She gave up only after that fateful, embarrassing day when Kara ceremonially presented her with the Crafty Case, saying, "Here, now you can play with it on your own, whenever you want."

At fifteen, Kara kept her hair dead straight and rimmed her eyes in thick black eyeliner. Some days she slouched for endless hours on the sofa, yawning hugely, like someone suffering from terrible jet lag. Other days she was flushed and glittery-eyed, almost maniacally happy. Her most treasured possession was her mobile phone, which beeped night and day with text messages from her friends.

Lyn watched as Kara opened the fridge door and stood with one hip at an angle. She stared vaguely into the fridge, swinging the door, and suddenly said, "When did you lose your virginity?"

"None of your business," answered Lyn. "Do you want something to eat? Have you had breakfast?"

Kara turned around with enthusiasm. "Was it really late? Like, embarrassing late? Why? Did no one want to sleep with you? Don't feel bad. You can tell me!"

"The apples are good. Have an apple."

Kara took an apple. She slammed the fridge door and swung herself up on to the kitchen bench, swinging her legs.

"Who did Dad lose his virginity to? Was it Mum, do you reckon?"

"I don't know."

Kara gave Lyn a sly, slanting look over her apple. "I'm going to lose my virginity by the end of next year."

"Are you? Good for you."

Lyn wasn't especially worried about Kara and sex. She was fastidious and easily revolted. Just last night Michael had said at the dinner table, "Lyn, I want to pick your brains about something," and Kara had exploded, covering her face, making him vow to never say anything so disgusting as "pick your brains" ever again.

Surely she wouldn't be interested in anything as messy as a penis.

Lyn opened the dishwasher and began rinsing that morning's breakfast dishes. Due to the distressing and frankly shocking news about Dan, last night's drink with Cat and Gemma had gone three hours longer than scheduled. That meant today's "to do" list was longer than usual. She'd been up since 5:30 A.M.

Dan was a truly horrible cheating sleaze . . . She must remind Michael to call his mother for her birthday . . . Why did Dan even tell Cat? What did it achieve? . . . If Maddie slept for another hour or so, she could prepare for tomorrow's meeting at the bakery . . . Cat could get so irrational. Would their marriage survive this? . . . Ten Christmas cards a night, starting from tonight . . .

And beneath all those thoughts was a flicker of concern, a long-buried, knotty little worry that she was refusing to bring out and dust off, just in case it looked really bad.

"It's going to be my New Year's resolution," Kara was saying, her mouth full of apple. "To lose my virginity next year. Are you going to tell Dad?"

"Do you want me to tell him?"

"I don't care."

"Fine. Shouldn't you be going?"

"So, but what do you think about me losing my virginity this year?"

"I think it's a very personal decision."

"So you think I *should*. Wait till I tell Dad you said I should lose my virginity next year. He'll go ballistic."

"I never said that."

"Out of all the men you've slept with, where would you rate Dad? Is he like—any *good*?" Kara's face contorted with delighted disgust. "Is he in your top ten? Have you got a top ten? Have you slept with more than ten men even?"

"Kara."

"Oh my God, don't answer. I just thought of you and Dad having sex. I'm going to throw up. Oh my *God*! I can't get it out of my mind! It's *revolting*!"

A miniature figure in pink pajamas toddled into the kitchen, sucking on an empty bottle like a cherubic wino. "Hi!"

Lyn nearly dropped the plate she was holding. "Maddie!"

"Hi!" Maddie politely acknowledged her mother and then immediately turned to Kara with worshipful eyes, offering her bottle like a gift to a goddess.

Kara graciously accepted the bottle. "Can she get out of her cot herself now?"

"So it seems," said Lyn, trying to readjust to a new world where Maddie could no longer be safely incarcerated in her cot.

The doorbell and the office phone began to ring simultaneously.

"Could you watch her for a minute?" asked Lyn.

"Sorry." Kara swung herself off the bench and handed the bottle back to Maddie. "I'm *really* late for school."

Carelessly, she ruffled Maddie's dark curly head. "Seeya, sweetie!"

Maddie's bottom lip quivered. She slammed the bottle down on the floor.

Lyn picked up Kara's half-eaten apple from the kitchen bench and threw it in the rubbish bin. She scooped up Maddie and walked toward the front door.

"Kara, Kara," Maddie sobbed pitifully.

"I know just what you mean, darling," said Lyn, holding tight to her squirming little body. "Kara, Kara."

To: Michael
From: Lyn
Subject: Please hurry home
Shocking day. Both your daughters driving me insane.
P.S. Who did you lose your virginity to?
P.P.S. Please pick up milk and cockroach baits on your way home.

To: Lyn
From: Michael
Subject: O.K.
Home at 6:30 at the latest.
Fish and chips on beach to make up for my daughters?
Lost my virginity to Jane Brewer on the way home from watching
Star Wars at the movies. The force was with me! HA!
P.S. Why?

It was past midnight that same day. Michael kissed her tenderly and said, "You did come, didn't you?"

"Yes, of course," said Lyn. "Ages ago."

She moved her hips. "Heavy."

"Sorry." He rolled onto his back with a sigh and reached across to the bedside table for a glass of water. "No need for me to pick up stray women in bars."

"Michael!"

"Just letting you know you're safe with me, sweetheart."

"Well, thanks, you big chauvinist pig."

He put down his glass of water and settled back down into bed, making contented purring sounds as he pulled up the quilt and curled his body around Lyn's back.

He was always so chipper after sex.

"Cat is devastated," said Lyn.

"Hmmm."

"You're not very sympathetic."

"Your sweet sister can be a real bitch."

"So can I."

"No you can't.

"We're identical. Remember?"

"No. You're my lovely little Lynnie."

Efficiently, he bundled her hair to the side so it wouldn't tickle his face, kissed her shoulder blade, and within seconds began to snore into the back of her neck.

Sex with husband. Check.

I absolutely did not think that, she thought.

She shouldn't have let Michael call Cat a bitch. She wasn't, for one thing, but more important, Cat never let anyone say a bad word about her sisters. Oh, *she* could say plenty of bad words about them but nobody else—not even Dan, Lyn would bet, in the privacy of their own bedroom. Cat's loyalty was fierce and staunch.

In their school days, Cat was their own personal hit man, their hired thug. When they were seven, for example, Josh Desouza spread a vicious rumor about Gemma. The rumor was that she'd shown him her underpants. (The rumor was true. He tricked her by accusing her of not wearing any. "But I am!" cried Gemma, devastated. "Prove it," he said.) When Cat heard about it, her face went bright red. She walked straight up to Josh in the middle of the playground and *head-butted* him. Head-butting hurt a lot, she confided to them afterward, but she didn't cry, well, only a little bit, when she got home and saw the red mark on her forehead.

Now they were in their thirties, Cat was still ready to spring to their defense, often unnecessarily. Just the other day she and Lyn went out to lunch. "Didn't you ask for a salad?" Cat said to Lyn. "Excuse me! My sister hasn't got her salad!"

"I am actually capable of asking myself," said Lyn.

"My sister." Cat said it with such unconscious pride. Even after she'd just been telling you what a complete loser you were for ordering a bocconcini salad, when everyone knew bocconcini was a conspiracy to make you eat rubber.

"I've got something to tell you," she said to them in the pub, as if they didn't already know *that* the moment they saw her face from the other side of the room.

Lyn fell suddenly, very deeply asleep.

The voice was teeth-jarringly sweet. "Lyn! Georgina! How *are* you?" Lyn's stomach muscles tightened in anticipation. She tucked the portable phone under her ear. "Hello, Georgina. How are you?"

She was in the middle of trying to undress Maddie for an unscheduled bath. Maddie had just spent five pleasurable minutes smearing herself with sticky black Vegemite and didn't want her handiwork removed.

There was only one person capable of leaving an open Vegemite jar sitting in the middle of the living room floor: Georgina's daughter Kara.

"To be honest, Lyn, I'm rather annoyed."

Maddie sensed her mother's attention slip and squirmed free. She escaped from the bathroom, chortling with wicked glee.

"What's wrong?"

Lyn turned off the bath taps and followed Maddie out into the hallway. Her sisters told her that she had well and truly paid her penance for breaking up Georgina's marriage by practically bringing up her daughter, leaving her free to lead a life of leisure. They also reminded her that not only had Georgina blissfully remarried some guy who looked like Brad Pitt and seemed bizarrely quite nice, but that she was a vindictive bitch from hell who *deserved* to have her husband stolen from under her nose.

But still, Lyn was always conscious of Georgina being the wronged party. And so she played her part in these terribly civilized, grown-up-about-it conversations and didn't even attempt to apply one of the four key techniques for dealing effectively with passive-aggressive behavior.

"Kara is very upset," said Georgina. "I'm surprised Michael allowed it, I really am. With respect, Lyn, I'm rather surprised at you!"

"I have no idea what you're talking about." Lyn watched Maddie pick up Kara's favorite T-shirt from the floor and hug it adoringly to her Vegemited body. There was really nothing she could do to stop her.

"I'm talking about the article in *She*," said Georgina. "Kara says you didn't even ask her permission to use her name! She's a sensitive child, Lyn. We all need to be a little careful with her feelings."

"I haven't seen the article." Lyn took a deep stress-management breath through her nostrils. She tried not to think of Kara's ten-year-old face crumpling each time Georgina called to cancel a day out. A little careful of her feelings, indeed.

"I understand of course. Your public profile is important to you," said Georgina. "Just be careful in future, won't you? How's that little ruffian of yours by the way? Kara seems to spend a lot of time looking after her for you. That must be a real help! Wish I had some help when Kara was little. Well, must fly!"

Lyn momentarily considered throwing the portable phone against the wall.

"Bitch," she said.

"Bitch," repeated Maddie, who had an unerring ear for inappropriate new words to add her to vocabulary. She applauded with chubby joyful hands. "Bitch, bitch, bitch!"

LOVE. KIDS. CAREER.
WOMEN WHO STRIKE THE "TRIPLE" JACKPOT!!!

While most of us find it incredibly difficult to juggle career and family, some women seem to have hit up upon that elusive magical formula.

At just thirty-three years of age, Lyn Kettle is the

founder and managing director of the hugely successful business Gourmet Brekkie Bus.

Brekkie Bus specializes in mouthwatering Sunday morning breakfasts delivered straight to your door. As every Gourmet Brekkie Bus fan knows (this reporter is one of them!), these breakfasts are to die for. Flaky croissants, eggs Benedict, freshly squeezed juice—and of course, those incredible pastries!

Lyn, a pencil-thin blonde (obviously she doesn't indulge too often in her own Brekkie Bus breakfasts!) first conceived the idea just three years ago, when she was managing a successful café. Since then, the business has gone from strength to strength with franchises across the country and interest from overseas buyers. Last August Lyn scooped the prestigious Businesswoman of the Year Award.

But running Gourmet Brekkie Bus doesn't stop Lyn from spending quality time with her husband, computer whiz Michael Dimitropolous, her eighteen-month-old daughter, Maddie, and her fifteen-year-old stepdaughter, Kara. Lyn works from home and her mother takes care of Maddie two to three days each week.

"My family is incredibly important to me," said Lyn from her exquisite harbor-side home. For the interview, she wore a beautifully cut suit, her blond hair elegantly styled, her makeup flawless.

A huge vase of roses adorned the dining room table. I asked if it was her birthday.

"No," said Lyn, blushing a little. "I'm very lucky. Michael often buys flowers for no particular reason."

But that's not all! She also finds time to teach aerobics two nights a week. "I love it," said Lyn, crossing her shapely legs. "It's my time-out. I couldn't live without it."

Lyn also loves skiing (Aspen this year!), reading (personal development books are always a fave!), and mountain biking (yes, really!)

And here's an interesting tidbit! Lyn is a triplet! Her sister Catriona, a marketing executive at Hollingdale Chocolates, is identical to Lyn. Gemma, who isn't identical (although she does bear a striking resemblance to her sisters!) is a primary-school teacher. The triplets are all very close.

"My sisters are my best friends," confided Lyn.

Their mother, Maxine Kettle, is president of the Australian Mothers of Multiples Association, a regular speaker at events for mothers of twins and triplets, and author of the book *Mothering Multiples: The Heaven, the Hell*, which has sold in countries around the world. Their father, Frank Kettle, is a well-known Sydney property developer. Their parents divorced when the girls were six.

"We had great childhoods," said Lyn. "We split our time between Mum and Dad and we were perfectly happy."

What next for Lyn?

Another baby might be in the cards, and she is considering expanding the Brekkie business to include Gourmet dinners and lunches.

Whatever she does next, you can be sure it will be a success for this remarkable young woman! What an inspiration!

To order your Gourmet Brekkie delivered straight to your door, call Gourmet Brekkie Bus now at 1-300-BREKKIE.

Lyn shuddered as she handed back the magazine to her mother. "Thank God she included the plug for the business. I don't know what Kara's problem is, I'm the one who looks like an idiot."

"I do," said Maxine. "It's the photo. Kara looks quite dreadful."

Lyn took back the magazine and looked more closely at the

photo. The photographer had caught Kara mid-grimace, her mouth pulled down sourly, one eyelid drooping unattractively. It wasn't the photographer's fault; Kara had scowled and sulked and sighed throughout the entire session. She was only there at her father's insistence.

"You're right," said Lyn.

"I know I am." Maxine looked at Maddie, who was chattering with animated delight to her own reflection in the china cabinet. "Lyn, what is on that child's face? She's filthy!"

"Vegemite. When Gemma and Cat read this, I'll never hear the end of it."

"Well, I don't see why." Maxine got down on her knees and held Maddie's chin firmly while she rubbed at the Vegemite with a handkerchief. Maddie kept her eyes fixed on the little girl in the china cabinet and smiled secretively. "You said they were your best friends."

"Exactly! And I never said any such thing."

She picked up her keys from the coffee table and looked at Maddie, who was now busily shredding pages from *She* magazine.

"Kiss for Mummy?" she asked, with little hope.

"No!" Maddie looked up, affronted. Lyn leaned down toward her and Maddie shook an admonishing finger. *"No!"*

"Oh well."

Lyn picked up her briefcase. "I'll be back around six. I've got to pick Kara up from her friend's place after the meeting at the bakery."

"You look absolutely *dreadful,* Lyn," announced Maxine.

"Thank you, Mum."

"You do. You're a skeleton, all pale and drab and miserable-looking. That color doesn't do you any favors of course. I've told you girls not to wear black, you refuse to listen. The point is, you do far too much. Why isn't Kara's mother picking her up? I mean *really,* why won't Michael put his foot down?"

"Mum, please."

Lyn could feel a scratchy tickle at the back of her throat. She put down her briefcase and sneezed three times.

"Hay fever," said Maxine with satisfaction. "It's that time of year for you three. I'll get you an antihistamine."

"I don't have time."

"It will only take a minute. Sit."

She disappeared down the hallway, heels tapping a brisk rhythm across the tiles, Maddie running along behind her. Suddenly exhausted, Lyn sat back down on her mother's puffy cream sofa.

She looked at the familiar photos that lined the walls. The traditional Kettle Triplet pose: Gemma in the middle, Lyn and Cat on either side. It pleased their mother's sense of balance to have the redhead separating the blondes. Identical dresses, identical hair ribbons, identical poses. Three little girls with crinkled eyes, laughing at the camera. They were laughing at their father of course. When they were children they thought he was the funniest man to walk the Earth.

She could hear her mother talking to Maddie in the kitchen. "No, you may not have one. These are not lollies. There is no point in looking at me like that, young lady. No point at all."

Some of Lyn's friends complained about their children being spoiled by doting grandparents. She didn't need to worry about Maddie missing out on her discipline quota with Maxine. It was like sending her to boot camp.

On the coffee table was a typed document Maxine was obviously in the middle of proofreading. Lyn picked it up. It was a speech for a parenting workshop her mother was running called "Triple the Heartache, Triple the Fun!"

"She's made a career out of being our mother," Cat always complained.

"So what?" Lyn would say.

"It's exploitation."

"Oh, please."

Lyn flicked idly through the speech. Most of it she recognized from previous speeches, articles, and her mother's book:

Sometimes you may feel like a traveling freak show. Eventually, you'll get used to the stares and the approaches by strangers. I remember once I counted the number of times I was stopped by well-meaning people wanting to look at my daughters as I walked through Chatswood Shopping Center. It was—

Fifteen, thought Lyn. Yes, we know, *fifteen* times!

It has been calculated that it takes twenty-eight hours a day to look after triplets. That's tricky, considering we only have twenty-four at our disposal! (Wait for laugh)

I'm not so sure you'll get one, Mum. That's not actually very funny.

Monozygotic twins—meaning one egg—share 100 percent of their genes. Dizygotic twins—meaning two eggs—share only 25 percent of their genes, like any normal sibling.

Gemma would be offended to hear herself described as a "normal" sibling. When they were in second class, Sister Joyce Mary chalked a picture of the three-leafed shamrock on the blackboard to illustrate how "the Father, Son, and Holy Ghost were three persons but one God." Gemma's hand shot into the air. "Like triplets! Like us!" The nun winced. "I'm afraid the Kettle girls are not like the Holy Trinity!" "Yes, but I think we are, Sister," said Gemma kindly.

When Gemma told the story to their mother, Maxine explained that her analogy might have been reasonable if they'd all come from the one egg. However, as only Cat and Lyn were identical and Gemma was a "single egg" they probably couldn't be compared to the Holy Trinity, which was a lot of nonsense anyway. "I don't want to be a single egg!" wailed Gemma. "What if we were *Siamese* triplets?" asked Cat. "With our heads all glued together?" But their mother had turned up the car radio to drown out Gemma.

Sibling rivalry is obviously a complex issue, which I will be discussing at length. On other hand, you may feel envious of mothers of "singletons" and worry that your babies are actually closer to each other than to you. This is perfectly normal.

That was a new one. Surely their profoundly practical mother had never worried about anything like that?

"Why did you tell that journalist Gemma was a teacher?" Maxine came back into the room and handed over a glass of water and a tablet.

"I think she might still do some casual teaching every now and then," said Lyn, putting the speech aside. "How was I meant to describe her?"

"Yes, well, that's certainly a point," said Maxine. "Odds-body! Jack of all trades! I called her the other day and she casually mentioned she was off to do *stilt walking* for some promotion at Fox Studios. Gemma, I said, are you actually capable of walking on stilts?"

"She wasn't," said Lyn. "She told me she kept toppling over. But apparently the kids in the audience all thought it was hilarious."

"Hilarious indeed. Gemma is a *drifter*. I read in the paper today about that murderer in Melbourne. They called him a drifter. I thought to myself, that's how people would describe Gemma! My own daughter! A drifter!"

"She doesn't drift far. At least she only drifts around Sydney."

"I'll grant you that." Maxine, who was sitting on the sofa in front of Lyn, suddenly took a deep breath and pressed her hands to her knees in a strangely awkward gesture. "Yes, well, I've been meaning to talk to you about something. A little issue."

"Have you really?" Her mother wasn't in the habit of *meaning* to say things; she generally just said them. "What is it?"

At that moment, Lyn's mobile began to ring and vibrate on the coffee table. She glanced at the name on the screen. "Speak of the drifter. I'll let her go to voicemail."

"No, answer it. I'll talk to you about it another time. You're in a rush anyway." Maxine stood up briskly and removed the glass of water from Lyn's hand.

"Tell Gemma to water that poor man's flowers," she ordered cryptically, and went tapping off again down the hallway, calling out, "Just what are you up to now, Maddie?"

"Cat Crisis!" announced Gemma happily. "Guess where she is!"

"I give up, where?"

"Well, all right then, I'll tell you. She's sitting in her car outside the *woman's* place!"

"What woman?"

"What woman, she says. *The* woman! The woman dastardly Dan had sex with! Cat is *stalking* her. I think Cat is perfectly capable of boiling a rabbit, don't you? Or a puppy. Even a kitten."

"Can you please be serious for once in your life?" said Lyn. "What's she doing there?"

"Wait till you hear how she found her! She was like an undercover detective."

"Gemma."

"I am being serious. Deadly serious. We have to stop her! She says she just wants to see what the woman looks like, but that sounds a bit passive for Cat, don't you think? She's probably planning to throw acid at her, something to horribly disfigure her. Can we drive there together? My air conditioning isn't working."

"I've got a meeting," Lyn looked at her watch, "in half an hour."

"I'll see you soon. I'll wait out front."

"Gemma!"

"Can't talk, going to sneeze!" Gemma hung up mid-sneeze.

Lyn put down the phone and rubbed her eyes with the heels of her hands, while she tried to remember where Gemma was living at the moment.

She thought of her meeting at the bakery. The rich fragrance that would envelop her, the respect that would greet her, the pleasure of dealing with efficient, professional, calm, *normal* people.

She called out to Maxine, "You'd better give me two more of those antihistamines."

She'd forgotten all about her mother's "little issue."

CHAPTER 3

"You stood me up."

"Did I?"

"Was it because somebody died?"

"Oh, I hope not."

Waking up was Gemma's least favorite thing. She resisted it daily. Even when she was woken up by a phone call, like now, she continued to fight consciousness by keeping her eyes squeezed shut, her breathing deep, and not concentrating too hard.

If she was lucky, the conversation would be short and she could slip straight back into lovely sleep.

"I was actually sort of hoping somebody did die. Somebody not that important. It would help my shattered ego." The voice was rather appealingly masculine but she had no idea who he was, or what he was talking about, and sleep was still a possibility.

"Yes, I see," she slurred politely.

"Did you get a better offer?"

"Umm." She breathed deeper and burrowed farther under her quilt.

"Are you still in bed? Big night last night?"

"Shh," said Gemma. "Stop talking. Sleep time. It's Saturday."

But there was something twitching urgently and irritatingly at the very outer corner of her consciousness.

"Exactly. It's Saturday. Last night was Friday night. I waited. And waited. Everyone in the restaurant felt sorry for me. I got free garlic bread."

"Who is this?" Like Frankenstein's monster coming to life, Gemma suddenly sat bolt upright.

"How many of us did you stand up last night? Is this like a regular Friday night thing for you?"

"Oh my God! You're the locksmith!"

She threw back her quilt and jumped out of bed, the phone to her ear. She bunched back her fringe with one hand. How could this have happened?

"I can't believe I forgot! That is so *rude.* So bad-mannered. I am *so* sorry. I had a family crisis. It was exciting, my sister turned into a psychotic stalker. Still, that's no excuse."

"Keep going."

"I feel terrible. Really."

She really did feel terrible. Not just because of hurting the locksmith's feelings but because if she could so completely forget something like that, something she was quite looking forward to, then who knows what else she'd forgotten in her life? Perhaps she'd forgotten other things and never remembered she'd forgotten them. Good things. Like lottery wins. Job offers. It was frightening.

"You should feel terrible," said the locksmith. "How do you plan to redeem yourself?"

Gemma sat cross-legged on the edge of her bed and pulled her T-shirt over her knees. He sounded quite sexy and stern. Perhaps she should make a habit of standing up first dates.

"Oh, *redemption,*" she said. "I'm a Catholic, we're right into it. What shall I do? Buy you breakfast?"

"No. I think you should *cook* me breakfast. Breakfast for you. Lunch for me. Brunch for the two of us. You can tell me all about your psychotic sister."

"I would, I really would, but I don't cook. So we'll have to think of something else."

"I'll be there in twenty minutes."

Gemma let her T-shirt spring back from her knees and cuddled them to her with pleasure.

"I don't cook," she repeated. "My sisters cook."

"Your sisters didn't stand me up."

He hung up without saying good-bye.

Well! He sounded *nice*!

Of course, they always did in the beginning.

Lyn believed that Gemma was addicted to a chemical called phenylethylamine. This was the chemical that flooded divinely through your body when you fell in love. Gemma had been in exactly fourteen relationships over the last ten years (Lyn was keeping count), and according to Lyn, it was starting to get beyond a joke, in fact it was becoming scary. Gemma was obviously breaking up with these perfectly nice men whenever the relationship moved from Stage 1—attraction—to Stage 2—intimacy—because of her addiction.

The good thing was that you could also get phenylethylamine from chocolate. Lyn said Gemma should therefore eat more chocolate and settle into a long-term committed loving relationship in Stage 3.

Gemma wondered what her chances were of reaching Stage 3 with—

With . . . ?

What the hell was his name?

Her mind was quite blank.

There was a peculiar significance to it, she knew that.

She remembered picking up her keys from the kitchen table and jangling them in a maternal "You silly things" fashion, as if it was their fault they'd got locked in the house. The locksmith smiled at her. He smiled straight into her eyes because he was exactly her height.

Gemma and her sisters had a strict "nothing under six feet" policy, but looking into this man's eyes had been rather pleasant, slightly shocking in fact, as if they were lying in bed together. Maybe, she thought, it was time for a change of policy.

"It's funny how people always want to show me the keys they've locked in their houses," he said.

His head was so closely shaven it was almost bald. He had wide shoulders, a slightly crooked nose, and . . . extraordinarily long eyelashes. They would have made a handsome man look effeminate. They made the locksmith a tiny bit beautiful.

Gemma said, "You have the most amazing eyelashes."

It was a bad habit of hers, complimenting strangers on their physical attributes. She once told a woman in an elevator that she had an especially lovely collarbone. The woman had looked panic-stricken and had begun jabbing at the elevator buttons.

"I know," said the locksmith. "I'm surprised you took so long to mention them." Gemma burst into surprised laughter as he leaned forward and furiously batted his eyelashes at her. Then he laughed too. He had the deep, comforting belly laugh of a much larger man. It made her laugh even more.

She was still chortling away when he told her his name and asked if he could take her out to dinner that Friday night.

His name was significant in a vaguely comical sort of way. Something made her think, well, I'll remember *that* name, ha ha. And there was also something that was just a tiny bit sad about it. Just a faint, delicate shadow of sadness. It was very odd. What could it be? What name could be funny and sad all at once? How fascinating! She couldn't wait to remember it.

She looked around her room for inspiration. The sun was streaming through the open window, a breeze gently lifting and dropping a faded lace curtain. It had been only a couple of weeks, but it looked like this could be one of her favorite houses. The solid, mahogany furniture seemed patient and wise and the clutter-filled drawers and shelves felt friendly and nonthreatening.

She'd just finished two months in a funky inner-city apartment. All that funkiness had started to give her a headache. Here, in the settled leafy suburbia of Hunters Hill, she would be serene and meditative. She might even learn to cook.

Gemma was a house-sitter. She had a bold, boxed ad in the Sydney House-Sitter's Directory:

> Single woman in her thirties with excellent references.
> Very responsible. Extremely security conscious. I take
> house-sitting seriously! Walk back in the door and
> feel like you've only been gone for five minutes! Your
> home, your pets, and your plants will receive my tender loving care!

This house belonged to the Penthursts, retired doctors, who were traveling around Europe for a year. Dr. and Dr. Penthurst, Mary and Don, had taken a liking to Gemma and had already sent her a postcard. "How are my African violets?" wrote Dr. Don from Venice.

Dr. Don had a collection of six African violets with fat, velvety leaves. "You need to talk to them for at least twenty minutes a day," he had told her. "You probably think I'm dotty, but it works. It's documented! It's on the Net! One theory is that it's the carbon dioxide. Anyway. Just have a little chat with them. Doesn't matter what you say."

"Just water them, dear," said Dr. Mary, out of his hearing.

"Oh no," said Gemma. "Your house has to feel as if you're still here."

Now she walked up to the row of pots on the windowsill and caressed their leaves. She called them all Violet, her own private joke. "What was that locksmith's name? Mmmm? Violet? Any ideas? What about you, Violet? Now, *Violet*, I bet you remember!"

The Violets were silent, as stumped as she was.

Gemma sat back down the bed and looked at her framed family photos on the bedside table. They were the only personal items she displayed when she was house-sitting. Otherwise she lived in their houses exactly as the owners left them.

Her photo collection was an eclectic mix, skidding without logic through the generations. There was her father grinning with evil black-and-white innocence at age five, next to a furious fifteen-year-old Cat, one obscene finger stuck up at the photographer. (Really, Gemma, why would anyone even *keep* such a dreadful photo, said their mother, let alone put it on public display? I'll give you fifty bucks for it, said Dan. Look at that chick! Nobody messes with my wife.)

Next to the photo of Cat was an old black-and-white one of their mother at around the same age. She was on a beach, her arm slung with casual abandon over her best friend's shoulder. It looked like they'd just come out of the water and collapsed on the sand. Maxine was smiling radiantly at the camera, her hair plastered to her forehead. It was hard to imagine that girl growing up into the immaculately irritable Maxine Kettle.

Gemma looked at the photo of her mother and the locksmith's name reappeared right where she'd left it.

Charlie. Of course it was Charlie. What a relief.

Charlie was a joke name because it was the name of Mum's boyfriend before Dad. The one she would have married, the one she *should* have married. Charlie belonged to the life their mother would have had if her ovaries hadn't betrayed her.

There were photos of him in the old albums from Maxine's nineteenth birthday. He was a smiley nerd with protruding teeth. Thank God you didn't marry him, we would have got those teeth, Gemma and her sisters told their mother. Maxine sniffed and looked at them with narrowed eyes, as if imagining the quiet, tasteful daughters she would have had (one by one, of course!) if she'd married Charlie Edwards.

So that's why the locksmith's name was funny. But why was it sad?

"Surely I don't feel sorry for you, Mum," said Gemma to her mother's photo. Maxine smiled back at her and Gemma pressed her face right up close to the photo. "Do I? Why would I?"

Enough! It was time to think about new Charlie. Charlie with the long eyelashes and perfectly adequate teeth! Charlie who was on his way over right now with the erroneous expectation of home-cooked food.

Gemma lay back down on the Penthursts' wonderfully comfortable king-sized bed and stretched luxuriously.

What could she possibly cook for her redemption breakfast? The answer was nothing of course. She didn't even have a loaf of bread in the house.

Twenty minutes later she woke with a start and a voice in her ear. "You're starting to seem a little unreliable."

She opened her eyes. A man was squatting by her bed, large hands dangling over skinny legs in blue jeans.

"How did you get in?" she asked, sleepily. He rolled his eyes. "Oh. Of course." Gemma lifted her arms above her head and yawned. She met his eyes and her yawn turned into a laugh of pleasure halfway through.

"Hello there, Charlie."

"Hello there, Gemma. Where's my lunch?"

The eyelashes were just as she remembered them.

To: Gemma Kettle
From: Gwen Kettle
Subject: Hello darling
Dearest Gemma,

Frank has wired me up to the World Wide Internet. It took him a long time and he swore a lot, as you can imagine. I think we are right now. I am sending each of you an e-letter. How are you? How is your hay fever? Better I hope. Frank says that you invest in shares on your computer and that you are doing very well. Congratulations, darling, and well done to you. I told Beverly next door about it but she did not believe me. She is a very annoying woman. With much love, your Nana

To: Gwen Kettle
From: Gemma Kettle
Subject: NANA IN CYBERSPACE! HELLO!
NANA!
CONGRATULATIONS and well done to you too! Dad never mentioned he was helping you get on the Internet and I was so excited to see your e-mail pop up. We can e-mail all the time now! It's true that I buy stocks on the Net and it's great fun, just like playing the pokies at the club, only not so many jackpots! I'll show you how. (It would be a good idea not to mention this to Mum if you are talking to her.) Beverly next door is a complete twit.
I am giving serious consideration to a new boyfriend. We had breakfast together this morning. (Now don't get any wrong ideas, please, Nana. It wasn't because he stayed the night.)
He is a locksmith. That could be handy, couldn't it? For example, if you needed your locks changed at any time. (Do you? How is security at your place?) He drives a motorbike and his family is Italian. Sexy, hey? I might bring him over to visit soon and you can tell me what you think.
Love from Gemma

"So, when do you think I should have sex with my locksmith?"

It was that same night, and Gemma lay immersed to her neck in a peachy-smelling bubble bath, talking to Lyn on the portable phone. She had turned the lights out and the bathroom was lit by dozens of perfumed, flickering tea-candles. A box of funny-shaped chocolates from Cat's work was in convenient reach. (Cat kept her in constant supply of rejected Hollingdale chocolates. It was a truly tragic occupational hazard that Cat was now repulsed by even the smell of chocolate.)

The Penthursts had a gigantic claw-foot bathtub, which was

wonderful, although it did remind Gemma of those movie scenes where the woman dreamily (so foolishly!) runs an extremely steamy bath while a knife-clutching villain creeps up the stairs. To ensure this didn't happen, she thought about it a lot. As an added security measure, she took the phone with her into the bath and telephoned no-nonsense people like her sisters and her mother.

"I'm thinking, controversially, the fourth date. Normally, I succumb on the third date." She lifted a foamy leg and watched the froth sliding back into the steaming water. "What do you think?"

Lyn's voice burst forth from the portable phone, spoiling the ambience quite considerably. "I don't know and I don't care," she said with an irritable clatter of crockery. Lyn always seemed to be packing or unpacking a dishwasher when she spoke on the phone. "I've already got one teenager in my life, thanks very much."

"Oh."

Gemma's leg splashed down into the water as she hurriedly tried to think of a breezy new topic of conversation to demonstrate that her feelings weren't hurt.

"For God's sake, Gemma, why do you always have to be so bloody *sensitive*?"

Too late.

"All I said was oh."

"I've got Maddie whining. I've got Michael stressed. I've got Kara threatening to sue me. I've got Christmas orders flooding in and staff flooding out. What do you expect?"

"I don't expect anything. It was just, I don't know, idle chat."

"I don't have time for idle chat. Have you talked to Cat since Friday's drama?"

"Yes," Gemma relaxed again. "Dan wants them to try counseling."

"He's a fuckwit."

That was strong language for Lyn.

"Yes, he is," said Gemma. "But only a temporary fuckwit, don't you think? They'll work it out. Dan just made a stupid mistake."

"I've always hated him."

A tidal wave of bubbles went flying over the side of the bath as Gemma sat up straight.

"Really?"

"Yes, really."

"I thought we all loved Dan!" Gemma felt slightly sick.

"It's not a group decision who we like and don't like."

"Yes, O.K., but I didn't know we—I mean you—*felt* that way."

"I have to go." Lyn's voice softened and a saucepan banged. "The locksmith sounds really lovely. Sleep with him whenever it feels right. Try not to break his heart. And don't take any notice of me. I'm just tired. I need more iron."

Gemma put the phone on the wet bathroom floor and used her big toe to dislodge the plug just slightly so she could put more hot water in. She selected a large warped strawberry cream.

Of course she was angry with Dan. She was furious with him. She wanted to punch him in the nose. She was looking forward to publicly shaming him on Christmas Day by not giving him a present. Not even a scratch 'n' win card.

But the cold hatred in Lyn's voice was way beyond what Gemma was feeling.

It made her feel left out.

She thought about Friday and pulling up behind Cat's blue Honda. For some reason it had wrenched Gemma's heart to see the lone little car sitting on the side of the road outside some strange block of units.

Lyn turned off the ignition with a grim flick of her wrist.

"This is ridiculous."

Together they walked over to Cat's car and tapped on the driver's window.

Cat wound down the window. "Get in, get in!"

Gemma hopped in the backseat, while Lyn went around to the front. There were spots of feverish color on Cat's cheeks. "This is fun, isn't it?" Her eyes were bright.

"Nope," said Lyn.

"Yep," said Gemma.

"It's O.K. It's fine. I'm not going to talk to her," said Cat. "I just have to see what she looks like. I can't bear not knowing what she looks like."

"Apart from the weirdness of this," said Lyn. "wouldn't this girl be at work?"

"Oh no, she's too *young* for work, Lyn!" said Cat. "She's studying law. Smart, as well as attractive. My husband doesn't have one-night stands with just anybody! Anyway, I've worked out her timetable. She had a lecture first thing and then nothing for the rest of the day."

"Oh. My. God." Lyn twisted around in her seat to look at Cat.

Cat turned and looked at her fiercely. "What's your problem?"

Gemma looked fondly at their identical profiles. "There's someone coming," she said.

Lyn and Cat turned their heads and Cat made a strangled noise. A girl was walking toward the car. She had long swinging dark hair and a knapsack.

"Is it her?" A bubble of schoolgirl hysteria was expanding in Gemma's chest. "Should we hide?"

"Yep, that's her," said Cat. She sat very still, looking straight ahead at the girl as she got closer and closer to the car. "That's Angela."

"How do you know?" whispered Lyn, beginning to sink lower in her seat.

"I made Dan describe her to me," said Cat. "I'm positive."

She put her hand on the door handle. "I'm going to talk to her."

"*No!*"

Lyn and Gemma both made a frantic grab for her arm as Cat purposefully got out of the car, slamming the door behind her.

Lyn put her face in her hands. "I can't watch."

Gemma stared, transfixed, as the two women got closer to each other.

"Should we go after her?"

"Just tell me if she starts to assault her," said Lyn in a muffled voice.

"She's walking up to her," said Gemma. "The girl's smiling at her."

Lyn took her face out of her hands and together they watched the girl talking to Cat. She was talking animatedly and pointing up the street, past the car, making twisting directions with her hands. Cat was nodding her head. After a couple of seconds and more pointing and head nodding, Cat turned around and began walking back to the car. Her face was impassive. She opened the car door and got back in behind the driver's seat. The three of them sat in silence.

Cat leaned forward and rested her forehead against the top of the steering wheel.

Lyn said, "It probably wasn't even her."

Gemma said, "She wasn't at *all* pretty," and then all three of them jumped at a sudden, urgent rapping on Cat's window. It was the girl, smiling, her head on one side as she bent down toward the car.

Oh dear, thought Gemma, holding her breath. She's gorgeous.

Cat clumsily wound down the window.

"Sorry," said the girl. "I realized I should have said first left, not first right. So it's left, left, then right."

"Ha!" said Cat, as if giving a polite response to a bad joke. Lyn leaned forward and gave an awkward little flutter of her fingers. "Thank you *very* much!" Gemma's stomach cramped as she tried to suppress a gigantic wave of laughter. "That's O.K.," said the girl. "Left, left, right." "Yep," said Lyn heartily. "Got it!"

The girl smiled and walked back toward her flat.

"She's nice." Cat's hands were clenched around the steering wheel. "The bitch is fucking *nice*!"

"It's not relevant," said Lyn.

"Actually, I don't think she was that nice," said Gemma. "She seemed a bit dull to me. Lacking in personality."

"Can we just get out of here?" said Lyn. "Please?"

That night, while Charlie was eating free garlic bread, the three of them watched videos at Lyn's place. Michael cooked them pasta. Cat cheered up a little after reading Lyn's mortifying *She* article. Maddie skidded maniacally back and forth among all three of them until her bedtime, when Lyn suggested they introduce her to the "igloo" game.

It was a game Cat created when they were little. It involved huddling under a white sheet and pretending they were three Eskimos in an igloo. It was extremely cold and icy in the igloo of course, so you had to put your arms around each other and snuggle close, shivering and trembling and making your teeth chatter loudly. Sometimes Cat would bravely venture out into the snow and catch a fish or kill a polar bear for their dinner. (Gemma and Lyn weren't allowed to go hunting because it was Cat's game, so she made the rules. They had to stay in the igloo and get the fire ready.)

It was their favorite game for when their parents were fighting. When the yelling started, Cat used to say, "Quick! Into the igloo!"

Maddie thought the igloo game was hysterical—and it was a good way for Lyn and Gemma to secretly give Cat a hug, while they huddled and trembled.

Gemma laid her head back against the rim of the bathtub and was suddenly intensely uncomfortable, too hot and headachy. Baths, she thought, were just like her relationships, all "ooh, ah" in the beginning and then suddenly, without warning, she had to get out, out, *out*!

She walked gingerly across the slippery tiles to reach blindly for the light. Rubbing steam from the bathroom mirror, she stood sideways and gave herself a sultry centerfold pout over one shoulder. It was her secret opinion that she looked sexiest when her hair was wet.

Sex.

It was such a funny thing. Sometimes, she found it amazing that she actually had sex with anyone. It was so, well, shocking.

"Ladies and men do *what*?" eight-year-old Gemma had exploded, when their mother sat all three of her daughters down to briskly and precisely explain the grisly facts of life.

Maxine sighed and went over the fundamentals one more time.

"I don't believe you!" Gemma was horrified.

"Neither do I." Cat folded her arms aggressively. She always kept a careful eye out for conspiracies, especially when it came to her mother. "You're making it up."

"I wish I was," said their mother.

"I think it might be true," Lyn said sadly. How did that girl come into the world knowing everything already?

Sometimes when Gemma thought about sex, sometimes even when she was *having* sex, she felt a faint echo of that horror she felt as an eight-year-old. My goodness, she'd think, looking up at the ceiling as some boyfriend earnestly scrabbled around her body, what in the world is he doing *now*?

It didn't stop her from having quite a lot of sex.

She rummaged through the bathroom cupboard for the Listerine and thought about Charlie, standing in the Penthursts' kitchen that morning. "This fridge is the saddest thing I've ever seen," he'd said, taking out a bottle of milk, sniffing it suspiciously, and then throwing it straight into the garbage. "You really don't cook, do you?"

"Nope."

He closed the fridge door and leaned back against it, folding his arms. "Well, what are you going to feed me, Gemma?"

He had a lovely, slightly wrong way of saying her name, a caressing emphasis on the second syllable. Gem*ma*.

She took him to a local café where they served breakfast all day and the patrons sat on low, cushiony sofas reading free magazines and newspapers, looking self-consciously relaxed over their Big Breakfast Specials.

As first dates went it was promising. There was a pleasing

crackle of sexual tension that caused their eyes to keep meeting and sliding away and meeting again. Charlie seemed slightly flushed and she felt a heightened awareness of everything: the smells of coffee and bacon, the edge of his T-shirt against the caramel skin of his neck, her own hand reaching across for the sugar. But there was also an odd familiarity, as if she already knew him, as if they'd been to this café dozens of times before, and this was just an ordinary Saturday. Instead of sharing vital information about jobs, hobbies, ex's, and families, they flicked through the magazines and shared stupid information about celebrities and diets.

"Did you know that the shape of Nicole's head proves that she could never have been happy with Tom?"

"Check out this woman. She lost over forty kilos by walking up and down her hallway. Now her husband says he liked her better when she was fat."

And then, when they were leaving and Charlie asked, "What are you doing tonight?" something about the slightly defensive way he was standing and the way his eyes grinned straight into hers, made her want to cry and laugh at the same time.

Wrapping a towel around her, her mouth minty with Listerine (tonight was most definitely first-kiss time) she went dripping down the hallway into her bedroom to choose her most unsexy, unmatching underwear so she wouldn't be tempted to sleep with him too soon.

Probably, she thought, it was always this good in the beginning.

She imagined her fourteen ex-boyfriends, all lined up one after the other in an orderly queue. The plumber who liked country music, that funny redheaded guy with the glasses, the graphic designer who talked too much in the movies, that big guy who was obsessed about losing his hair. At one end was Marcus, grinning a bit contemptuously, the farthest away, but still clearer and sharper than the rest of them. And, now right up front, chuckling his belly laugh, was Charlie. The queue dipped suddenly in height. He was at least a head shorter than the rest of them.

Would Charlie one day be giving her that puzzled, hurt look? "But why? I thought we were going so well?"

At least, thought Gemma, Cat knew exactly what she wanted. She wanted Dan and she wanted a baby. She also wanted a Ferrari, a house by the beach, Lyn's Italian leather jacket, and for some man at Hollingdale Chocolates to get run over by a bus.

And that was it. No doubts. No confusion. No lying awake at night trying to work out the magic formula for happiness. Even if she didn't exactly have what she wanted at the moment, at least she knew what it was. Gemma couldn't imagine a feeling more peaceful, or exotic.

The doorbell rang in an impatient way, as if it had already been rung once. She threw on some clothes over her unsexy underwear and went running down the stairs to stop him from breaking in again.

Perms and the Pill

It must have been in the late sixties. I remember I was wearing my mauve miniskirt, long yellow socks, and platform shoes. Paula and I were off to the hairdressers for our first ever perms.

We had to walk through that park on Henderson Road and we saw this girl about the same age as us. Tall, with gorgeous long red hair. She was running around after these three adorable little girls. All identically dressed in little yellow sundresses with their hair up in top knots. At first, we thought she was just minding them. But then we could hear them calling out, Mummy, watch me! Mummy, come here! The poor girl was running this way and that, trying to keep them all happy.

Paula said, "Triplets! Aren't they sweet!" And at that very moment, one child grabbed another one and sank her teeth into her bare arm! The bitten child screamed blue murder! And the mother said, very firmly, something like, "I said no biting today! That's it! We're all going home!" Pandemonium! They scattered, like a bomb had fallen, pelting off in different directions! How that poor girl managed to get them home I don't know.

Well, Paula and I were gob-smacked. We had no idea children bit one another, like savage little animals! You know what we did straight after our perms? We went to the new Family Planning Clinic in the city and got ourselves prescriptions for the Pill. We did! Perms and the Pill on the same day. I've never forgotten it.

CHAPTER 4

"My Wife is a triplet, you know," Dan said chattily. He leaned back against the squeaky vinyl sofa and crossed his arms comfortably behind his head. Cat watched him suspiciously. He was finding marriage counseling far too enjoyable for her liking.

"Really!"

The counselor wriggled with delight. Her name was Annie and she was a bubbly ball of spiritually advanced energy and positive new age vibes. Cat couldn't stand her. She could feel her sulky teenage self reemerging in the hard line of her jaw. It was like religion classes when soft, oozy Miss Ellis made them share their *feelings* with the class. Gemma adored her, obligingly spilling her soul, while Cat and Lyn listened, appalled, at the back of the classroom. Cat would have taken a double period of calculus with psychopathic Sister Elizabeth Mary over one squirmy religion class with pink-fluffy-cardigan Miss Ellis.

"And are you close to your siblings, Cat?" beamed Annie. Her green dress was covered in a diseaselike rash of sunny yellow polka dots. No doubt there was a pink fluffy cardigan in her wardrobe. She leaned forward, presenting them both with an uninterrupted view of endless freckled cleavage.

"Not really." Cat concentrated hard on Annie's forehead.

"Are you *kidding*?" Dan, who had been observing Annie's breasts with awe, took his hands out from behind his head. "She adores her sisters! They're unhealthily close if you ask me."

"Except no one did ask you, Dan," said Cat. Annie sat back in her chair and tapped her pen against her teeth with gentle empathy.

"The three of them are like this exclusive little club," said Dan. "And they're not taking any new members."

"I want to talk more about Dan's *infidelity*." Cat shifted noisily on the green vinyl.

Dan looked irritated. "I don't think it's constructive to keep going over and over it." He looked at Annie for approval.

"Cat has a need to work through her feelings about this, Dan," replied Annie. "We probably should respect that, yes?"

Ha! Annie was on her side! Cat gave Dan a triumphant look, and his eyes glinted back at her.

"Annie, you're right of course," he said admiringly and gently patted Cat's thigh.

Competition was an aphrodisiac for Cat and Dan. Their relationship was all about smart verbal jabs and wild wrestling for the TV remote and flicking each other with tea towels. Whether they were skiing or playing Scrabble or avoiding each other's cold feet in bed, they were both equally, aggressively, in it to win.

They had fun together. Sometimes, just for the pleasure of it, they went through all their friends, trying to pick a couple who had more fun than they did. No one came close. They were the winners!

Not any more though. Now they were the losers. The couple going through a "rough patch."

To her disgust and horror, Cat heard a sad, strangled little sob come out of her mouth. With practiced soothing murmurs, Annie nudged the discreetly placed box of tissues across the coffee table.

Cat grabbed a handful, while Dan cleared his throat and ran his hands up and down his jeans. "I went to see her, you know," said Cat, looking at them both above her tissues, snuffling noisily. "She gave me directions back to the Pacific Highway."

"Who?" asked Annie.

"Angela. The girl Dan slept with."

"Goodness me," said Annie.

"Fucking hell," said Dan.

To: Lyn; Gemma; Catriona
From: Maxine
Subject: Proposal for Christmas Day
Girls:

It seems to me that it is quite ridiculous and inequitable that I am always responsible for cooking a hot Christmas lunch. I have done so for the last thirty years and it is becoming tiresome. This year I would like to propose a cold seafood picnic somewhere by the water. Everybody could contribute. Your thoughts, please?

To: Maxine
cc: Cat; Lyn
From: Gemma
Subject: Proposal for Christmas Day

MUM! You have made exactly the same proposal every Christmas for the last five years. Every year we ACCEPT your proposal with enthusiasm. Every year you IGNORE us and continue to cook a hot XMAS lunch. You are so funny! This year I would like to make a counterproposal. Let's have Christmas lunch at Lyn's!! She has an exquisite harborside home as we all know. That way we could all swim in her exquisite harborside pool and enjoy observing her shapely legs as she brings us drinks. We'd be lovely and cool and polite to one another. It would be fun! We could all contribute something. I will contribute my potential new boyfriend, Charlie. He is delicious.

With much love, Gemma

To: Gemma

cc: Maxine; Cat

From: Lyn

Very funny G. But a good idea. I will have a seafood lunch for Christmas at my place. Better for Maddie anyway. Everybody can bring something. We'll give you Christmas off this year, Mum. I shall e-mail more details. O.K. with you, Cat?

To: Maxine; Gemma; Lyn

From: Cat

Re: Christmas

Fine with me.

To: Gemma; Lyn; Cat

From: Maxine

If you would all feel more comfortable at Lyn's place then I won't raise any objections. I do apologize that past Christmases have obviously been so unpleasant for you all. I shall bring a turkey and roast potatoes, Lyn. Otherwise there are sure to be complaints. Gemma, Lyn has a lot on her plate! She certainly won't be serving you drinks on Christmas Day. Everybody will have to roll up their sleeves and pitch in! As for bringing a new boyfriend, who we've never met, please don't be ridiculous.

To: Maxine

From: Gemma

Subject: Christmas Day

You're a classic, Mum.

Love, Gemma

"You look very nice," said Dan.

They were crossing the Harbour Bridge in the back of a cab, an hour late for Dan's Christmas party in the city. "Thanks." Cat smoothed down her skirt and scraped at her lipstick with her fingernail.

It was her fault they were late. Over the last few days her body had become a leaden weight that needed to be dragged around from place to place. It was a tremendous effort to do anything at all.

Dan had sat silently on the end of their bed while she paused to rest and sigh after doing up each button on her shirt, his feet tapping a violent rhythm on the carpet. He liked parties.

Cat watched the lights of the city reflecting red and blue on the harbor's murky depths. She liked parties, too. In fact, December was normally her favorite time of year. She loved the way Sydney become all giggly and light-headed. She loved the way nothing mattered quite so much and work deadlines lost their power. Of course we can't even *think* about that until after Christmas, people said happily. But this December didn't feel special at all. There was no special December smell in the air. It could just as easily have been March, or July, or any boring old month.

The car careened across two lanes as they took off from the tollgates and Cat fell against Dan's shoulder. They both laughed polite-stranger laughs and Dan looked at his watch. "We're making O.K. time, we won't be that late."

"That's good."

They sat in silence while the cab headed toward the Rocks. Cat spoke to the window. "Do of any of your friends know, you know, about . . ."

"No."

He took her hand and put it in his lap.

"Of course not. Nobody knows."

Cat looked out at George Street. Traffic had slowed to a jolting stop-and-start crawl. Horns tooted. Men and women in business suits spilled out of the pubs and their laughing faces seemed hard and strident. People in the distance kept seeing Cat and Dan's cab, throwing one arm in the air and then dropping it with

aggressive disgust when they saw it was taken. Sydney wasn't giggly and light-headed at Christmastime; Sydney was just drunk and
sordid.

"I wish you'd got the Paris job," she said.

"Yeah, well, I didn't."

Ever since Dan had started working for the Australian branch
of a French company, they had dreamed of a transfer to Paris. The
Christmas before, he had made it onto the short list for a management position and the dream got so close they could touch it.
They even enrolled themselves in a Beginner's French course at
the local evening college. In France, they would be themselves,
but better. They'd wear French clothes and have French sex, while
still, of course, maintaining their fundamental Aussie superiority.
They'd be more worldly, more stylish, and in years to come, they'd
say, "Oh yes, we both speak fluent French! *Naturellement!* We had
a year in Paris, you see."

But he'd missed out, and it had taken weeks to recover from
the sour disappointment. And now here they were trapped in
their stale, same-old Sydney lives. The only difference was a girl
with shiny black hair and fresh young skin.

Cat turned away from the window to look at Dan. "Did you
kiss her good-bye?"

He let go of her hand. "Oh, Cat, please no more, not tonight."

"Because you called a cab, didn't you? What did you do while
you waited for it? Did she stay in bed or did she get up and wait
with you?"

"I don't understand why you can't leave it alone," said Dan. He
was looking at her as if he didn't know her, as if he didn't even
particularly like her. "You're actually getting pretty fucking boring, Cat."

"*What?*"

The rage was a glorious relief after the apathy. It went straight
to her head, like tequila.

"I can't believe you said that."

She had a vision of his head snapping back as her fist slammed into his chin.

In a sudden rush of movement she leaned forward, so that her seat belt pulled tight against her and tapped the taxi driver on the shoulder.

"Can you believe he said that?"

"I was not listening, sorry." The driver cocked his head politely toward her.

"Oh, Jesus, Cat." Dan bunched his body up into the corner of the cab, as if he were trying to disappear.

"We've been married for four years," she told the taxi driver, becoming more exhilarated with fury with every word. "Everything's going well; we're even trying to have a *baby*. And then, what does he do? He goes out and has *sex* with some strange woman he picks up in a bar. He tells me this while we're eating *spaghetti*. So, fine. That's fine. I'm trying to deal with it. He's sorry. He's very fucking sorry. But you know what he just said to me?"

The cabdriver had pulled up at a red light. The streetlights illuminated his face as he twisted around from the steering wheel to contemplate Cat. He had a black beard and smiling white teeth.

"No, I do not know," he said. "You tell me."

Dan groaned quietly.

"He said I was boring because I keep asking questions about it."

"Ah, I see," said the driver. He glanced over at Dan and back at Cat. "This is very painful for you."

"*Yes,*" said Cat gratefully.

"The lights have changed, mate," said Dan.

The driver turned back around and accelerated. "If my wife unfaithful to me, I kill her," he said enthusiastically.

"Really?" said Cat.

"With my bare hands, I hold them to her neck and I squeeze."

"I see."

"But for men, it is different," he said. "Our biology, it is different!"

"Oh, for God's sake!" Cat put her hand on the door handle. "Stop the car. I can't stand either of you."

"Pardon me?"

She screamed at him, "Stop the car!" and opened the car door to reveal the ground rushing by beneath them. Dan reached over and clenched her upper arm painfully hard. He told the driver, "You'd better pull over!"

The driver swung the steering wheel and slammed on the brakes to an enraged chorus of horns.

"You're hurting my arm."

Dan loosened his grip. "Do what you want. I give up."

Cat climbed out of the car, while Dan looked straight ahead, his arms folded, and the cabdriver watched with wary eyes in the rearview mirror. Gently, precisely, she closed the door behind her.

She wondered if she was going mad.

It felt like a decision she could make. One small step over an invisible line and she could choose lunacy. She could lie down right now in the middle of Sydney and scream and kick and throw her head from side to side like Maddie having a tantrum. Eventually someone would call an ambulance and stick a needle into her and she could sink into a mindless sleep.

The cab pulled away from the curb in a mature, sober fashion so Cat could see just how childishly she'd behaved.

It was like every fight she'd ever had with her sisters. A wave of rage would sweep her up and carry her high and righteous until she did something embarrassingly excessive. Then it would dump her, *splat,* leaving her stupid and small.

Maxine's voice sharp in her head: *If you don't learn how to control that temper of yours, Catriona, you'll pay the price. Not me! You!*

No doubt Dan and the cabdriver were chuckling and shaking their heads over the amusing, probably premenstrual hysteria of women. Dan would make up some excuse about her nonappearance at the party, get drunk, and not even spare her a thought until he was unsteadily aiming his key at the front door.

Or of course, he could find some other woman to sleep with. It would be understandable. Not only did his wife not understand him, she was fucking boring too.

An excited babble of Christmas-drinks noise was coming from a bar directly behind her.

"Got any ID, love?" asked a bouncer who seemed to be having trouble balancing the top half of his body. Any minute he would topple forward from the weight of his muscles.

"Yeah, I need ID like you need more steroids," she told him and walked past him into the bar.

Men. What was the *point* of them?

Expertly, her elbows vicious, she ducked and wove her way through the crowd to the counter and ordered a bottle of champagne.

"How many glasses?" asked the girl. Her roundly innocent eyes made Cat feel like a wizened old crone.

"One," she snapped. "Just one."

With the ice bucket and champagne cradled brazenly under one arm, she walked out of the bar and onto the street. The top-heavy bouncer didn't try to stop her. He was distracted by some more appreciative thirty-plus patrons who were gigglingly presenting their ID.

She walked down George Street toward the Quay.

"Merry Christmas!" A group of drunken office workers in witty Santa Claus hats danced around her.

She kept walking.

Why did everyone have to be so inanely happy?

She continued on past the Opera House and finally into the Botanical Gardens. Hitching her $200 Collette Dinnigan skirt up to her thighs, she settled down cross-legged on the ground, her back up against a tree. She poured herself a glass of champagne and let it slosh all over her hand and onto her skirt. "Cheers."

She toasted the harbor and drank thirstily. Boats strung with colorful lights slipped across the water, throbbing with music and the shouts and cries of overexcited party people.

If she drank this whole bottle she'd have a hangover for tomorrow morning's counseling session. Now that would really add to the whole experience.

Tomorrow they were discussing their childhoods. Their "homework"—Annie's plump fingers formed exaggerated inverted commas in the air—was to think of a memory from their childhood when they had observed their parents dealing with conflict. "We're going to look at the role models in your life!" cried Annie.

Cat was looking forward to submitting the famous story of Kettle Cracker Night 1976. There was no material in Dan's boringly happy childhood that could possibly match it. She would win the battle for most psychological damaging childhood hands down.

Cat, Gemma, and Lyn, six years old, wearing identical blue hooded parkas and brown corduroy pants. Everyone in the street had come to a Cracker Night party in *their* backyard. There was a towering, noisy bonfire and its crimson glow made everyone's faces shadowed and mysterious. The kids were waving sparklers that fizzed and crackled white-hot silver stars. Their father, a cigarette held rakishly in the corner of his mouth, kept making all the men laugh, big booming bursts of raucous laughter. Their mother, in a short green dress with big gold buttons down the middle, was handing around a big platter of prunes wrapped in bacon with little toothpicks. Her hair was still long then, a smooth auburn sheet that stopped in a neat straight line just past her bottom.

At *last,* after endless hours of lobbying the slow-moving parents, it was time for the real fireworks. Beer bottle in hand, their father strolled theatrically to the center of the yard, pulled at his trouser knees, squatted down, and did something mysterious and clever with his cigarette lighter.

"Wait till you see this one, girls!" he said to his daughters. Seconds later—*bang!* The air exploded in color.

"Oooh!" exclaimed everyone at each new firework. "Aaaaah!"

It felt like their dad was creating the fireworks himself. It was wonderful. Cat was pretty sure that it was the best night of her entire life. So it was *typical* that Mum had to try and ruin it.

"Let one of the other men have a turn now, Frank," she kept saying, and Cat hated her mother's hard, whiny tone and the way it was getting sharper and sharper. She was probably just jealous of Dad for having the fun job, while she was stuck handing around cups of tea.

"For God's sake, *hurry,* Frank!"

He stood grinning in the center of the yard, challenging her with his chin, taking a slow, deliberate sip of his beer. "Relax, Max babe."

And then it happened.

Frank lit a Roman candle and was still on his knees, unsteadily peering down at it. "Frank!" their mother warned. This time Gemma caught her mother's fear. "Hurry, Daddy!" she called, and Lyn and Cat gave each other looks that said, *She's such a baby!*

Frank stood up, took a step back, and the Roman Candle exploded. The beer bottle fell to the ground as he held out his hands, palms down, as if he could stop the firework from exploding.

Cat, Gemma, and Lyn watched their father's ring finger get blown cleanly off his hand. It went hurtling through the air illuminated in sharp detail by a flash of brilliant purples and greens.

He collapsed backward into a silly sitting position, like a clown, clutching his hand. There was a strange sweet fragrance in the air, the smell of their father's sizzling flesh.

"You stupid, *stupid* man!" Their mother's voice was a furious wail. She stalked across the yard toward him, her high heels sinking into the grass.

"Girls. Inside, *now!*" And they all had to go inside to the TV room and sit with Pop and Nana Kettle. Sammy Barker got to find their father's finger where it had fallen into the rosebush underneath their parents' bedroom window.

Cat never forgave her mother for that. *She* should have been the one to find her dad's finger, not snotty-nosed Sammy, who gained instant celebrity status at St. Margaret's Primary.

It was only a few months later that their dad packed his things and moved into a flat in the city. They couldn't save his finger. He kept it floating in a jar of formaldehyde. It was brought out from his bathroom cupboard with much ceremony for especially privileged guests.

Now *that* should keep Annie satisfied. And how pleasingly symbolic! It was their father's *ring* finger that got blown off! A symbol of their parents' explosive marriage.

Of course it was one of Dan's favorite family stories too. *"Awesome!"* he said when he heard it for the first time. At dinner parties, he told the story as if he'd been there too.

If Dan had been one of the neighborhood kids, Sammy Barker would have had *no* chance at finding that finger.

Lifting the champagne bottle from the ice bucket, she held it by the neck and refilled her glass. She hiccuped as she settled herself back against the tree.

Maybe she should just forgive him. Maybe she *did* forgive him.

After all, didn't she herself have fantasies about Dan's uni friend, Sean? Every time they went out with Sean and his irrelevant wife, Cat would feel her cheeks start to go pink after her third glass of wine, as shocking images popped unbidden into her mind.

It was alcohol. Alcohol was a terrible, terrible thing, she thought and held up the champagne bottle to look at it accusingly.

Perhaps she could just *choose* to stop being angry, as recommended by Lyn's self-help gurus.

She felt a sense of wonderful well-being at the thought. It was like recovering from the flu, when you suddenly realized that your body was functioning normally again.

Her mobile phone beeped. It was a text message from Dan:

Where R U? Did not go to party. Waiting at home 4 U.
Sorry. Sorry. Sorry. XXX

Carefully, Cat got to her feet, pulled her skirt back down to her knees, and, leaving the empty bottle and ice bucket on the ground, began to walk toward the ferry.

"Well! Here we are again!" Annie had gone for a nautical theme today. She wore a blue-and-white-striped shirt and a little red scarf tied jauntily around her neck. Her eyes were clear and dewy. Cat and Dan regarded her with bleary awe. They'd been up all night, drinking and crying.

"Now, you're a *triplet,* Cat!"

"Yes!" said Cat, failing to match her enthusiasm.

"Now, a lot of triplets have unusually strong relationships with their siblings. Yes?" said Annie.

Oh, Christ. Annie had obviously been foraging through her old textbooks since their last meeting.

"Now, what I'd like to look at today is *Dan's* relationship with your sisters!"

"What about our homework?" asked Cat.

Annie looked confused. She obviously didn't remember the homework.

"Well, yes, but first let's look at this. I think it's important. Dan?"

Dan smiled.

"I get on well with her sisters," he said. "Always have done."

Annie nodded encouragingly.

"Actually," said Dan. "I even dated one of them before Cat."

An invisible fist punched the air from Cat's lungs.

"What are you talking about?"

Dan looked at her. "You knew that!"

"No, I didn't."

"But of course you did!" said Dan nervously.

Cat's heart was hammering. "Which one?" Gemma. It would be Gemma. Dan was looking at her beseechingly, Annie was quivering with professional pride at this breakthrough.

"Which one?" insisted Cat.

"Lyn," he said. "It was Lyn."

CHAPTER 5

"But Surely She knew that!"

"I never told her."

"Why not?"

"It was complicated." Lyn buttered Michael a piece of raisin toast and put it on his plate. "She's not eating anything, you know."

"Isn't she?"

Michael looked at Maddie, who was sitting in her high chair next to him. Maddie dimpled flirtatiously at her father with blissful unconcern for the applesauce dripping from her face. She slammed both hands in the gooey mess in front of her.

"More!" she demanded and leaned forward, opening her mouth wide.

Lyn watched as Michael held the spoon high, made "clack, clack, clack" helicopter sounds, circled it around her head, and zoomed it toward her mouth. At the very last instant Maddie snapped her mouth shut and shook with silent hilarity as Michael tried to wedge the spoon in between her pursed lips.

Maddie might have inherited her father's black curly hair and dimples, but her sense of humor was pure, unadulterated Kettle.

"She hasn't had one mouthful," said Lyn.

"She'll eat if she's hungry." Michael put down the spoon and picked up his coffee mug. "Kara used to do the same thing. She never starved."

Lyn privately suspected that Maddie was much smarter than Kara would have been at the same age. "Oh, she's just average," she told the other mothers at play group, without believing a word of it. She felt sorry for them, Maddie's superiority was so embarrassingly obvious. "Maddie is perfectly capable of not eating when she's hungry. She thinks it's funny."

"Ah, mothers, you're all the same!" said Michael comfortably. "Georgina used to get herself in a state with Kara. It's obviously innate, this desire to see your children eat."

Lyn squeezed the bridge of her nose hard between her thumb and forefinger. She didn't want to be in any category that also included Georgina.

Michael pointed his piece of toast at her and spoke with his mouth full. "Your sisters do exactly the same thing with their noses when they're annoyed. I noticed Cat doing it Friday night. Had a little laugh to myself."

Lyn let go of her nose. "Did you now." She stood up and shoved hard at his shoulder. "Swap places please. I'm going to indulge my strange desire not to see my child starve."

Michael circled one arm around her waist and pulled her down onto his lap. Lyn picked up the spoon and the jar of baby food and sized up her daughter. "Do you want your breakfast?" she asked. Maddie opened her mouth to say "no" and Lyn shoved in a laden spoon. Maddie swallowed, licked her lips, and opened her mouth to bellow at these deceitful tactics. With unerring accuracy, Lyn jammed in another mouthful.

"Your mother has incredible reflexes," said Michael admiringly. Maddie didn't look impressed.

"Better than bloody Georgina, I bet," said Lyn as she wiped Maddie's glowering face with her bib. "Oh *much* better than Georgina!" Michael jiggled her up and down on his lap suggestively. "In *every* respect."

"What's better than Georgina in every respect?" Kara came into the dining room, pulled out a chair so that it screeched horrendously across the floorboards, and sat down at the table in front of them. She picked up a box of cereal and looked at it with disgust. Michael and Lyn froze.

"Kara!" crowed Maddie and clapped her hands, showering her parents with applesauce.

"Lyn, I bet," said Kara. She put on a prissy voice. "Your lovely Lynnie is so much better than Mum, isn't she?"

Michael cleared his throat. "Good morning, sweetheart!" he said hopefully, while Lyn extricated herself from his arms. "I made scrambled eggs," she said to Kara. "Want some?"

Kara made retching noises.

"Don't do that please, Kara," said Michael.

"What? Scrambled eggs make me sick. So what?"

"You're being rude and you know it."

Lyn said mildly, "You liked scrambled eggs yesterday."

Kara ignored her. She was looking mutinously at her father. "Oh. And it's really polite comparing Lyn to my mother in front of me, isn't it? How do you think that makes me feel?"

"Sweetheart, I was not comparing Lyn to your mum. I was just being silly."

"Yeah, what*ever*, Dad. I'm not stupid."

"No, darling, you're not. You're very intelligent. Speaking of which, I've been keeping my eyes peeled for a good laptop for you—"

"Oh! Now you've made me feel sick! I can't *stand* it here!" Kara threw down the box of cereal so that Sultana Bran went flying and stormed out of the room.

Michael raised baffled hands at Lyn.

"Eyes peeled," she explained. "You shouldn't have said you were keeping your eyes peeled."

"My God," Michael shook his head slowly back and forth.

"What do you think of that, Maddie?"

Maddie looked at him in solemn agreement.

"My Dod." She frowned heavily and shook her head vigorously back and forth. "My Dod."

TO DO
WORK
  Sign off New Year promotions.
  XMAS Day staff roster
  Staff bonuses
  Ring back M.
  Accounts!!!
FAMILY
  Book M.'s swimming lesson.
  XMAS gifts still to buy: Mum, C., K.
  Menu for XMAS Day
  Appointment for K. with Dr. Lewis
  Talk to C. re D.
FRIENDS
  Call Yvonne for birthday.
  E-mail Susan.
MISCELLANEOUS
  Query gas bill—why so high?

"Cat. It's me. Please don't hang—"

The phone clicked and beeped ponderously in her ear.

Oh, for God's sake, thought Lyn, as she replaced the phone. Each time Cat hung up on her, it felt like a stinging slap across her face. It was so childish! So unproductive!

She doodled an asterisk next to *Talk to C. re D.*

Fine then, she would move on to another priority. She looked at her list, sighed, checked her watch, and considered her half-full coffee cup. It was still hot. She couldn't even pretend she felt like another one.

Get a grip, she told herself. It wasn't like her to procrastinate like this. Come on, remember the third habit: First things first.

When Lyn was in her final year at university, she had a pro-found, almost religious experience: She read *The Seven Habits of Highly Effective People.*

Every page brought a new epiphany. Yes! she kept thinking, as she highlighted another paragraph in fluorescent yellow and felt herself expanding with potential. It was such a relief to discover that she wasn't at the mercy of her unfortunate Kettle genes or her overly dramatic Kettle childhood. Unlike animals, she learned, human beings could choose how they responded to stimuli. She could change her programming, with a simple paradigm shift. She didn't have to be a Kettle girl! She could be whoever she wanted to be!

Her sisters, of course, refused to be converted. "What crap," sneered Cat. "I hate those sort of books. I can't believe you're falling for it."

"It's weird," said Gemma. "Every time I tried to read about the first habit, I just fell into the deepest sleep."

So Lyn became a highly effective person on her own—and it worked. It worked like a charm.

"Oh, you're so lucky!" people said of her success. Well, she wasn't lucky. She was *effective.* Ever since then, she had begun each day with a strong cup of coffee and a brand-new "to do" list. She had a hardbound notebook especially for the task. At the front was her "principle-centered personal mission statement" and her long-term, medium-term, and short-term goals for each of the key areas of her life: work, family, and friends.

She loved that notebook. It gave her such a soothing sense of satisfaction as she drew a neat, sharp line through each new priority—check, check, check!

Just recently however, she'd noticed the tiniest, quickly sup-pressed blip of panic whenever she began a new list. She found herself thinking unproductive thoughts like, What if it was simply physically impossible to do everything? Sometimes it felt like all the people in her life were scavengers, pecking viciously away at her flesh, wanting more, more, more.

A friend from university had called recently, complaining that Lyn never kept in touch, and Lyn had wanted to scream at her, I have no time, don't you see, I have no time! Instead, she had done a spreadsheet and listed all her friends, categorized by importance (close friend, good friend, casual friend) with columns for dinners, lunches, coffees, "just called to see how you are" phone calls and e-mails.

If her sisters ever discovered the existence of her "friend management system" they would be merciless.

She looked out her office window at the dazzling expanse of turquoise water and thought about herself through the eyes of the *She* journalist. When she'd walked into Lyn's elegant home office with its harbor views, her lip had curled with envy. In some ways, Lyn agreed with her. She did have it all—adoring husband, gorgeous child, stimulating career—and she damn well deserved it. She worked hard, she was good at what she did—she was effective!

But some days, like when Gemma telephoned from the bathtub, water sloshing in the background, Lyn wondered what it would be like to be a little less effective, with nothing more to worry about than when to sleep with a new boyfriend.

And some days, like today, it felt like there was a band of pressure squeezing tightly around her skull. *Talk to C. re D.* Oh God.

No paradigm shift could eliminate a good strong dose of Catholic guilt.

The year Lyn turned twenty-two someone switched her life over to fast-forward and forgot to change it back again. That's how it felt. When people said to her, "Can you believe how fast the year has gone? Christmas again!" she replied too fervently, "I know! I can't believe it!"

Sometimes she'd be doing something perfectly ordinary, sitting at the dinner table passing Kara the pepper and without warning, she'd feel a strange, dizzy sense of disorientation. She'd look at Michael and think, Surely it was only a few months ago that we got married! She'd look at Maddie and think, But you were a tiny baby, only a few days ago! It was as if she were being picked up and put down again in each new stage of her life like a chess piece.

She could pinpoint the moment her life switched over to fast-forward. It was the day she got the phone call in Spain. The phone call about Gemma.

"It's bad news," said Cat, her voice echoing hollowly down the line and Lyn said "What?" even though she heard her perfectly well, just to put it off, just to annoy Cat, because she didn't really believe it was anything bad.

"Bad news!" Cat repeated impatiently. "It's something really, really bad."

Lyn had spent the last ten months working in a London hotel and hating every minute of it. Now she was making up for it with eight long weeks of carefree summer travel around Europe before returning home in time for Gemma's wedding.

Lyn had met an American boy named Hank in Barcelona. They caught the train together down the Costa Brava and stopped at a little town called Llanca. Each day lasted a lifetime. Their balcony looked right out on sparkling sea and hazy mountains capped with snowy white buildings. She and Hank weren't sleeping together yet, but it would take only couple more jugs of sangria. Sometimes as they walked through sunlit cobbled streets he'd grab her and push her up against a wall and they'd kiss until they were both breathless. Lyn felt like she was living in an Audrey Hepburn movie. It was laughably romantic.

"What bad news?" asked Lyn calmly. She looked down at her sandy feet on the white tiles of her hotel room and admired her tanned, pink toenails. No doubt it was the bridesmaids' dresses. Gemma probably wanted them to look like fluffy meringues, or more likely, something strange, like Gothic witches or flower-power hippies.

"Marcus is dead."

Lyn watched her toes curl in surprise.

"What do you mean?" she said.

"I mean he's dead. He got hit by a car on Military Road. He died in the ambulance. Gemma was with him."

It was like being winded. Lyn grabbed at the telephone cord.

"It's O.K. She's fine. Well, she's not fine. Her fiancé is dead. But she's fine. She's not hurt or anything."

Lyn let out her breath. "My God. I can't believe it."

"She says you're not to come home. She doesn't want to ruin your holiday."

"Don't be stupid," said Lyn. "I'm coming now."

There was the tiniest tremor in Cat's voice. "I said you probably would."

Hank came into the room while she was calling the airline and sat by her feet on the tiled floor, dripping from his swim. He took hold of her ankle. "What's the deal?"

"I'm going home."

He was sitting right next to her, touching her, but already he felt like a memory. His wet hair and tanned face seemed frivolous and insubstantial.

And that was when things switched to fast-forward.

She caught a train to Barcelona and managed to get on a flight to Heathrow, where a man at the Qantas counter upgraded her to business class, clucking sympathetically and tap-tapping conspiratorially at his keyboard. He handed her the boarding pass with a beatific smile, as if he knew he was handing her a brand-new destiny.

She had the window seat next to a man in black jeans and T-shirt. As they were putting their seats into an upright position for takeoff, he asked her if she was from Sydney.

"Yes," she said in an exasperated tone, without looking at him. He was irrelevant. Didn't he see that? He was completely irrelevant.

"Ah," he said sadly, and she was suddenly disgusted by her unnecessary rudeness.

"I'm sorry. I'm going home for a funeral. It's been a bit stressful."

"Of course," he said. "I'm sorry. How awful for you." He was a long, lanky man with a mop of black curly hair and serious eyes behind John Lennon glasses.

It was his voice that did it. Maybe if he'd just had an ordinary voice, they would have spent the rest of the flight in silence. But he had "the voice." Ah, the voice, her sisters said with understanding when they heard. Not that they went for it themselves, they just recognized it on Lyn's behalf.

Gemma would say, "The mechanic who serviced my car had that sort of voice you go on about. I gave him your number. He has a girlfriend, but he kept it just in case things didn't work out. He said it's good to have a backup."

She first heard it from her Year Eight Geography teacher. Mr. Gordon was bearded and paunchy, but he spoke about rivers and mountain ranges in a voice with an underlying sweetness. It was perfectly masculine but somehow gentler or softer than the average man's voice. It made her feel safe.

"My sister's fiancé was killed in a car accident," she explained. "They were getting married in six weeks. The invitations were just about to go out."

He made a "tsk" sound. "That's terrible."

Lyn came from a family of poor listeners. If you had something to say, you had to battle constant interruptions, challenges, outright boredom—*get on with it* —and loud triumph over any trip-ups—*Ha! You just said the opposite two seconds ago!*

Michael listened to Lyn with unhurried, flattering interest. It was a brand-new experience for her. It made her eloquent.

It was why she fell in love with him, the pure, almost physical pleasure of their conversation—listening to him and having him listen to her.

Not that she fell in love with him immediately. There wasn't a hint of inappropriate flirtation in their first conversation. He spoke about his wife and little girl and Lyn told him about Hank. But still, it was quite an intimate conversation for two strangers. Perhaps, Lyn always thought afterward, it was the environment— that strange roaring vacuum suspended high above the planet, that peculiarly familiar feeling that you'd always been on this plane and you always would be.

She told him how angry she felt with Marcus for dying so stupidly, so thoughtlessly, so close to the wedding—ruining her sister's life! Why wasn't the fool looking when he crossed the road?

"You must think I'm terrible," she said to Michael, snuggled under her airline blanket, feeling a little drunk on too many liqueurs.

"No," said Michael. "How hard is it to cross a road?"

"Exactly."

She told him how weirdly nervous she felt about seeing Gemma, a strange sense of resistance even as she rushed home to be with her. It felt as if Gemma had moved up to a higher, more complex level of human emotions that Lyn couldn't even hope to understand. She didn't know the rules. She didn't know the right thing to say to make it better. It was like Gemma possessed a secret, terrible knowledge that Lyn could only clumsily guess at.

"I've always known the right thing to say. I'm *good* at making people feel better. But nothing is really going to make her feel better, is it? Not for a long, long time. It's not fair."

"A friend of mine lost his little boy to leukemia," said Michael. "I was so frightened of calling him up, I got a migraine. I almost chickened out."

"But you did it."

"Oh yeah, I did it."

And for a minute they both sat silently, trying out other people's pain, until Michael said, "Mmmm, I think another liqueur might be in order, don't you?"

Eventually, they both fell asleep, waking up rumpled and

sticky-mouthed to the stomach-churning aroma of airplane breakfasts and Australian sunshine streaming through the plane.

They promised each other they'd get together for a drink sometime. He gave her his business card, and she wrote her number on the back of one of his cards.

Lyn looked at the name on the card, as he stood in the aisle reaching easily into the overhead locker for his bags.

"Um," she said, looking up at him from her seat. "Aren't you . . . someone?"

He smiled down at her. She noticed the faintest suggestion of a dimple creasing his left cheek, like an innocent memory from his childhood. "Yup," he said. "No question about that. I am definitely someone."

When Cat saw the card, she told Lyn that he was an up-and-coming computer genius, with stacks of money and an ex-model for a wife.

They met for their drink about a month after the flight. Lyn arrived at the city bar with low expectations. No doubt they would find it impossible to replicate the easy intimacy of their conversation on the flight and there would be lots of awkward pauses and a sense of why did we bother?

Instead, the conversation flowed just as seamlessly. She told him about the funeral and Gemma's strange, white face, how she didn't want to say one word about how she felt about Marcus. Not one word. And this from a girl who normally shared her innermost thoughts as casually and often as most people talked about the weather. Lyn had bought a book on the Stages of Grief to try to understand.

He told her about taking his daughter kayaking on Middle Harbour and how his wife was renovating their house for the third time, which Michael was doing his best to understand too.

She told him about an idea she had for home delivering gourmet breakfasts.

He told her how he was planning to get in on the ground floor with some computer networking phenomenon they were calling the "Internet."

When they stood up to say good-bye, Lyn thought to herself with satisfaction, Well, it just goes to show it *is* possible to have a friendship with an interesting, intelligent (actually rather attractive) man without that distracting sexual element.

Next thing she knew Michael had his arms around her and they were kissing in a way that had a very distracting sexual element.

Lyn had become the Other Woman—an event not listed on her five-year plan.

To: Lyn
From: Nana
Subject: A little suggestion
Dearest Lyn,
I hear that you're having Christmas lunch at your place this year. Well done to you, darling. I wonder if your father and I could come too. He seems to have broken up with that little foreign girl and he is very down at the moment. He's not like himself. I hear you're planning a seafood theme. That sounds lovely. I could bring a nice leg of lamb for you. I'm not sure how your mother would feel about Frank coming, but he assures me they are on good terms these days. What do you think? How is Maddie? Gemma tells me she can sing all the words to the Kentucky Fried Chicken commercial. She is a very intelligent child. She takes after you and your sisters. With much love from Nana

To: Nana
From: Lyn
Subject: Christmas Day
Dear Nana,
Of course you and Dad can come to Christmas lunch. The more the merrier! (I checked with Mum and she agrees that she and

Dad can speak civilly to each other these days. Miracles will never cease!) You will be pleased to learn that Maddie can now sing all the words to the Pizza Hut commercial as well. She's working her way through all the major fast-food groups. Mum is horrified.

Love from Lyn

To: Cat
From: Lyn
Subject: The Dan Issue
Hi Cat,

I wish you would stop hanging up on me. We can't avoid each other for the rest of our lives. I don't know what Dan has told you but here are the facts.

1. After we left the pub that Melbourne Cup Day you said kissing that boy was like kissing an ashtray and if he called you there was no way you would go out with him.

2. I met Dan again by accident two days later at the Greenwood with Susi. (He thought I was you at first.) Dan asked me to go out. I said yes. I THOUGHT YOU WEREN'T INTERESTED—see above.

3. I didn't tell you because we weren't talking at the time. I can't remember why. (Some fight about money on the way home in the cab from the Cup? Gemma's fault probably.)

4. We went out about three times. It was only a couple of weeks before I was leaving for London. It was certainly not a relationship.

5. The first time I realized you two were serious was at Marcus's funeral, which was hardly the right time to say anything.

6. Then I got all distracted with Michael and next thing I knew, you and Dan were engaged and it just seemed so irrelevant and stupid.

It was over ten years ago, Cat. I am really, really sorry that you're upset. But it meant nothing. Can we just forget about it? Can you call me? What do you want for Christmas?

Lyn

To: Lyn
From: Cat
Re: The Dan Issue
I want something very, very expensive for Christmas.
Cat

Lyn looked at her computer screen and smiled. Good. Cat was sounding like herself again. She drew a straight line through *Talk to C. re D.*

Hopefully that was it. In a strange way, it had made her feel as if she was somehow involved in their marriage problems, as if she and Dan had cheated on Cat, which was ridiculous of course.

It was just three dates. Three dates, a long time ago, in another world, another time. All was fair back in the early nineties. Before the AIDS prevention ads started to seem scary, not funny, before the Kettle girls started settling down.

Lyn had a sudden, unexpectedly vivid memory of lying on Dan's bed, in his messy, boy-smelling room. "Do you like it when I do this? Seems like you do, huh? What about this?"

Did she like it just that bit more because she knew deep down Cat had been lying when she said wasn't interested? Who wouldn't be interested? He was gorgeous. No long-term potential, of course, but very sexy.

God, she hadn't thought about that for years. She'd better stop it, or she'd blush next time she saw the cheating bastard.

It was later that night and Lyn stood at the bathroom mirror applying her moisturizer with upward patting motions. She looked straight ahead at her own reflection, trying to avoid the sight of Michael cleaning his teeth. It baffled her how much it annoyed her. He was just so *enthusiastic* about the whole procedure, sawing vigorously away at his gums, toothpaste frothing over his upper lip. For the first time it occurred to her to wonder whether it had irritated Georgina too.

"Do you know we've been together now for as long as you and

Georgina were?" she said, as he bent down, mercifully finished, to rinse his mouth.

"Have we?" Michael dried his mouth with a towel.

"Yes," said Lyn. "So are you going to be unfaithful to me now?" There was a harder note in her voice than she'd wanted.

Michael put down the towel. "No," he said carefully. "No, that wasn't actually my intention."

"Pfffff," said Lyn. "I guess it wasn't your *intention* to be unfaithful to Georgina either."

Michael leaned against the bathroom door. "Is this to do with the whole Cat and Dan thing?" She didn't say anything. "Is it Kara? This morning's teenager from-hell-performance?"

"It's nothing. It was a joke."

"Didn't sound like one."

Lyn put away her moisturizer and Michael's toothpaste. She walked past him into their bedroom. He snapped off the light and followed her.

Without speaking, they pulled back the quilt, climbed into bed, and took their books from their bedside tables. They lay side by side on their backs and held their books in front of them.

After a few seconds, Michael suddenly put his book flat down on his chest.

"Do you remember the first time we went camping together?"

Lyn kept looking at her book. "Yes."

"I remember waking up that first morning and seeing you next to me in your sleeping bag, all curled up, and I felt so . . . so pleased to see you. It was like the feeling you got when you were a kid and you had a friend stay the night. While you were sleeping you'd forget he was there and then you'd wake up and see him sleeping on the mattress on the floor and you'd remember and you'd feel all happy. You'd think, Oh that's right, good old Jimbo's here—we're gonna have fun today!"

Lyn went to speak and he put his hand on her arm to stop her.

"My point is I can't remember ever *once* feeling that way with

Georgina. Even during our supposedly good times. Our very worst times are still ten times better than the very best times I had with Georgina. When you and I first got together, I remember thinking, Bloody hell, why did nobody tell me it could be this good?"

Michael picked up his book again. "So that's why I'm not going to be unfaithful to you."

Lyn blinked and watched the words on her page dance and dissolve.

"Because you remind me of my mate Jimbo."

She closed her book and used it to whack him on the stomach.

CHAPTER 6

"Lord God, Lamb of God, you take away the sins of the world, have mercy on us. You are seated at the right hand of the Father, receive our prayer. For you alone are the holy one, you alone are the Lord—"

"Remind me to tell you about water aerobics!"

"What?" Gemma bent her knees and dropped her head down to her grandmother's height.

"Water aerobics!" hissed Nana Kettle into her ear. "I don't want to forget!"

"O.K." Gemma stifled a giggle and Nana gave her a naughty look.

When the Kettle girls were little, their grandmother used to take them to Sunday morning Mass and sit with a ramrod-straight back, monitoring their every move with flinty eyes. The stealthiest pinch of a sister's thigh didn't escape her. Now, Gemma took Nana to church every few weeks. Her grandmother still dressed as piously as ever—buttoned-up cardigan and skirt—but her standards of behavior seemed to have slipped. One Sunday the two of them got the giggles so bad, Gemma worried that Nana would choke to death right there in the pew.

"I don't know how you stand it," said Cat. "Why do you go? It's not like you believe in *God* anymore, do you?"

"I don't know," said Gemma, which infuriated Cat.

"Do you have an opinion on anything?"

"Not really."

It was true, in a way. Opinions were for other people. It was fascinating how upset they got about them.

"Please be seated."

The congregation shuffled, coughed, and sighed as they settled themselves down for the sermon. Nana dropped her chin on to her chest for a nap.

Gemma watched the people in front of her. She loved secretly spying on people, observing their little dramas. There was a couple today with a tiny baby. At the beginning of Mass, their baby had cried and they both became cross and irritated, mouthing panicky instructions at each other. Now, the baby was sleeping, and Gemma watched the man's hand reach across and pat the woman's knee. The woman slid slightly on her seat so that her shoulder pressed forgivingly against his. Ah. Lovely.

The man had very thick brown hair. Marcus had had hair like that. Actually the back of his head was remarkably similar to Marcus's.

Don't, Gemma told herself sternly. He doesn't look at all like Marcus. Think about Charlie's head! Charlie's adorable, balding head!

But it was too late. Marcus had elbowed Charlie right out of his way.

"What the fuck are you doing?" was the last thing Marcus said before he dropped Gemma's hand, stepped off the curb, and died instantly.

It was an unfortunate choice of last words. After all, he had said much nicer things to her in his lifetime. He'd said lovely things. Romantic things. Passionate things.

It was just that now, before Gemma could remember a single *"I love you,"* she first had to remember, *"What the fuck are you doing?"*

What the fuck she was doing was leaning over to pick up the wedding invitation that had mysteriously slithered out of the satisfying square bundle held firmly in her hand.

"Oh!" she said. Had she been shedding invitations the whole way from the car?

Marcus let go of her hand. Gemma reached down for the envelope. There was a shrieking squeal of brakes, like an animal's frightened scream.

She looked up and saw Marcus flying. He was a big man, Marcus, and he was flying like a rag doll in the air, his limbs flailing loosely in a horribly undignified manner.

He didn't fall like a rag doll. He collided violently with the road, slamming lumpily against the concrete.

Then he was still.

"Oh, Jesus." Gemma heard a man's voice.

Run. She knew she was meant to run to him.

Car doors were opening. People were pounding across the pavement, calling urgent, important instructions to one another.

Within seconds Marcus was surrounded by a group of people and still Gemma stood, with their wedding invitations in her hand.

This was something quite big. This was something for grown-ups to fix. This was something for strong, fatherly men and efficient, motherly women. Capable people.

Carefully, she put the pile of envelopes down in the gutter and stood with her hands hanging limp and heavy by her side, waiting for somebody to tell her to what to do.

Then her body started moving on its own, running across the road, and her hands were pushing rudely at people's backs and shoulders to make them get out of the way. She could hear herself screaming "Marcus!" and his name sounded strange to her, as if she were making it up.

Two weeks after the funeral, she went back to work. It felt like she'd been away visiting a different planet. She was teaching second grade at the time and when she walked back into her classroom, she was greeted by an eerie sight—twenty-four seven-year-olds sitting upright in their seats, hands flat on their desks, big eyes watching her every move.

Even the naughty ones were quiet. Not a peep from Dean the Attention-Deficit Demon. Then one by one they began to walk up to her desk, to silently hand her gifts. Mars Bars. Bags of chips. Hand-drawn cards.

"It made me very sad that you were sad, Miss Kettle," said Nathan Chipman, a trifle accusingly, as he handed her a soggy Banana Paddle Pop. He leaned over and whispered confidentially in her ear, his breath warm against her neck. "I even cried a little bit."

Gemma put her head down on the desk and felt her whole body torn by wrenching sobs, as feet pattered across the room and dozens of little hands patted her consolingly on the back and stroked her hair.

"Don't cry, Miss Kettle. Don't cry."

There's something wrong with me, she thought. There's something very badly wrong with me. She was twenty-two and she felt all used up, a dried-out old husk, a dirty old rag.

After school that day, she obeyed a sudden weird impulse and went to confession, fascinated by her own behavior. It had been so long, and she and her sisters had shrugged off their Catholic educations so effectively, it felt like she was taking part in a bizarre, cultish ritual.

But as soon as she knelt down in the dusty-smelling, terrifying little cupboard and the window slid across revealing the priest's shadowy profile, she automatically crossed herself and chanted in that secret, trembly whisper of years ago, "Bless me, Father, for I have sinned, it has been six years since my last confession. Here are my sins."

And then she stopped and thought, Dear Jesus, what the hell am I doing here?

"Um. Here are my sins. Yes."

Oh my. Now she was going to laugh.

"Take your time, my dear," encouraged the priest, and she didn't want to let him down because he sounded so nice and normal and she did want absolution and she thought about Marcus's father at the funeral, sobbing so hard he could hardly stand, and there was an undigested lump of guilt lodged in her throat making it difficult to breathe.

"I'm sorry," she said. "I'm very sorry for taking up your time."

She got up from her knees and walked straight from the confessional, and out of the church and into the sunshine.

After a year or two she stopped feeling guilty.

Sometimes she wondered if she stopped feeling anything at all.

After Mass, as per their routine, Gemma took Nana home for a cup of tea and a manicure.

The Kettle girls had inherited responsibility for Nana's nails from their grandfather. Every Sunday night, for forty-three years, right up until the week before he died, he had given his wife a beautiful manicure, lining up nail polish, nail file, and polish remover on the dining room table with the same professional precision as the tools in his shed. "Oh don't worry, love, that looks perfect," Nana would say impatiently as he held up her little finger to the light and frowned critically. "If a job's worth doing," Pop would mutter.

Gemma doubted that Pop would have approved of Gemma's work. Although she hunched with concentration over each finger, swearing under her breath and twisting around in her seat, the polish still formed peculiar ridges and lumps.

It didn't seem to matter. Nana really just wanted an excuse to sit and chat. Today, she was telling the story of Pop's promotion to supervisor and how he wore a tie to work for the first time.

"So off he went, proud as punch with his lovely striped tie!" Gemma put the nail brush back in the bottle and shook it with hopeful vigor while she listened.

"And when he came home that night I could see he was a little down but he didn't say a word. The next morning, I said to him, Les, aren't you wearing a tie today? And he said, Oh, Bob had a word with me. Said the men were having a bit of a joke about it and it wasn't really necessary to dress so formal, seeing as he wasn't one of the big managers. Oh, he was so hurt, Gemma, that they would laugh like that. He never wore a tie again."

Gemma sniffed loudly. That particular story always made her ache with sadness. She thought about how Pop must have got that horrible feeling of embarrassment, that shoved-in-the-stomach feeling when Bob called him over to have his "word."

"I hate Bob," she said.

"Yes, well, he was a funny fellow. Long dead now of course. Prostate cancer."

"Serves him right," Gemma said with satisfaction, blowing on her grandmother's fingers to dry them. "I hope it was painful."

"You've got your pop's lovely sweet nature," said Nana, seemingly oblivious to all indications to the contrary.

Gemma snorted and used her thumbnail to try and scratch paint away from her grandmother's cuticles. "I do not. None of us take after Pop. We're all bad-tempered, like Mum, and competitive, like Dad. Actually, now I think about it, we're quite awful."

"Oh, don't talk such silly talk! You do all drive too fast, I must say. You get that from your father."

Gemma chortled. "*Lyn* has got the most tickets at the moment."

"That's because she's always rushing around. Mathew should help her more."

"Michael, Nana."

"Yes, Michael. That's what I'm saying, darling. He doesn't help enough with those breakfast trucks. She seems to have to do it all herself."

"Well, of course she does. That's because it's *her* business."

"Don't be silly, darling," said Nana vaguely. "Now tell me about this new young man. He's a locksmith, is he? Your grandfather would have liked that, he would have been so interested!"

Gemma bundled up the bottles and cotton buds from the table and walked toward the bathroom. "He's lovely," she began.

"Your grandfather never liked Marcus, you know," said her grandmother suddenly. "He said, I don't like that bloke!" Gemma stopped at the doorway. She couldn't believe it. "Nana?"

"Mmmm?" Nana was admiring her nails, holding them up to the light.

"Didn't Pop like Marcus?"

Her grandmother put her hands back on the table in front of her and began to push herself up to a standing position. "I do hope Maddie doesn't grow up looking too *Italian,*" she said, with one of her baffling leaps to a new topic of conversation.

"Nana! For one thing Michael is Greek, not Italian, and what if Maddie *did* grow up looking Italian? What have you got against Italians? Charlie is Italian!"

"Charlie," said Nana thoughtfully. "Your mother had a boyfriend called Charlie. Frank used to make terrible fun of his teeth. I don't think he was Italian, though."

Gemma groaned with frustration and went into the bathroom. She opened the mirrored cabinet to see shimmering clean shelves instead of the normal overflowing jumble of ancient bottles and jars.

"I see Lyn's been here!" she called out.

Pop never had a bad word to say about anybody. It couldn't be true.

She walked back into the dining room. "Pop liked Marcus didn't he, Nana?"

Her grandmother beamed. "Oh *yes*! Your grandfather had a lot of time for Mathew. They used to talk about computers."

Gemma sighed. Perhaps Mum was right. It was best to take Nana Kettle in small doses.

The Ferry

When I was nine, my parents took me on holiday to Australia. I loved it! I can even remember the exact moment when I decided, yep, this is where I'm going to live one day.

We were on the Manly Ferry after a day at the beach. It had been one of those long, hot, typical Aussie summer days, the sky at sunset looked like pink cotton wool and the cicadas were screeching. We were sitting on the wharf side of the ferry and the guy had already hauled in the little walkway, when my mother said, "Look at these people, they'll never make it!" It was a man and three little girls about my age, and they were running like mad, yelling out, "Wait for us!" One of the girls was ahead of the others. She was running so fast, arms pumping, looking back over her shoulder at the others. I saw the man swoop the other two girls up by their waists, one under each arm, like sacks. The girls were giggling their heads off, legs dangling, and the man's face was bright red with effort.

I think the ferry guy would have ignored them, but passengers started calling out, Wait, wait! So he rolled his eyes and put the walkway back out again and they all came clattering on, laughing and panting. Some of the passengers even cheered them. It looked like they'd just come straight out of the ocean. The little girls all had dripping wet ponytails sticking out of the back of baseball caps and bare feet caked in sand. The father had their beach towels over one shoulder and he said, "Thanks, mate!" and slapped the guy on the shoulder.

They walked right by us and I could hear them saying, "That was so funny, Dad!" "Let's have an ice cream now, Daddy!" I realized they must have been sisters. Well, being only an only child living in sad, sodden old Manchester, it seemed to me that they led dream lives.

I thought, I bet you girls have no idea how lucky you are.

That's when I decided I was going to come and live here when I grew up. It felt like the first grown-up decision I'd ever made. I remember looking at my parents and feeling sorry for them, because they'd miss me when I moved all the way to Australia.

They do too.

CHAPTER 7

Gemma skidded wildly through the crowded shopping center, dodging and weaving past Christmas shoppers. "The problem with families is they typecast you," Charlie had said the night before with the tips of his fingers light against the back of her neck. "I'm the voice of sanity. Sometimes I wouldn't mind a turn as the voice of insanity."

"Yes!" Gemma agreed too violently because his fingers were making her shiver and she still had one date to go before she succumbed. "You're exactly right!"

Today, just for fun, she was going to break free of at least one stereotype. For once she was going to be right on time to meet her sisters. It had been a Herculean effort, but it looked like she was going to make it. (How did they manage their relentless punctuality? You had to plan everything so far in advance! It was exhausting!)

She pounded to the top of the packed escalator, apologizing as bag-laden shoppers moved aside for her. As she reached the top, her unzipped handbag flew upward and its entire contents went cascading in a noisy clatter down the escalator. Gemma watched in horror as the crowd bent as one to scrabble for her things. As they stepped off the escalator she accepted each new item they handed her. Handfuls of loose change. Purse. Mobile phone. Lipstick. Scrunched-up tissues.

"Thank you," she said. "Oh, thank you. Thank you so much."

A little old lady carefully pressed a tampon into her hand. "Thank you, I appreciate it."

Sweet Jesus, please don't let there be a condom.

Finally, her entire, thankfully condom-less, bag was restored to her, and she ran breathlessly to the designated coffee shop, now five minutes late. Neither Cat nor Lyn was there. She was first! Triumphantly she sat down at a table and ordered a pineapple juice.

They were shopping for a combined Christmas present for their mother. It was their annual challenge to find something she might actually keep. Maxine consistently returned every gift she received. "Yes. Well. That's lovely, girls," she would say as she unwrapped their agonizingly selected gift and doubtfully turned it back and forth. "Perhaps you could give me the receipt, just in case."

Sipping her juice, Gemma contemplated the woman at the next table, snapping irritably at a little boy of about Maddie's age. Gemma wrinkled her nose at him over the edge of her glass to try and make him feel better. He stared back at her, seemingly stunned. Idiot child. Wait till Maddie and Lyn arrive, she thought, they'll show you two.

Gemma was in awe of Lyn's mothering ability. The day they took Maddie home from the hospital for the first time, she couldn't believe that Lyn was allowed to actually keep this real, live baby. Her own sister, walking out of the hospital, holding that fragile little bundle, chatting away to Michael, even occasionally taking her eyes *off* the baby! Gemma kept expecting some official to tap them on the shoulder and say, Now wait just a minute there, where do you think you're going with that!

If Gemma had a baby she'd be terrified she'd accidentally drop it or feed it something poisonous. What if she simply forgot she even *had* a baby and then remembered days later?

She had a sudden image of herself running up the escalator

and a baby flying from her clumsy hands, hurtling through the air, shoppers looking up with mouths agape, the tampon lady tossing aside her walking stick to hold out both hands to catch it.

She snorted through her straw.

She remembered the first time she and Cat baby-sat Maddie for Lyn. Cat was lying on her stomach on the floor reading a magazine, while Gemma sat on Lyn and Michael's bed cradling the warm, sweet-smelling swaddle against her shoulder. It suddenly occurred to her that the baby had gone extremely still.

She carefully turned Maddie over.

"Oh my God," she said. "I've killed the baby."

Cat didn't look up from her magazine. "Well, Lyn's going to be really mad at you."

"Cat! I'm not joking!"

Cat threw aside the magazine and bounced to her feet. Together they stared at Maddie's flushed, creased face. Cat poked her gently in the stomach. The baby didn't move. Gemma pressed her hand to her mouth. "What have I done?"

Cat poked again, harder—and Maddie's face crumpled as she erupted into a scream of rage. Cat picked her up and began to jiggle her. "Yes, I know, darling, we won't let that murderous Auntie Gemma hold you anymore."

It had been the most terrifying moment of Gemma's life.

"Gem! Gem! Oh! Gem!"

Gemma looked up to see Maddie running through the coffee shop to her, followed by Lyn pushing an empty stroller. Maddie was wearing blue denim overalls and a gaudy pink and silver tiara in her hair. Gemma had bought her the *Little Princess* tiara, secretly coveting it for herself.

"Over there! Gem!" called Maddie to the little boy at the next table as she went running by, pointing her out, as if to say, Are you mad? How could you have missed seeing this extraordinary person sitting right next to you!

Gemma swooped her onto her lap, and Maddie placed both

her tiny starfish hands firmly on Gemma's cheeks and immediately launched into an incomprensible story.

Lyn remained standing, clutching the stroller handles. "What's the matter?" she demanded.

"What do you mean?" asked Gemma, turning her head and letting Maddie turn it back again.

"Why are you so early? What's wrong?"

"Nothing's wrong! Why are you so late?"

"I'm not," Lyn maneuvered the stroller out of the way and sat down. "I'm right on the dot. We always tell you a time half an hour earlier than the actual time."

"Your Auntie Gemma is typecast," Gemma told Maddie. "Just like Meg Ryan. That's why nobody believed she was a brain surgeon in that movie."

"City of Angels," said Lyn. "Shocking movie. Michael and I walked out of it."

"Nobody would believe I was a brain surgeon either."

"Probably not. You'd keep dropping your instruments."

"I think I would make an excellent surgeon. I'd be very calm and cool."

"You've got something on your cheek. Mascara, maybe." Lyn licked her finger and reached over for Gemma's cheek.

Gemma recoiled. "I'll do it myself!"

"It's only saliva. When you become a brain surgeon, you'll have to touch mushy, bloody brains."

"Dirty," said Maddie sympathetically. She put her own finger into her mouth and began to rub away at Gemma's cheek.

"Where's the waitress?" Lyn swung around in her chair and tapped her fingers on the tabletop. "I need caffeine to help me cope with Cat. This is the first time I've seen her since the Dan thing."

"Oh yes! I knew there was something I was looking forward to! The biggest family scoop of all time."

"Stop it, please. It was a long time ago. I can hardly remember it."

"Oh, come on. Explain yourself. I don't get it. Why didn't you just tell her at the time?"

Lyn pushed her hair back behind her ears and leaned forward with her elbows on the table.

"Why didn't *he* just tell her is more to the point! I was on the other side of the world. By the time I got back they'd already been seeing each other for months. Obviously I should have said it right away. But she was so happy and they were all over each other, remember? It seemed cruel to say, Oh by the way, I dated him too. And besides—"

"Yes?" said Gemma benevolently. She was feeling especially affectionate toward Lyn today, she looked so uncharacteristically uncertain.

"I never thought it would last. I didn't think Dan was the commitment type. Every week I expected it to end. Next thing you know, you and I are both walking down the aisle in purple taffeta."

"And why didn't you tell me?"

"You?" Lyn looked at her with disbelief. "You can't keep a secret."

Gemma's affection levels plummeted. "That is *so* not true!"

"That is so not true," repeated Lyn thoughtfully. "You talk like a fifteen-year-old. Kara says that. That is *so* not true, Lyn, I do pick up my own washing."

Gemma gritted her teeth and went back on the attack. "So, did you sleep with Cat's husband too?"

"Gemma! He wasn't Cat's husband at the time."

"Did you?"

"What if I did?'

"Nothing if you did. I'm just wondering. Did you?"

"I lost my virginity to him."

"You *didn't*!" Gemma allowed Maddie to slither from her lap. "Your first time was with Hank in Spain!"

"Well, it wasn't."

"But it was!"

"I guess I might be just a little more qualified to speak on the subject."

"I can't believe it."

Gemma and Lyn watched Maddie trot over to the little boy at the next table and put her face right up close to his so their noses were practically touching.

"So." Gemma didn't look at Lyn. "Dan, hey? Any good?"

Lyn didn't look at her. "Yes. Very."

Gemma's mouth dropped. For some reason this seemed incredibly shocking. Lyn looked at her sidelong with a glint of pride, and the two of them began to rock with wicked laughter.

"Stop it," said Lyn helplessly. "It's not funny."

Gemma grabbed a napkin to wipe her eyes. "No, it's terrible. You're terrible. I didn't know you were so terrible."

"Cat! My Cat!"

Pushing the little boy unceremoniously to one side, Maddie went running through the coffee shop toward Cat. Gemma smoothed both her hands down her cheeks as if to wipe away the laughter, and Lyn sat up very straight.

"One word and you're a dead woman," she said as she held up her hand to wave at Cat.

"Get a grip."

Cat walked toward them with Maddie clinging to her hip. The woman with the little boy had stood up and was gathering together her shopping bags. When she saw Cat, she did a little start and straightened.

"Hello!" she said. "You're Lyn Kettle, aren't you? The Brekkie Bus business! What a coincidence, I was only just reading about you in *She* this morning."

Cat shifted Maddie to the other hip.

"I'm her sister. The unsuccessful version. But Lyn's right there." She pointed at Lyn and the woman did a double-take as Lyn gave her an embarrassed little wave.

"That's right! You're triplets! Oh, you can *really* tell!"

The woman was swinging her head back and forth observing the three of them with satisfaction.

"And you're just the same as the other two, except your hair is red!" she said to Gemma.

"That's right!" Gemma praised her.

"Good Lord, we'd never noticed!" Cat said.

The woman's smile became a little fixed. "Well, it was a pleasure to meet you all!" She held out a hand to Lyn. "I really admire what you've achieved."

"Thank you." Lyn shook her hand graciously.

"Bye now," said Cat, and she buried her face in Maddie's stomach and growled, so that she gurgled with delight.

"What are you doing here?" Cat asked Gemma as she pulled out a chair and sat down with Maddie on her lap.

"She's refusing to be typecast," said Lyn. "Do you both want a coffee? I'm going to order one at the counter."

"How are you?" asked Gemma, as Lyn went for their coffees. The dark shadows under Cat's eyes reproached them for their laughter.

"Fine," answered Cat. "Never better. I stopped by at Nana Kettle's on the way here. She says you're going to do water aerobics with her. You're a glutton for punishment."

"I think it will be fun. Want to come?"

"Yeah, right. You made a shocking mess of her nails last week."

"Thanks," said Gemma. A sudden thought occurred to her.

"You know something weird Nana said?"

"Everything she says is weird."

"She said Pop didn't like Marcus."

An expression of nervous caution immediately crossed Cat's face. Cat and Lyn both became peculiarly polite whenever Marcus's name came up.

"Did *you* like Marcus?" asked Gemma. "You can say if you didn't. He's dead, you know."

"I know he's dead. Of course I liked him."

"Did you think we had a good relationship?"

Cat shifted around in her seat, looking for Lyn. "Um. I really don't know. I mean, yes. You did. You were getting married."

Maddie banged her hands on the table and Cat handed her the salt and pepper shakers. Pleasantly surprised, Maddie immediately turned them both upside down.

"I do remember something," said Cat suddenly. "I remember when you came back from skiing in Canada. The holiday you got engaged. Marcus said something about you being *timid* on the slopes. I said, What the hell are you talking about, timid? I've seen Gemma ski double black diamonds at a million miles an hour. You looked really strange, I thought maybe you'd had a big fight."

Gemma opened her mouth and waited for something to come out.

Cat looked at her crossly. "See! Now I've upset you."

"I'm sorry."

Abruptly Cat changed the subject.

"So did *you* know about Dan and Lyn at the time?"

"No," Gemma said definitely.

"Well, thank God they never had sex. That would have been too revolting."

There was no time for Gemma to prepare her face. Cat looked at her. "But Dan said—"

Lyn came back to the table with two coffees. She removed the salt and pepper shakers from Maddie and firmly placed her in the stroller, distracting her with a spoonful of cappuccino froth.

"What?" she said, as she sat down and saw Cat's face. "What now?"

Immediately, she looked with furious accusation at Gemma.

"What did you say?"

Gemma woke to the smell and sound of the sea. Through the open doorway of the bedroom she could see straight down a short, beige carpeted hallway to a small balcony with a table and two chairs. The screen door was wide open, and without lifting her head from the pillow she could see a sliver of ocean sparkling in the morning sun.

She kept still, enjoying the sensation of Charlie's back warm against hers. She wondered if he was pretending to be asleep.

Every move was so significant, every word loaded, the morning after you had sex for the first time.

She could see her underwear strewn down the beige hallway in pleasingly provocative satin crumples. "Look! Matching underwear!" she'd slurred proudly through a red-wine induced haze the night before. "Well done!" Charlie had said, although he didn't waste much time looking at it.

There was movement next to her, a hand reaching for her hip

"Good morning."

"Good morning."

She wondered how his postsex personality was about to manifest itself. You never could tell. She hated it when they woke up wary, with that now-don't-you-be-thinking-this-is-a-relationship look in their eyes. If she saw even the slightest hint of that sort of look, she'd dump him on the spot.

"That was very lovely," she said, watching 8:31 snap over to 8:32 on his bedside digital clock. "Last night, I mean."

Most men, Gemma knew, were convinced they were extraordinarily talented lovers and simultaneously terrified that maybe they weren't. It was important to pay them lavish compliments about their abilities. It put them in a good mood.

Actually, now she thought about it, it *had* been very lovely. Quite surprisingly lovely.

"That second time," she continued thoughtfully. "I had a rather startling orgasm."

There was a dry chuckle from next to her, and suddenly she found herself flipped over and enveloped in a gigantic bear hug, her face pressed against Charlie's wide chest. He had a body like a footballer, except for his legs, which were heartbreakingly skinny. She breathed in the faint leftover scent of his aftershave.

"A *startling* orgasm, did you? Why, did you feel it in your left ear?"

"No. It was just startlingly delicious."

"And why the surprise? I'm a locksmith. I have trained hands. Trained to unlock delicious orgasms. You should have been lying there thinking, Yep, just as I thought."

Thank God! Postsex Charlie was still presex Charlie.

"I like to keep my expectations low to avoid disappointment."

He reached over for the blind by his side of the bed and pulled hard at the cord so that sunlight instantly flooded the room. Gemma put her hands over her eyes. "Bright light! Bright light!"

"Perfect weather," he said, uncovering her eyes. "Now. Gemma Kettle. Sweet Gemma Kettle. Here's my proposal for the day. First, I think I'd better give you another startling orgasm. Then I think I should make you breakfast while you're in the shower. Then you'll be so turned on by my cooking skills—especially in light of your own shameful efforts last week—you'll probably want to seduce me back into the bedroom. Then I think we should go down to the beach and have a boogie board. I've got a spare one. Can you boogie board? Then back here for a siesta and more startling sex. Then maybe a movie?"

Gemma stared at him. "Goodness."

"Not enough sex?"

"No. That seems like quite a substantial amount."

Charlie's face changed. "Or you might have plans, of course. You probably have plans. My little sister tells me I'm too domineering. So you know, that's fine, off you go to your plans, I don't mind."

He smiled at her, lines deepening on either side of his brown eyes with their ridiculous eyelashes. "I've got plans myself actually. Now I think about it."

It seemed like everything he was feeling was right there in his eyes—a hint of nerves, a touch of laughter.

No secrets. She hated secrets.

"Sisters," she said, pulling him to her. "Who cares what *they* think."

They followed Charlie's proposal to the letter.

To: Cat; Gemma
From: Lyn
Subject: XMAS

1. I bought Mum a David Jones voucher for Christmas. You both owe me $50.

2. Please do not get Maddie anything edible. She'll be sick.

3. Could you both bring salads and wine on Christmas Day? Can you confirm what sort of salads?

4. Gemma—are you really bringing your new boyfriend? Can you confirm?

To: Gemma; Lyn
From: Cat
Subject: XMAS

I confirm that I'm not coming Christmas Day.

To: Lyn
From: Gemma
Subject: XMAS

OH MY GOD! Does she mean it?

P.S. I confirm I will bring a VERY SPECIAL, VERY EXOTIC SALAD. I confirm that Charlie will just drop by quickly so you can all admire and gasp at his eyelashes but then he has to go to his own family lunch.

To: Gemma
From: Lyn
Subject: XMAS

If she means it, it's your fault. You fix it.

To: Lyn; Cat
From: Gemma
Subject: XMAS
Excuse me but YOU did it. You're the one having multiple orgasms with her husband.

To: Lyn; Gemma
From: Cat
Subject: XMAS
IS THIS LIKE SOME SORT OF SICK JOKE???
"Multiple orgasms with my husband"?
GEMMA: YOU'RE STUPID. LYN: YOU'RE A BITCH.

To: Gemma
From: Lyn
Subject: XMAS
YOU FIX IT.

"Nope. Won't do," Charlie announced as they sat down opposite each other in a café. "You're too far away."

He moved his chair from the opposite side of the table, so he was close enough to entwine his legs around Gemma's.

He could make her melt like warm caramel.

Three weeks since she met him. Six dates. Two nights at his place. Two nights at hers. A lot of kissing. A lot of fine-quality sex. A lot of stupid jokes.

She knew it was always good at the start of a relationship, but was it always *this* good?

Yes, probably.

"No sticky date pudding," she said sadly, looking at the menu. "It's gone out of fashion."

"We should make our own," Charlie said. "Let's make a sticky date pudding together tomorrow night. Not that you'll be any help. But you can stand around and look pretty and pass me things."

"First I have to see my sister. I have to fix things."

"I'm sure it's not your fault."

"Well. It is a little bit."

"Do you fight a lot? Do triplets fight more than normal?"

"The Kettle triplets do. But I don't think we're normal. Mum used to take us to a club for triplets when we were little and some of them adored one another. We were so disgusted, we threw rocks at them."

"Little savages." Charlie stroked her wrist with his thumb.

"We got expelled from the Triplet Club for a whole month. Do you fight with your sisters? When I was little I used to have fantasies about having a big brother."

"My sisters would have paid you to take me. I used to beat them up. I specialized in vicious Chinese burns."

"No!"

"Yep. Then I went through my juvenile-delinquent stage and ignored them."

Gemma was rather aroused at the thought of Charlie as a juvenile delinquent. She imagined him in a black leather jacket, striding in slow motion down a dimly lit street.

"Then once I got bored with delinquency, I suddenly became friends with them. It was nice. Like getting bonus friends overnight. Now we give each other relationship advice."

"Really. What do they tell you?"

"Oh stupid things, of course. I don't listen to them. But I give them very wise advice."

"Like what?"

"Well, the other day one sister happily announced she's seeing a married man, for Christ's sake. So my advice was to stop it."

"Oh, very wise. It might be a bit more complicated than that."

"It's not." Charlie was looking around for the waitress. "Why are these women all avoiding eye contact with me do you think?"

"My sister fell in love with a married man. It was their destiny to be together. His ex-wife was a witch."

"Mmm," began Charlie disapprovingly, when a waitress finally appeared, fumbling in her apron for a pen.

"Before we order you have to tell us what happened to your sticky date pudding. My girlfriend is still recovering from the shock."

The sweet, teenage pleasure of hearing herself described as Charlie's girlfriend made her forget all about defending Lyn's destiny.

It was 3 A.M. that same night and Gemma burst gasping into consciousness, as if she'd been drowning in a deep, dark pool of sleep.

She'd forgotten something. Something very important.

What could it be?

Then it hit her and she screamed, "Charlie!"

He woke with a gasp and leapt straight out of bed, bouncing on his toes like a boxer, jabbing wildly at the air around him. "What? Where? Stay back!"

Gemma rolled out of bed, her legs trembly with fear. "We forgot! Charlie, how could we!"

She ran to the chest of drawers and began scrabbling wildly through her clothes, throwing them on to the floor. "We forgot we had a baby! We left it in the drawer!"

It would be too late. The baby would be dead. Babies needed *food,* or milk, or something! She imagined a tiny, shriveled-up corpse with accusing eyes. How terrible. How could they have forgotten? They were murderers.

Charlie was behind her, enfolding her in his arms. "We don't have a baby, you fruitcake," he said. "Come back to bed. It's just a dream."

"No, no." She opened a new drawer. "We have to find our baby."

But even as she was saying the words she was starting to doubt herself. Maybe there was no baby?

She turned to face Charlie. "We don't have a baby?"

"No, we don't have a baby. It's a dream. Jesus. You frightened the hell out of me."

"Sorry." Now she felt a bit stupid. "Did I tell you that I sometimes have nightmares?"

"No, you didn't." He put his arm around her shoulders and guided her back toward the bed. "Just as a matter of interest, how often do you have them?"

CHAPTER 8

"This is going to sound bad," said Dan, with the courageous expression of a bloody-lipped boxer stumbling back to his feet for another round. "But I sort of—forgot."

"You forgot you slept with my sister."

"I forgot."

"You *forgot.*"

"Yes."

"How is that possible?" Cat felt insulted on Lyn's behalf. "She lost her virginity to you!"

"I hadn't even thought about it for years," confessed Dan, "until Annie asked. All I remembered was going out with her a few times. But if Lyn says we did, then we did. I wouldn't argue with Lyn. She probably records every shag on a spreadsheet."

Cat refused to smile.

"I was young, I got around. It feels like another world."

"You still get around."

He flinched and took it like a man.

Cat believed him. He could remember rugby league grand final scores from fifteen years ago and quote whole slabs of *Simpsons* dialogue, but his memory of personal events was notoriously shocking. It hadn't mattered before. If this revelation had come before Angela (*long black hair tumbling, black bra strap sliding, stop it, stop it, stop it*) maybe she would have laughed. Yes, she probably would have laughed. She would have exaggerated her shock, milked it, but not really cared, because she took Dan's faithfulness for granted. Everything else in her life could and probably would go wrong, but she thought she and Dan were a given.

Naive. Pathetic.

"I would never have gone out with you if I'd known. Do you know that? Lyn's leftovers. You would have had no chance."

"Just as well I didn't tell you then."

"Is it?"

She could have had a different life.

Once, when she was waiting for a leg wax, Cat read a magazine article about a study of identical twins separated at birth. When they were reunited years later, they discovered amazing similarities in their lives. In spite of very different upbringings, they had ended up with the same jobs, hobbies, habits, pets, cars, and clothes, even the same names for their children! This proved, according to the author, that personality, just like the color of your hair, was decided at conception. Your destiny was indelibly carved in your genes.

Bullshit, thought Cat, flipping the page irritably and wondering how much longer the bloody beautician would keep her waiting. Look at Lyn and me! Look at those whatsits name twins from school. But the author was ready for her. The reason that identical twins brought up together were different, he retorted, was because they *deliberately* set out to be different from each other.

"Hmmmph," muttered Cat. It seemed to her that there was a fundamental contradiction in his argument. If environment didn't matter for the separated twins, why did it matter so much for the poor twins forced to live side by side with their doppelgangers?

But while the beautician ripped hair from her calves and tried to sell her moisturizer, Cat buried her nose in a lavender-smelling towel and wondered whether it was she or Lyn who was leading the "right" life, the one they were predestined to lead. Nana's next-door neighbor once said to her, Are you the one that's done so well for herself? Bev! cried Nana. This is *Cat*! She scuba dives!

Or were they both leading hybrid versions of the right life? Perhaps Lyn should have married Dan? And what about Gemma? How did a shared fraternal twin muddle the formula?

"There you go, my dear! All defuzzed!" The beautician patted Cat's legs with uncalled-for intimacy. "I bet you feel like a new woman!"

And Cat had said ungraciously, "I bet I don't."

It was still light on a Monday evening and Cat had just pulled into her driveway after work, when she saw Gemma's battered green Mini come screeching around the corner.

The Kettle girls were all speed freaks, but Gemma combined her need for speed with a spectacular lack of ability. She regularly drove into things—other cars, walls, the occasional telegraph pole.

Cat dropped her briefcase, pushed her sunglasses up onto her head, and leaned back against her car with folded arms to enjoy watching Gemma reverse park across the street.

After four bizarre attempts that each ended with the car crunching straight into the curb, Cat finally pushed her glasses back down onto her nose and walked across the road.

As she got closer to the car, the nasal whine of a scratchy cassette tape assaulted her ears. One of the multitudes of ex-boyfriends had been a country music fan and left Gemma with an unfortunate passion for Tammy Wynette. It was like, Cat thought, he'd given her herpes.

Gemma smiled radiantly when she saw Cat. She was singing, thumping her hands on the steering wheel in time to the music. *"Stand by your man!"*

"Get out and let me do it," yelled Cat above the music.

Gemma switched off the tape. "How are you?"

"Fine." Cat pulled on the door handle. "Come on."

Gemma hopped out of the car holding a bottle of wine in a brown paper bag.

This was clearly a peacemaking mission.

"Shall I direct you?"

"No." Cat got behind the wheel and pulled on the handbrake. "There's room enough to park a truck here, let alone this matchbox."

She parked the car in two moves. (You drive like a guy, Dan always said. It's very sexy.)

Cat slammed the car door shut and handed Gemma her keys. "You give women drivers a bad name."

"Yes, I know. I'm very ashamed. How are you?"

"You already asked me that. Was there a message in that song for me?"

"What do you mean?" Gemma looked alarmed.

"Stand by your man."

"Oh. Goodness. No. I mean, stand by him if you want—it's really up to you."

"Gemma!" Cat had glanced down to see her own black summer sandals on Gemma's feet. "I was looking for them just the other day!"

"Oh! Sorry. Are you sure they're not mine? I seem to have a memory of cleverly bargaining for them at the Balmain Street markets."

"I bargained for them at the Balmain markets. Help yourself to my memories, why don't you, as well as my shoes. I let you wear them to Michael's fortieth, remember?"

"Oh dear, this isn't going too well," said Gemma. "I'm meant to be fixing things. I've got a whole speech ready."

Cat took the bottle of wine from her. "You'd better get me drunk first."

They went inside, and Cat went to the bedroom to change out of her work clothes while Gemma opened the wine.

"There's some good Brie in the fridge," Cat called out. "And some olives."

She came out buttoning up her shorts to find Gemma staring reverently at the fridge door.

"What are you doing?"

"You've got Charlie's number here." She peeled off a colorful advertising magnet in the shape of a key and held it out to Cat. "I forgot it was thanks to you that I met him. Remember, that day when I got locked out watering the garden and I called you? How did you get this magnet? It was the hand of fate!"

"More likely a letterbox drop. Or the hand of Dan. How is your luscious locksmith anyway?"

"He's wonderful."

"You say that every time."

"This one's different."

"You say that every time too."

Gemma pulled the cork from the bottle. "Do I? I guess I do."

Cat wondered if her fifty dollars was safe. As soon as Charlie had arrived on the scene, she and Lyn had followed their normal routine of putting money on how long he'd last. Cat had him off the scene by March. Lyn had him lasting till June. A closet romantic, that girl.

"In a funny way, he reminds me of Pop Kettle," said Gemma. "There's something sweetly old-fashioned about him."

"God. That doesn't sound very sexy."

"Everything seems very simple and uncomplicated when I'm with him."

"Ah. A bit thick, eh?"

"Shut up." Cat watched as Gemma automatically poured exactly the same level of wine in each glass. She did it herself. It was the legacy of a childhood spent sharing cakes and chocolate bars and lemonade with two eagle-eyed sisters.

"You'll meet Charlie," said Gemma. "He's going to stop by at Lyn's and say a quick hello on Christmas Day."

"I'm not coming on Christmas Day," said Cat, wondering if she meant it.

"Of course you are," said Gemma. "You haven't heard my persuasive speech yet. Where's Dan tonight?"

"Out picking up another slut in a bar."

"That's nice for him."

"He's playing squash. I think. The worst thing about this is he's turned me into one of those suspicious wives. Noticing what time he gets home. I hate it. I'm not like that. I've never been like that. All of sudden I'm a cliché."

"You'll be O.K." Gemma ate an olive and spat out the seed into the palm of her hand. "Dan adores you. He does, I know he does! The thing with Lyn was just nothing, and the thing with that girl was just a stupid mistake. You and Dan have always been the best couple. Everybody says that."

Cat held the stem of her wineglass firmly. Jesus. She'd done more crying over the last few weeks than she'd ever done in her whole life.

"I never thought this could happen to me," she said with difficulty. "It's so sordid. So tacky. You know what I mean? I thought I was too good for it."

"Oh, Cat!" Cat felt her body become stiff and awkward as Gemma put her arm around her shoulder and she breathed in her familiar soft, soapy Gemma smell.

Lyn had a clean, citrus fragrance. Was there a "Cat" fragrance? Probably not. She probably smelled like a cardboard box.

Cat shrugged Gemma's arm away. "It's O.K. I'm fine. Come on, let's drink our wine on the balcony. Enjoy my *marvelous* view."

"I like your view," said Gemma loyally.

Cat and Dan lived in a renovated 1920s apartment, with high, ornate ceilings and polished floorboards. Their view was a sliver of bay, a sweeping arc of the Anzac Bridge, and a lot of gum trees.

On summer mornings they ate breakfast with an audience of brilliantly colored rosellas quivering busily on their railing.

They had bought before the last boom and had built up enough equity to buy an investment property a year ago. According to the standards of property-obsessed Sydney for a hip, professional young couple, they were doing O.K. In fact, they were right on track.

Gemma and Cat sat down and rocked back on their canvas chairs, balancing themselves by entwining their big toes around the railings of the balcony fence.

Cat said, in honor of their mother, "Sit like that if you want to break your neck, young lady!" Gemma responded in perfect Maxine-pitch, "You'll be laughing on the other side of your face when you're in a wheelchair, miss!"

"I wonder if we'll say things like that to our own kids," said Gemma after a minute. "I heard Lyn ask Maddie if she wanted a smack the other day. Maddie shook her head in this patronizing way, as if to say, Really, what a stupid question!"

Cat could visualize the exact expression on Maddie's little face. It was amazing to her, how a toddler could already be such a little *person*. Sometimes just looking at Maddie twisted Cat's heart. She was the one thing Lyn had that Cat couldn't even pretend not to want. Lyn had got pregnant the very moment, the fucking *month,* she scheduled it. Why hadn't Cat's identical womb responded to orders? The injustice of it. Month after month, you're not a mother, you're not a mother, and once again, you're not a mother.

Her period must be due any day now, just to add a final touch to the general gloom and doom.

Gemma rocked her chair back onto all four legs and gulped a mouthful of wine. She put the glass down at her feet. "Right," she said with a deep breath. "I'm ready to do my speech."

Cat swirled her own glass reflectively. When *was* her next period due?

Gemma stood up and opened her arms wide, like a politician

behind a podium. "Cat. This has been a difficult, terrible time for you—"

"My period is three weeks late."

"What?" Gemma plunked herself back down and picked up her wine again. "Are you sure?"

Cat could feel a strange shivery tremble in her lower stomach.

"It was due the day Dan told me about his one-night stand. I remember. I had a pimple. Right here on my chin. I thought it meant my period was coming. That's what it normally means. But it didn't come. And I didn't think about it like I normally do."

Gemma was jiggling up and down in her chair, wine sloshing all over her hand.

"You're pregnant! You're having a *baby*!"

"I might not be. I might just be late." It seemed so improbable, as if just by remembering her period was late, she could instantly make herself pregnant.

"Let's see your stomach!" Gemma reached over for Cat's T-shirt and pulled it up. They both contemplated her stomach and Gemma poked it gently with her finger.

"Hello, little baby," she said. "Are you in there?"

"I don't think it shows after three weeks," said Cat.

Gemma put one hand flat against Cat's stomach and one hand against her own.

"Ooooh, I think you're fatter!"

"I've got one of those pregnancy kits in the bathroom." Cat tried to keep her voice casual. "From the last time I was late. That was the time my period arrived as soon I got home from the chemist."

She watched Gemma waver at the possibility of a definite answer. She knew exactly what she was thinking: *I don't want to be here if she finds out she's not pregnant.*

"I bet I'm not," said Cat. "It's probably just stress."

"Come on." Gemma stood up. "Let's do it."

They sat on the edge of the bath and read the instructions together.

"It sounds a bit complicated," said Gemma, but Cat had just been thinking the opposite. It was too simple, too matter-of-fact. How dare this smug little plastic stick have the power to decide her future?

"Two blue lines I'm pregnant, one blue line I'm not. Can't get much simpler than that. You can give me some privacy now thanks."

Gemma closed the bathroom door behind her and then quickly opened it again to vigorously wave a hand with tightly crossed fingers.

Cat looked at herself in the mirror and felt strangely disoriented. *Are you a mother?* For a minute she saw Lyn's face looking calmly back at her.

Lyn said more than once she'd had the experience of being in a shopping center and waving hello to Cat, only to feel like an idiot when she realized she was waving at her own reflection.

It had never happened to Cat. She knew her own reflection perfectly well, and she hated it. She disliked nothing more than accidentally catching sight of herself in a mirror, especially if she was smiling. There was something so naked and pathetic about that unexpected sight of her foolishly happy face.

They weren't identical. Lyn had something indefinable, something special, something Cat had missed out on.

"Are you done yet?" called Gemma.

"Give me a minute."

Cat looked at the little plastic stick. Let's see what you've got to say for yourself.

She and Gemma sat on the cold bathroom tiles with their glasses of wine and their backs propped against the bathtub, while they waited for the stick to make up its mind.

Cat took off her watch and set the timer. "You can look for me," she said. "I can't look."

"O.K." Gemma hugged her knees to her. "This is very exciting. I feel like I'm practically part of the baby's conception!"

"Well, I hope that doesn't mean you've slept with Dan too," said Cat.

"No. Actually, I've never been the slightest bit attracted to him."

Cat felt unreasonably miffed at this. "I don't see why not. He's good enough for me. Good enough for Lyn. Good enough for what's-her-face, *Angela.*"

"Well, if you're *offering* him. I mean, I'd choose him over Michael, any day."

"Oh, God yes," said Cat with satisfaction. "He'd be terrible in bed. All eager and skinny."

Gemma hooted. "Yes, poor Lyn. I bet when he comes he does that little triumphant punch-in-the-air thing he does when we're playing tennis."

Cat snorted so hard her wine went up her nose and Gemma had to slap her on the back.

Cat picked up her watch. Only a minute to go. She was feeling a little hysterical. "Dan's sexually *skilled,* you know," she said. "It's like he's got a talent for it."

"Yes, so I've heard."

Cat looked at Gemma, who had her head tipped back and seemed to be swilling her wine at a remarkably fast pace. "I beg your pardon? Is that what Lyn said?"

Gemma put down her glass and wiped the back of her hand across her mouth. "I always remember the first time you slept with Dan you actually snuck out of bed to call me," she said. "You told me it was the most incredible experience of your entire life. Marcus and I had a big fight about it."

"That's right."

Cat had a sudden memory of herself, the sleeves of Dan's football shirt dangling sexily past her wrists, whispering into the phone. Tender lips from too much kissing. Sticky thighs.

"But why did you and Marcus fight about it?"

Gemma looked away. "I don't remember. Is it time?"

Cat looked at the watch. "Yes," she said. Now she was coldly calm. "Two lines I'm pregnant, one line I'm not. Don't stuff it up."

She stayed sitting while Gemma got to her feet and picked up the stick from the cabinet. Cat looked at her hands. There was silence. Gemma sat back down on the floor next to Cat.

"It doesn't matter." Cat felt tears blur her eyes. "It's fine. It doesn't matter."

Gemma reached over for Cat's glass and poured the remaining wine into her own. "No more of that for you."

"You're kidding."

Gemma shook her head and smiled goofily, widely, her eyes shiny. "Two lines. Two very, very pretty blue lines."

For the first time in her life, Cat threw her arms around her sister with complete, involuntary abandon.

To: Lyn
From: Gemma
Subject: Cat
I FIXED EVERYTHING!

The Magical Caramel Sundae

It must have been nearly a year after we lost her. I'd stopped by at a McDonald's in between appointments. It was about four o'clock in the afternoon and the place was overflowing with school kids. I had a table next to three girls—they were maybe fourteen or fifteen. Tall, gangly, and beautiful in that schoolgirl way.

The tables were so close together, I could hear every word they were saying. One of them was obviously upset about breaking up with a boy and the other two were trying to cheer her up, all to no avail. So one girl pulled out a notepad from her schoolbag and said, "Right, let's write down a list of everything that was wrong with him, that will make you feel better!" The miserable girl, slumped over her cheeseburger, said, "No, no, it won't, that's the most stupid idea I've ever heard."

But the girl with the notepad was relentless. She said, "Number one, he had disgusting eczema." The miserable girl said furiously, "He did not!" But all the girl writing could think about was how to spell eczema!

Then the other one of them went off to the counter and came back with a caramel sundae. In a very dramatic voice, she said, "This sundae has magical healing properties. Just one mouthful and you will be cured!" She tried to force the spoon into the sad one's mouth and they all three started to laugh. The girl finally took a mouthful and the other one slapped her across the forehead like a faith healer, and said, "Be gone, sadness demon!" They just had such infectious giggles, all of sudden I surprised myself by laughing out loud.

It was the first time I had laughed, properly laughed, since she died. It felt like a turning point, realizing I could still laugh.

It's funny. I bet those girls don't even remember that day. But for me, it really was a magical caramel sundae.

CHAPTER 9

Dan couldn't seem to take it in at first. He stood in their living room staring at her, the ends of his hair still damp with sweat from his squash game.

He seemed bewildered. "A baby," he kept saying slowly. "We're going to have a baby."

"Yes, Dan, a baby. You know—floppy head, makes a lot noise, costs a lot of money."

And then finally he seemed to get it and let his squash racket fall to the floor and hugged her hard around the ribs, so that her feet almost lifted off the ground.

Rob Spencer caressed his tie lovingly. "Masturbation. Interesting."

"The message is pleasure," responded Cat. "Self-indulgent pleasure."

"Yes, but she's masturbating, isn't she? I mean what we have here is a woman in a bath, mas-tur-bat-ing."

People began to shift uneasily in their chairs. Marianne, who was taking the minutes, threw down her pen and put her hands over her ears. "Could you please stop saying that *word*, Rob!"

It was the last day before Hollingdale Chocolates closed for the Christmas break, and Cat was giving a presentation on a new advertising campaign for the following year's Valentine's Day. A full-page ad was projected via her laptop onto a large screen at the end of the room. The ad showed a woman lying in a bath, smiling wickedly, her eyes closed. One languid hand was allowing an empty Hollingdale Chocolate wrapper to flutter to the floor. The other hand wasn't visible. The headline read, *Seduce someone special this Valentine's Day.*

Cat was pleased with the campaign. She'd got the idea after Gemma told her how decadent she felt eating Hollingdale Chocolates in the Penthursts' bath. Some guy at the agency contributed the "self-pleasure" element. (What a lovely idea! said Gemma when she heard, looking rather inspired.)

"The focus groups loved it," said Cat.

"Oh yes, and they're never wrong, are they? Ha!" Rob looked jovially around the meeting room. He lowered his voice. "Two little words: Hazelnut Heaven."

"Arrggh!" People clutched their chests as if they'd been shot. Others buried their heads in their hands. Sidelong glances were shot down the end of the table where the CEO of Hollingdale Chocolates, Graham Hollingdale, chewed a pen lid and looked bored out of his mind.

Hazelnut Heaven had been last year's new-product disaster. When it happened, the entire company ducked wildly for cover, hurling blame like hand grenades over their office cubicle walls. They passed the buck so furiously and successfully that it stopped nowhere. Twelve months later, recalling the experience created a warm glow of camaraderie.

Cat gave the obligatory rueful chuckle. "You're right, Rob. There are no guarantees. But I do think we've got all the right elements for our target audience."

"Love your work, Cat!" said Rob. He leaned forward and pressed a finger to his lips. "But to be frank, I have some real concerns about this one."

Aha. It had been a few weeks since she'd pointed out his error in the Operations Meeting. Rob had been biding his time, cradling his wounded ego, waiting to pounce. If this had happened yesterday, her adrenaline would have been pumping. Today, it all seemed like an amusingly childish game. It was only a job—a means of making money. *And she was having a baby*. At the thought of the baby magically curled in her womb, Cat felt an exquisite burst of joy.

"We agreed on this concept over a month ago," she said calmly. "You loved it, Rob."

"Hey, I hate to admit it but I can be wrong! This has got to be an open forum, Cat. No finger-pointing. No politics. Just honest opinions."

Cat swallowed a guffaw.

"O.K. then," she said. "Let's look at the creative rationale again. We wanted something strong enough to break through the clutter. It does. We wanted something to appeal to single women in their thirties. It does."

Rob held up his palms like he was testing the weight of two things. "Masturbation. Hollingdale Chocolates. Anyone else worried about what this says about our brand values, our brand *heritage?* Graham?"

Rob swiveled his chair to face the CEO. Graham sighed in an exhausted fashion and chewed harder on his pen lid. He was a strange, inscrutable man, with a disconcerting habit of allowing his eyelids to droop, turtlelike, whenever any of his staff spoke. The longer they spoke, the more it seemed he was drifting into a deep, comfortable sleep.

Rob stared at him for an agonizing few seconds and then swiveled his chair back to Cat. "I'm just not convinced you've cracked it this time, Cat. I know you're the creative genius. But just run with me here while I throw a few ideas around. What if she was lying in the bath dreaming of her *lover*? You could have one of those little bubbles coming out of her head, you know, to show she was dreaming."

"Yeah, now that sounds like a good compromise, folks!" contributed Derek, who was a moron. "Give her a lover!"

"She doesn't want a lover," said Cat. She doodled "July 23" on her notepad. It was the date her baby was due.

"Why not?" asked Graham suddenly. "Why doesn't she want a lover?"

Everyone turned in surprise to look at him. Cat looked at the slightly awkward jut of his chin. Perhaps, she thought, Graham Hollingdale was just shy. Perhaps his eccentricity wasn't arrogance after all. Maybe it was just plain, old-fashioned, teenage-boy gawkiness disguised by the authoritative uniform of a balding, middle-aged business executive.

She smiled at him—a Gemma smile—open, radiant, and guileless.

"She might like a lover at some point, but the message of the ad is that you don't need a lover to give yourself pleasure on Valentine's Day. All you need is a bath and Hollingdale Chocolates."

She looked at Rob. "There's no need to feel threatened by it."

Rob rolled his eyes. "I'm thinking about the impact on the *brand*—"

"Run it as is," said Graham. "I like it."

"Great." Cat slammed shut her laptop. "I'll e-mail you all PDFs."

"Fine." Graham subsided sleepily back into his chair.

Rob didn't look up. He was using a gold ballpoint to jab a straight line of vicious little blue dots across his notepaper. No revelations there. He was still the slimy prick he'd always been.

"Happy Christmas, everybody!" said Cat warmly.

She and her baby sailed from the room.

It was the night before Christmas Eve, and Annie the marriage counselor was celebrating with gigantic Christmas trees dangling from her ears. They had red and green lights that flashed disconcertingly on and off, on and off.

"Love the earrings, Annie," said Dan. He was holding Cat's hand as they sat thigh to thigh on the green vinyl sofa.

"Thank you, Dan." Annie gave her head a merry little swing. "Now, if you don't mind me saying, you two seem a lot cheerier than when I saw you last."

"We've had some news." Dan squeezed Cat's hand.

"I'm pregnant," said Cat.

"Oh!" Annie clasped her hands together. *"Congratulations!"*

"It's not like that means everything is suddenly O.K.," said Cat. She didn't want Annie thinking they were going to fork out one hundred and twenty bucks for an hour's worth of trilling and cooing.

"Of course not!" Annie's smile disappeared in tempo with her flashing lights. "But it is wonderful news after you've been trying for so long."

"Yes." Cat leaned forward to look at Annie seriously. "I want us to fix everything before the baby's born. I hated having divorced parents. I *hated* the way they spoke about each other. I'm not putting my child through that."

She sat back, embarrassed by her intensity. She hadn't even realized she felt that way until the words came out of her mouth. In fact, up until now, she'd always told people the opposite—that she couldn't care less about her parents' divorce.

Now their marriage was something they needed to fix before the baby was born. It was a task that had to be ticked off the list some time over the next nine months, like transforming the study into a nursery and installing a baby capsule in the car.

Annie was the expert. That's what they were paying her for.

"I still feel angry with Dan about what he did," said Cat. "Sometimes I can't even bear to look at him I feel so angry. Actually, sometimes I feel sick when I look at him."

"Are you sure that's not morning sickness?" asked Dan. "Because that seems a bit extreme."

Cat and Annie ignored him. "Obviously," said Cat, "I need to stop feeling that way before the baby is born."

She looked at Annie expectantly. Dan cleared his throat.

Annie opened her manila folder in a businesslike manner. "Well, I think this all sounds very constructive, very positive. Let's get started, then."

"Yes, let's."

Cat held on tight to Dan's hand and didn't look at him.

On Christmas Eve, Cat offered to baby-sit with Maddie while Lyn and Maxine went to the Fish Markets.

She arrived to find the two of them walking around the house on exaggerated tippy-toes. "We just got her down," explained Lyn. "It was a nightmare. The girls at play group say you only miss one or two and that's it, afternoon naps finished for good—never to return!"

It seemed to Cat that Lyn was speaking to her about Maddie in a more relaxed, mother-to-mother tone, now she was pregnant. It made Cat feel both humiliated and grateful to think that Lyn had been consciously—or perhaps subconsciously—curtailing her conversation.

"Have you told Mum yet?" asked Lyn, while their mother disappeared into the bathroom to reapply her lipstick.

"No. I'm going to make a family announcement at lunch tomorrow."

"Cat! Dad knows, Nana knows—you can't make a family announcement when the only one in the family who doesn't know is Mum!" said Lyn. "Tell her now."

Cat sighed. Every conversation with her mother was fraught with danger. It was as if they were former players from competing teams who shared a long and violent history. Sure it all seemed a little silly now but all the old antipathies about unfair penalties were still there just beneath the surface.

Throughout the seventies, until their peace treaty in the eighties, Maxine and Frank had fought, and their three little daughters had fought loyally and bravely alongside them. Lyn took Maxine's side. Cat took Frank's side. Gemma took everyone's side. It was hard to put a decade-long battle behind you.

Maxine reappeared, smelling of *Joy* and hairspray.

"The Smith family might appreciate receiving that shirt soon," she remarked to Cat, who was lying on Lyn's sofa, bare feet dangling off the end.

Cat looked down at her faded T-shirt. "I think they've got higher standards."

Lyn pinched her on the arm.

"I'm pregnant, Mum," said Cat to the ceiling.

"Oh!" said Maxine. "But I thought you and Dan were having problems."

Lyn said in an anguished tone, *"Mum!"* while Cat pulled a cushion out from under her head and held it over her face.

Maxine said, "Well, I am sorry, Lyn. I thought they were. Gemma mentioned something about *counseling."*

Cat didn't need to see her mother's face to know the lemony expression of distaste that would be pulling at her mouth as she said the word "counseling." Counseling was something other people did.

Cat took the cushion off her face and sat up. "People get pregnant from having sex, Mum. Not from a perfect marriage. You ought to know that."

Maxine's nostrils flared, but she drew herself upright, manicured nails digging into the strap of her handbag. It always astounded Cat—this ability of her mother's to pack away unsightly emotions, in exactly the same way she transformed unwieldy bed sheets into sharp-edged squares for the linen cupboard.

"I'm sorry, dear. It was just the shock, hearing you say it like that, just lying there on the sofa. It was odd. I'm very happy for you. And for Dan, of course. When are you due? Here, let me give you a kiss."

Cat sat upright, hugging the cushion to her stomach like a

recalcitrant teenager while Maxine pressed cool lips against her cheek.

"Congratulations, dear," she said. "You've cut back on your drinking, I hope."

As Lyn and Maxine closed the door behind them, Cat lay back on the sofa and thought about the announcement of Lyn's pregnancy. A special family dinner with Maxine practically gurgling with delight and pride, raising her champagne glass to Michael's camera, a proud, maternal arm around Lyn's shoulder.

Cat pressed her palms tenderly against her stomach.

"You and I are going to get along so much better, aren't we?"

Christmas Day. It began with such promise.

They slept in till ten. Cat could feel the heat in the air when she woke.

Secretly, like she did every morning now, she patted her belly. Good morning, baby. Happy Christmas.

"It's going to be hot," she said out loud, stretching and kicking off the sheet. Dan lay on his stomach, his face squashed into his pillow, his arms looped around it.

"Lucky we're going to the mansion," he said, his voice muffled. He half lifted his head from the pillow and opened one eye to look at her.

"Happy Christmas, Catriona."

"Happy Christmas, Daniel."

It was their thing, calling each other by their full names, whenever they wanted to be funny or portentous or especially loving. It started after their wedding, remembering their wedding vows. "I, Daniel, take you, Catriona, to be my wife . . ." except on their honeymoon it was more likely to be, "I, Daniel, take you, Catriona, to fuck your brains out."

No one's brains had been fucked out lately, of course. She'd let him back into the bedroom after three nights on the sofa bed, and ever since the news about the baby she'd stopped flinching violently every time his arm accidentally brushed against hers, but there was still an invisible, uncrossable line down the middle of their bed. Well, not quite down the middle. Cat's half—the wronged-party half—was a touch more generous.

They did what they always did on Christmas morning and stayed in bed to exchange their Christmas presents.

He gave her a delicate gold bracelet and the new *Marie Claire* recipe book and a "make your own herb garden" kit. She gave him aftershave and a new squash racket. They were just a little too effusive about each other's gifts.

"I'll let you open this one," said Dan, once the bed was covered with wrapping paper. He pulled an extra package from his bedside drawer.

Cat read the gift tag out loud: "To my new little baby girl or boy. Happy Christmas. I love you and I love your mum. From your dad."

Normally Dan's cards read, *To: Catwoman. From: Batman.*

The present was a miniature furry football.

"Boy or girl, they need to learn how to kick a ball properly," explained Dan. He bent his head down and spoke to Cat's stomach. "Did you hear that? No sexism in this family."

Cat looked at the top of his head, and her mind did one of those strange little shifts, a mental double-take. *He's going to be someone's dad.* There's my dad, their child would say one day and the other kids wouldn't bother looking up from their game because fathers were all pretty much the same really and this *dad* would be walking toward them—and the dad would be *Dan.*

For some reason, this thought was very, very sexy.

As Dan sat back up she pushed him by the shoulders and rolled herself on top of him, to sit astride his stomach. The Christmas paper crackled beneath them, and Dan looked up at her with narrowed green eyes, an unshaven jaw. "She's crossed the line."

"Yeah, I'm crossing the line." Cat pulled off her T-shirt and bent toward him. "And you'd better not cross it again, mate."

"Never," he mumbled, his tongue already in her mouth, his hands running up and down her spine.

She had thought sex would be ruined forever—but they were too good at it for it to be bad. The hurt of the last few weeks seemed only to make it more intense; it gave her a feeling of exquisite fragility, as if at any moment she would cry. She came fast and hard and that thing happened, the phenomenon that had only happened twice before and both those times she'd been smoking pot. It was like a stained-glass window shattered in her head and every fragment was a different memory or thought or feeling. There was the plate of spaghetti smashing against the wall and there was Gemma with shiny eyes saying, "Two very, very pretty blue lines," and there was Dan walking toward a child looking up to say, "That's my dad," and there was the Christmas tree of Cat's childhood, glittering with gold and silver tinsel in the morning light, surrounded by presents that had magically materialized overnight.

It took them a few seconds to catch their breath.

"Wow."

"Yeah, wow."

"So, this should make Christmas less stressful," Dan said as they drove toward Lyn's place. "Getting your parents over and done with in one go, instead of driving all over Sydney to see them."

Dan had a low-maintenance family. His parents had considerately moved up to Queensland a couple of years ago, and he had an enviably casual relationship with his only sister, Mel. Christmas was all about the Kettles, which was fortunate because they didn't leave much energy for anyone else.

"It will be more stressful," said Cat. "I think it's a bizarre idea having the parents together for Christmas. Mum will be even more uptight than usual, and Dad will be showing off. It will be painful to watch."

"And you can't drink yourself into oblivion anymore."

"I assume you're going to give up alcohol in sympathy with me."

"Enjoy your little fantasies, don't you?"

"You're still on probation. Don't get all cocky just because you got lucky this morning."

"Ooh, I got lucky all right."

As they waited for the traffic lights to change Cat looked out the window and watched a family who had just pulled up outside someone's house. A group of kids were running helter-skelter into the house, and a man was standing with his arms outstretched while a woman loaded him up with presents from the car. He pretended to stagger under their weight, and the woman flicked him on the arm.

The lights changed and Dan accelerated.

"You know, I might forgive you, one day," she said. "I might."

"The air conditioning isn't working," said Michael as he ushered them into the house. "My wife is not happy. Merry Christmas."

He had a screwdriver in his hand, which he handed to Dan. "It's time to initiate you into one of the great joys of fatherhood, mate."

Dan stared at the screwdriver.

"You get a picture on a box, a thousand little screws, and instructions entirely lacking in logic. Oh, it's fun. Today, we're working on a three-story cubby house. Santa Claus must have been out of her mind. Come on. You're not escaping."

"A drink?" asked Dan a touch desperately, as Michael led him off by the elbow.

Cat mouthed the word "probation" at him.

She found Lyn in the kitchen, wearing a sleeveless sundress that made her shoulders look too thin. The gleaming granite bench tops were covered with orderly rows of chopped ingredients. She was standing at the kitchen sink washing lettuce leaves.

"You're the most organized cook on the planet," said Cat. "What is that *noise?*" She bent down to see Maddie sitting under the table, frowning heavily, while she banged away discordantly on a tiny xylophone.

"My Cat!" cried Maddie and banged even harder to celebrate. "Look! Maddie noisy! Shhhh!"

"Ooh, can I see?" asked Cat hopefully, but Maddie was way too smart for that.

"No!"

"It's no use." Lyn wiped the back of a wet hand against her forehead. "It's her favorite present. You know who it's from— *Georgina*. The bitch. She must have combed the shops looking for the loudest toy she could find. I've had the worst morning. First the air conditioning. We can't get anybody out to fix it and they're forecasting thirty-four degrees. Nana will be complaining all day. Michael has spent two hours on that stupid cubby house. Mum's setting the table on the veranda, and she's so tightly wound up you can see the static crackling. You'd better keep away from her. Kara is upstairs, refusing to come out of her room. Gemma just called, all dreamy and idiotic, asking how to make a potato salad. Dad and Nana are late. Oh no, you *disgusting, vile creature!*"

Lyn did a strange little flapping dance on the spot and pointed at a cockroach in the middle of the kitchen floor. It seemed to have caught Lyn's panic and kept changing its mind about which way it should go.

"The spray! It's right there next to you. Stop laughing and kill it!"

Cat grabbed the spray. "Die, you little motherfucker," she said and blasted it.

"Yucky," observed Maddie, who had come out from under the kitchen table and now stood with her hands on her hips like a disgusted little housewife.

"That's exactly what *I* say when I kill cockroaches," said Lyn, as she scooped up the cockroach with a paper towel.

"Yucky?"

"Die, you little motherfucker. In exactly that tone of voice. I'm pretending to be Arnie Schwarzenegger."

"Yeah. Me too."

They grinned, pleased with themselves.

"We'll have to ask Gemma if she does it too," said Lyn.

"She probably doesn't know you're meant to kill them. What shall I do to help now I've got rid of your vermin?"

"Can you extricate Kara from her hovel? She listens to you. Thinks you're cool."

"O.K."

"You're glowing by the way," said Lyn as she returned to her lettuce leaves and Maddie returned to her xylophone. "Pregnancy must suit you."

Cat smiled widely. "Cool and glowing. Glowing coolly."

"Yeah, yeah. Go away. Maddie, I'm *begging* you to be quiet!"

Cat knocked once on Kara's door and walked into her dark bedroom, which smelled of perfume and illicit cigarette smoke. The floor was layered in discarded clothing.

It was Cat's own teenage bedroom. The one she got for four months of the year before she had to move out and let a sister take a turn at a room of her own. Kara was lying facedown on her bed, and Cat could hear the tinny beat of music from her headphones. She sat down on the end of the bed and grabbed her ankle.

Kara's shoulder blades twitched angrily and she turned over, revealing blotchy mascara tearstains.

"Oh," she said, pulling her headphones around her neck. "It's you."

"Yep," said Cat. "Happy Christmas. What's wrong?"

"Nothing."

"So why the suicidal look? Did you get really bad presents?"

"You wouldn't understand."

"No. Probably not. Try me anyway so you can prove yourself right."

Kara sighed dramatically.

"O.K., so this morning right, Mum gives me these shorts for Christmas and she goes, Try them on, try them on! I didn't want to try them on in front of everybody but she wouldn't shut up, so I did and I had to do this embarrassing, like *fashion parade,* with my gran saying Ohhhh, isn't she sweet? and then do you know what Mum said, really loudly, in front of everybody?"

Kara's voice quivered and Cat thought, You bitch, Georgina.

"What?"

"She said *they didn't really suit me!"*

Kara's face crumbled. "Can you believe she said that?"

"Mmmm. Well, I guess—"

"She means I've got fat, ugly, disgusting legs!"

"No, I don't think she did mean that actually."

"You don't understand. You've got great legs!" Kara pinched viciously at the flesh on her own thighs. "And don't you *dare* say there's nothing wrong with my legs because if you do, you're just a liar. I know there is, because at the swimming carnival, Matt Hayes pointed at me and said he'd seen better legs on a table, and all his stupid friends laughed through their noses, like they agreed!"

It was no wonder that teenagers ended up going on shooting rampages, thought Cat. She herself could cheerfully fire off a few rounds at Matt and his pathetic, pimply little mates.

"And don't talk to me about how the media tries to make women feel bad about their bodies and it's a feminist issue and blah, blah, blah. I know all that stuff! It doesn't make any difference."

Cat shut her mouth quickly. Kara lay back down on her bed and they sat in silence for a few seconds.

Cat tried frantically to think of something cool to say.

"I really hate my breasts," she offered finally, lamely.

"What?" Kara snorted.

"The Kettle girls missed out on breasts. You should hear the jokes boys have made about us over the years. They thought they were so witty. So hilarious."

"To Lyn, even? Did Lyn get upset?"

"Of course. Once a boy told Lyn she had two mozzie bites instead of tits and she cried for a whole week."

"Really? Did she?" Kara sat up, invigorated. "I can't imagine her, young, and getting all upset."

"And you obviously don't have any worries in that department."

"Shut up." Kara pulled at her T-shirt. "Boys don't care about breasts."

Cat stood up. "No. Of course not. Boys never think twice about breasts. Come on, you idiot, I'm sweltering in here. Are your legs capable of getting us downstairs?"

"Oh, all right. I'm starved to death, anyway. So what did that boy say again? Two mosquito bites, huh?"

"Don't ever mention it to her, will you?"

Now Kara looked positively delighted. "I won't. It might be a traumatic memory."

"Probably."

The sounds of "Rudolph the Red-Nosed Reindeer" floated up the stairs, and Kara winced painfully. "Oh no." She clattered down the stairs, two at a time, yelling out, "Dad! Stop embarrassing yourself! Turn it off!"

Cat followed her, wondering if that mosquito bite thing happened to Lyn, or herself. Oh well. The year she turned thirty she had finally made peace with her breasts.

Gemma, Nana Kettle, and Frank were sitting around Lyn's kitchen table shelling prawns and drinking champagne. The three of them all had tinsel bows tied around their heads, which were no doubt Gemma's creations.

"I wish you'd all go outside on the balcony," Lyn was saying.

"We're helping you," said Gemma.

"You're not. You're annoying me."

Frank stood up and grabbed Cat around the waist, swinging her around.

"*There* you are! The mother-to-be! Happy Christmas, angel! Sit down and put your feet up. That's what you do when you're pregnant. I hope Dan knows that. I hope he's waiting on you hand and foot. I'll have to have a word with him." He sat her down in his chair and began to pull at her protesting feet to put them on the table.

"Not on the food!" warned Nana.

Lyn said, "I'm sure you waited on Mum hand and foot when she was pregnant, Dad."

The doorbell rang. "That will be Charlie," Gemma happily popped a peeled prawn into her mouth. "He's come to let you look at him."

Lyn said, "Could you please stop eating the prawns!"

"Oh. Isn't that what they're for?"

"Why don't we ask this Charlie fellow to take a look at the air conditioning?" Nana fanned herself with a napkin.

"He's a locksmith, Nana."

"I expect he's handy, though. That's our problem. None of the men here are at all *handy.*"

"Gemma!" Maxine came into the kitchen followed by a man and woman. "Your friend is here."

"Everyone! This is *Charlie!*" Gemma waved her champagne glass rapturously and threw an arm around his shoulder.

He was a stocky man with a barrel chest, exactly the same height as Gemma. She hadn't mentioned he was short. Sort of attractive, thought Cat, for a short man. She leaned forward as she shook his hand to check out the famous eyelashes. They looked perfectly ordinary to her.

"And this is my sister," Charlie said to the room. "Her Vee-dub conked out this morning. So I'm the designated driver to our family lunch."

Cat turned her attention to the sister. She had long dark hair scraped back off her face and a red T-shirt with a scooped neck-line, revealing the cupped together curves of a luscious cleavage. She was beautiful. Model beautiful. She was also familiar.

"Hi." She smiled. There was a buzzing sensation in Cat's ears.

"I'm Angela."

Lyn had appeared from nowhere to rest her hand gently on Cat's shoulder.

"Hi, Angela," said Gemma, and as her smile slid away from her face, her champagne glass slid from her hand to shatter on the floor.

I have mosquito bites for breasts, thought Cat.

CHAPTER 10

Lyn's Christmas Day started in the gray half-light of 5 A.M. when she woke to see a pair of unblinking brown eyes only inches away from her own. Maddie was standing next to their bed, sucking her thumb, staring at Lyn as if she were hypnotized. It gave Lyn such a fright she banged her elbow on the bedside table.

"Shit!" She sat up straight, cradling her elbow. "How long have you been there? You're not meant to wake up for three hours yet!"

Maddie carefully unplugged her mouth and began to wail.

Michael woke up, instantly alert and cheery. He lifted his head from his pillow to observe Maddie. "Someone looking for Santa Claus?"

"She's too young for Santa Claus. She hates him, remember?"

"Merry Christmas to you too."

"I hurt my elbow."

"Ah."

He threw back the quilt and walked around the bed to pick up Maddie. Lyn watched his long skinny brown body in the Mickey Mouse boxer shorts Kara had given him for his fortieth. He had a new haircut—it made his head look smaller, shorn and vulnerable, like a schoolboy who got teased on the bus.

"Mummy hurt her elbow," he said to Maddie. "Did you hurt your elbow too?"

Maddie stopped crying and nodded her head tragically, pointing her finger at her own elbow.

Michael was delighted. "Did you see that?"

"She's a little liar," said Lyn proudly.

Michael climbed back into bed with Maddie in his arms and tucked her in the middle of them.

"She won't sleep," said Lyn.

"Your mummy is a pessimist."

But within minutes the three of them were sound asleep, Lyn and Michael curled on their sides facing Maddie, who lay flat on her back, star-shaped, a thumb-sucking sunbaker.

It seemed like only seconds later when the strident demands of the telephone woke them. Lyn answered it, her mind fuzzily clutching at a dream.

"You weren't asleep, were you?" Maxine's voice was tinny with distress. "It's nearly *nine o'clock.*"

"It's not. Is it?" Lyn was remembering her dream in alarming detail. She was eating mangoes, naked, in a bath with . . . with . . . with *Hank.*

Sticky. Sweet. Slippery. His tongue circling her nipple.

Oh dear. She'd been sleeping with her husband and daughter on Christmas morning and having erotic dreams about an exboyfriend. She looked at Michael, who had woken up and was contentedly scratching his stomach, his new haircut squashed flat on one side

"It *is* Lyn!" said Maxine. "Is everything under control? Is the turkey in the oven?"

There was something a little sad about having erotic dreams when you led such an unerotic life.

And what was she trying to prove by doing the Christmas lunch this year, right down to the bloody turkey? She wasn't depriving her mother of stress. She was giving her *more* stress, cruelly removing control from a control freak. "You like it," Cat always said. "You've always liked being the martyr. So go ahead. We won't stop you."

She could have spent the morning eating mangoes in the bath.

"It's only family," Lyn told her mother. "It's only us. Nobody's going to care if we're not sitting at the table right on the dot."

"Have you got a summer cold, Lyn?" asked Maxine, meaning, "Are you delirious?"

"I'm perfectly fine, Mum. I'm just saying we don't need to stress."

"Of course we need to 'stress,' as you put it. If we eat too late everybody drinks too much, you and your sisters start fighting, your grandmother falls asleep at the table, your father becomes morose, and Maddie gets overtired and eats too many lollies."

These were all valid points. "Besides which, I've got something I want to tell you all at lunch," continued Maxine. "I'm a little tense about it."

"You're tense about it? What's wrong? What's the matter?" "I'm a little tense" was a deeply personal revelation for her mother. It must be something terrible. It would be just like Maxine to announce terminal cancer over Christmas lunch.

"It's something good—I think. I'm happy about it."

Happy about it? That was even more worrying. Lyn pressed two fingers to her forehead. She could sense the beginnings of a vicious headache: a tribal thump in the distance.

Michael sat up in bed and flapped his arms like a chicken to indicate Maxine in a flap.

Lyn nodded.

"Talk!" demanded Maddie, reaching for the phone.

"Maddie wants to talk to you. I'll see you at lunch," said Lyn. "Don't you dare come early." She handed the phone to Maddie and then grabbed it back.

"Happy Christmas, Mum."

"Yes, dear."

A door slammed downstairs.

Michael raised his eyebrows. "That doesn't bode well."

Kara had spent Christmas Eve with her mother. She wasn't due back till lunchtime.

A minute later Kara stuck her head in the doorway.

"Happy Christmas, honey," said Michael and leaped up with arms outstretched. "You're early!"

Kara looked revolted. "Dad, you're not *dressed.* Anyway, I just wanted to say, I'll be in my room. I don't want anything to eat. I don't have anything to say. Just . . . leave . . . me . . . alone. Is that too much to ask?"

Michael stuck his thumbs awkwardly into the elastic of his boxers and held them out slightly from his concave stomach. "Ah."

"Dad, what are you *doing*?"

"I don't know," said Michael miserably, letting his hands drop.

"I *hate* Christmas!" exploded Kara, and she walked off down the hallway to her bedroom.

Lyn said, "So do I."

Michael looked at her.

"Not really." Lyn headed for the shower. "I just don't trust it."

The first Christmas after Frank and Maxine separated was the first Christmas the Kettle girls were separated from each other.

It began with a brochure—a glossy, seductive brochure.

"What do you think of this, girls?" asked Frank.

He laid the brochure on the red laminated table at McDonald's and flourished his hands back and forth just like the TV ladies on *Sale of the Century.*

Oh, he was hilarious, their dad.

They were six years old, full of the confidence of conquering kindergarten. At St. Margaret's Primary they were famous, just for being triplets. At Little Lunch and Big Lunch there was always a group of maternal sixth-grade girls lined up together on a long wooden bench who had come to watch the Kettle triplets play. "Oooh, they're so cute!" "Is that one Cat or Lyn?" "It's Lyn!" "No, it's Cat!" "Which one are you, sweetie?" Cat exploited them terribly, telling them stories about how poor they were, and how they had to share just one lamb chop for dinner. She collected at least fifty-cents charity money every day.

Oh yes. School had turned out to be a snap.

And now here they were in the brand-new McDonald's store with Dad, eating sundaes, turning their spoons upside down, and lingering their tongues over creamy cold ice cream and hot sugary caramel. Their father's dislike of sundaes was really quite extraordinary. "Just try one teeny mouthful, Daddy," Gemma was always encouraging. "Because I *know* you would love it. It's like eating a *cloud*. Or *snow*."

Maxine didn't let them eat McDonald's. They didn't tell her that Daddy let them eat all the bad-for-you food they desired. They didn't tell her that every second weekend was like a magical mystery holiday, with surprise after surprise on the itinerary and not a rule or a vegetable in sight.

But they just bet she suspected.

"You know what this is," said Dad, sliding the brochure over to them. "This is *the fastest water slide in the whole world.*"

"Really?" breathed Cat. "Truly?"

They stared at the brochure in awe. It showed a photo of a little girl hurtling out the end of an enormous funnel, carried along by a frothy rush of water. Lyn wanted to go on that water slide so badly. For an instant, she *was* that little girl with her heart pumping and her hands flung high in a perfect, flat blue sky.

"Whoosh!" said Gemma, running her fingers down the curling funnel of the slide.

"I think you'd go faster than a car," said Cat.

"Not faster than Daddy's car," said Lyn. "No, I don't think so."

"You *would*!" said Cat, pinching her hard on the leg with her fingernails. "Yes, you would!"

"Whoosh!" said Gemma again. She trailed her sundae spoon through the air. "You'd go *this* fast!"

"This water slide is in a special place called the Gold Coast," said Dad. "And you know what?"

"What?"

"I'm going to take you there for the Christmas holidays!"

Well! The excitement! Gemma's sundae spoon went flying in the air. Cat slammed both her hands triumphantly on the table. Their father smiled modestly and allowed his cheek to be kissed by each of them.

All the way home in the car they talked about it.

"I'm going to make myself go faster by pushing myself along," said Lyn. "Like this with my hands."

Cat said, "That won't work. I'm going to put my hands out in front like this, like an arrow."

Gemma said, "I'm going to do a special magic trick to make me go faster."

"Stupid, stupid, stupid!" chanted Cat and Lyn.

When they got home, Dad came inside to tell Mummy about the holiday.

Lyn was in the kitchen getting a glass of water. So she was the only one to see their mother's reaction.

She looked surprised, like Daddy had slapped her across her cheek. "But Christmas Day?" she said. "Can't you take them on Boxing Day?"

"It's the only time I can get away," said Dad. "You know the pressure I'm under with the Paddington project."

"I'd like to be with them on Christmas Day. I don't see how one day can make such a difference."

"I thought their welfare was your first priority. Your words, Max."

"I'm not saying that they shouldn't go, Frank."

Lyn watched as Mummy's eyes looked up to the ceiling. She took a deep breath as if she were going to do a gigantic sneeze, but then the sneeze didn't come.

It was odd.

Lyn stared at her mother over the rim of her glass.

It looked almost as if she were trying not to cry. As soon as the thought came into her head, Lyn knew it was true. She felt something click and slide into place. There was her mum, her normal, annoying, bad-tempered mum, and fitted neatly over the top of her was a new version—a version who got upset just like her daughters did.

"I want to be with Mum on Christmas Day," she said, and she had no idea why she said it because she didn't want that at all; the words had tripped straight out of her mouth without her permission.

Her parents acted as if they hadn't even realized she was in the kitchen. "Don't be silly, Lyn," said Mum. "You're going on a lovely holiday with your father."

Lyn looked at her father. "Why can't we go after Christmas Day?"

He reached for her and pulled her onto his lap, smoothing his hand over the top of her head. "That's the only time Daddy's work will let him go, darling."

Lyn ran her finger around the edge of his shirt button. "I don't believe you."

She wriggled off his lap as Cat and Gemma came running into the kitchen brandishing a Barbie doll's dismembered limbs.

"Lyn wants to stay here with Mummy for Christmas," said Dad. "What do you two want to do?"

Cat looked at Lyn as if she'd lost her mind. "Why are you being stupid?"

"Why can't Mummy just come with us?" beamed Gemma.

"Mum and Dad are *divorced,* spastic-head," said Cat. "That means they're not allowed to do things together anymore. It's a rule. It's the *law.*"

"Oh." Gemma's lower lip trembled. "Oh, I see."

"I'm going on holidays with Daddy," said Cat.

"I'm staying here with Mum," said Lyn. This was being *pure* and *good,* just like Sister Judith talked about in religion classes.

Lyn could visualize her own shimmering sin-free soul. It was heart-shaped and sparkly like a diamond.

Tears of panic slid rapidly down Gemma's face. "We have to be together when Santa comes!"

They weren't together when Santa came.

Over the next week Lyn and Cat campaigned aggressively for Gemma to join their side. Underhand tactics were used on both sides.

"Mummy will be so sad if we don't have Christmas here with her," said Lyn. "She'll cry and cry and cry."

"She won't," said Gemma in alarm. "Mummy doesn't cry. You won't cry, will you, Mum?"

Mum was cross. "No, I certainly won't, Gemma. Don't be so silly, Lyn."

"We'll go on the fastest water slide in the whole world and *Daddy* will cry if you don't come!" said Cat. "Won't you, Dad?"

He sniffed loudly and pretended to wipe his eyes. "Oh yes."

Lyn didn't stand a chance.

The problem was it didn't seem as if Maxine even noticed Lyn's saintly behavior. She was just as cross and annoying as ever. After a while Lyn realized that she didn't have a sparkly diamond for a soul at all. Deep down she felt *angry* with her mother, not pure and good and loving.

The thought of missing out on that water slide made her sick—but so did the thought of her mother sitting at the kitchen table with the tea towel over her shoulder.

So there you had it. She missed out on both the water slide and a gold star from Jesus.

That was the Christmas Lyn discovered the horrible pleasure of martyrdom.

Lyn knew she knew Angela as soon as she walked into the kitchen. She had the sort of face you remembered. Almond-shaped eyes. Exotic thick black hair. Caramel-colored skin.

Lyn's mind jumped from Brekkie Bus circles to play-group circles to Michael's work—to sitting in Cat's car watching Angela tap on the car window, her face bent down, her ponytail falling to one side.

Oh God. Oh God. Oh God.

How had Gemma managed to orchestrate this disaster? Quietly, she maneuvered herself behind Cat and placed one protective hand over her shoulder. Had she recognized her yet?

"I'm Angela."

Lyn felt Cat's shoulder become rigid and her own chest constrict in sympathy.

Gemma, of course, had no control over her emotions and quite unnecessarily dropped a full glass of champagne on the floor.

Lyn stared stupidly at the broken glass and tried to think calmly. This was a genuinely appalling situation. Three women in the one room who had all slept with Daniel Whitford.

It was all so . . . unhygienic.

"I'll get a dustpan," said Maxine as Charlie and Angela simultaneously bent down to begin picking up shards of glass in careful cupped hands. The rest of the Kettle family watched with interest.

"Butterfingers!" Nana Kettle leaned over to tap Charlie on the shoulder. "Gemma is such a butterfingers! That's what we call her! Butterfingers!"

"I'm sorry," Gemma stood staring fearfully down at Angela, as if she was some sort of awful apparition.

"It's only a glass, sweetheart," said Frank, his eyes appreciative on Angela's legs. "I'm sure Lyn doesn't mind."

Lyn took a breath. She couldn't see Cat's face, only the top of her head. "Of course not. Please. Leave it. Charlie . . . Angela. I'll look after it." It felt like a betrayal to use Angela's name. She needed to get these people out of her house.

"We're admitting defeat on the cubby house." Michael appeared in the kitchen, followed by Dan. "Time for a drink."

"Have we had our first breakage?" said Dan. "Let me guess the culprit."

Angela looked up from the floor. "Danny!"

Danny?

Cat shrugged away Lyn's hand, stepped over the glass, and walked out of the kitchen, her face averted from Dan.

"Crosspatch!" Nana Kettle informed Charlie triumphantly. "That's what we call that one!"

Dan backed himself up against the fridge. He looked nauseous. "Hi there."

"So you two know each other, eh?" said Michael. Understanding swept his face as his eyes met Lyn's and his words trailed lamely. ". . . how about that."

Gemma looked imploringly at Lyn. Lyn massaged her forehead and watched Kara carefully pouring herself a very full glass of wine, one eye monitoring her father.

"Swim!" Maddie came running full tilt into the kitchen. She was stark naked and wearing her yellow plastic floaties on each arm.

"Lyn—bare feet!" warned Maxine at the same instant as Charlie swooped Maddie into the air away from the glass.

"Thank you."

"My pleasure."

Maddie patted the top of Charlie's closely shaven head approvingly, as if he were a furry animal. "Swim?" she inquired brightly, tipping her head birdlike to one side. "Come swim?"

"Maybe another day, sweetie," said Charlie.

Angela had gathered her composure. "I know Dan from the Greenwood pub," she told Charlie. "I got chatting to him that night Bec and I handed out your fridge magnets."

"Oh!" said Gemma. "That must be . . . oh."

"Yes?" Charlie put a hand on Gemma's shoulder and looked at her with gentle bemusement. Maddie tapped her finger on the end of his nose and giggled.

"I rang Cat the day I got locked out of the house," explained Gemma. She gave Cat's empty chair a nervous glance. "She said, There's a number for a locksmith right here on the fridge."

"Ha!" Dan was obviously trying to follow Angela's jolly lead, but he was looking slightly manic, punching his fist into his palm. "I remember. It was shaped like a key. I stuck it on the fridge when I got home from the pub. Didn't even think . . . about it. Good idea, magnets. Yep. Get your name in front of people. Well. You owe me, Gemma!"

Lyn wanted to smack him.

"Not as much as I owe you," said Charlie, jiggling Maddie in one arm and putting his free arm around Gemma. He gave Dan a thoughtful, appraising look and then turned back to Nana Kettle. "Gemma is the best thing that's ever happened to me."

Nana Kettle beamed up at him, her eyes shining though her glasses. "What a lovely young fellow! Isn't he, Frank? Maxine?"

Maxine straightened up from the floor with the dustpan full of broken glass. "Very lovely," she said. Her eyebrows were question marks. "You certainly saved Maddie's feet from getting cut to pieces."

"Good reflexes," contributed Michael overheartily.

There was a contemptuous "pfffff" sound from Kara's direction.

"Well. We'd better make a move." Charlie handed Maddie over to Lyn. "It was great to meet you all."

"Bye everybody," said Angela. For a moment her flawless performance seemed to falter. "Bye, Dan."

"Yeah." Dan examined his hands. "Yeah. Bye then."

"I'll see them out," said Gemma.

There was a moment's silence in the kitchen. The central characters had left the stage, leaving the supporting cast without a script.

"What was that all about?" asked Maxine, shaking glass into the rubbish bin. "You were all behaving like lunatics. And have you noticed your daughter is drinking like a fish, Michael?"

Michael looked with confusion at Maddie.

"I think she means me, Dad," Kara raised her wineglass cheerily. "Remember. You've got *two* daughters."

"Dan, shouldn't you be finding out what's wrong with Cat?" Maxine commanded.

"Yeah." Dan seemed to be suffering from post-traumatic stress syndrome. He opened the fridge door and stood staring at its contents. "I'll just take her up a beer."

"What?"

"Oh. Yeah. I'll just take one for me then."

He ambled from the kitchen, nearly colliding with Gemma, who looked up at him with something approaching hatred.

"Can I talk to you for a sec, Lyn?" she said in a strained tone. "Now?"

Lyn leaned up against the desk in her office. "Well. That was fun."

"I feel terrible." Gemma slumped into a chair and sat on her hands.

"It's not your fault. It's just bad luck. Although, of course, if you could have found a locksmith for yourself instead of calling Cat—"

If you weren't always so bloody helpless.

"Yes, I know. This is terrible."

"Yes."

"Charlie was talking the other night about his sister. He said she's been seeing—no, he said she's *involved* with a married man. That doesn't sound like a one-off."

"Maybe it's another married man. Maybe she makes a habit of it."

"She called him *Danny.*" Gemma shuddered.

Lyn picked up her container of paper clips and rattled it, hard. "Why would he tell Cat about Angela in the first place if he was going to keep seeing her?"

"I don't know."

"I could kill him."

"I know. When I saw him coming out of the kitchen then, I thought, I could punch you, I could close my fist and punch you properly."

Lyn looked down at her in-tray. There was a yellow Post-it note with a frantic message from her marketing coordinator—*Lyn! Problem! Please look at before Christmas!* She hadn't even seen it until now. Her stomach clenched instinctively.

"Lyn?" Gemma looked up at her trustingly and swiveled her chair back and forth. "What will we do? Do we tell her?"

Lyn twisted her head from side to side. I am suffering from stress, she thought. I am suffering from profound stress.

The thought made her feel better for some reason.

"What do *you* think we should do?"

Delegate, Michael was always saying. You've got to learn to delegate.

"I don't know."

This was why delegating didn't work.

Lyn said, "I think we should worry about it after Christmas. You can find out more from Charlie."

"O.K."

"What's going on in here?" Cat came into the study, flinging back the door and coming to lean against the desk next to Lyn. She took the jar of paper clips out of Lyn's hand and rattled it aggressively. The strands of hair around her face were damp. She must have washed her face, scrubbing away all the radiant happiness of that morning. The skin under her eyes looked sad and raw.

"Are you O.K.?" asked Gemma.

"Yes." Cat took a paper clip and bent and straightened it between her fingers. She didn't look at Gemma. "You'll just have to break up with him."

"Sorry?" Gemma stood up from her chair.

"You'll break up with him sooner or later anyway."

"But I like him. I really sort of like him."

"He's a locksmith, Gemma."

"So?"

"So, for some reason you get off on sleeping with, I don't know—*blokes.* But it's not like you're going to marry one of them."

"Oh my God," said Gemma. "I can't believe you said that. That's so snobbish! You sound like . . . you sound like Mum!"

The ultimate insult.

"I'm not saying you're better than them, I'm saying you're smarter than them."

"Cat." Now Lyn could feel stress, like a toxic chemical, flooding her bloodstream. "You can't expect her—"

"She'll find somebody else in five minutes. Somebody better. He's too short for her. He's not good enough for her. Besides which, she only *met* him because of Dan."

"Yes, but—"

"I want to forget about it. I want to forget about that girl. How can I forget about it when Gemma's dating her brother? The whole thing's a joke."

On the word "joke," there was a break in Cat's voice.

A tiny fracture of grief.

For a moment there was silence in the room.

"I'll think about it," said Gemma.

Lyn put her knuckle to her mouth and breathed in deeply. "But, Gemma—"

"I said I'll think about it." Gemma pushed her chair back in toward the desk. "She's right. We would have broken up eventually anyway. I'm going to take Maddie for a swim."

She left the room.

"It's too much to ask," said Lyn. "What if he's the one?"

Cat flicked the mangled paper clip across the room. "I can assure you, there is no such thing."

CHAPTER 11

I've ruined Cat's Christmas, thought Gemma, changing into her swimsuit in Michael and Lyn's bathroom. I am a bitch, a witch, a klutzy butterfingers.

"The problem with you, Gemma," Marcus used to say, "is you don't *concentrate.*"

She pulled up the straps of her swimmers and looked in Lyn's cupboard for sunscreen. The house was becoming hotter and hotter. Nana, to Maxine's disgust, had stripped down to her petticoat. Gemma's own face in Lyn's bathroom mirror was bright pink. She still had the piece of tinsel tied lopsided around her head, giving her a dopey, hopeful look.

Charlie, she realized now, had talked about his sister Angela, but she hadn't even mentally noted that the names were the same. They didn't feel the same. There was Angela, Charlie's younger sister, whom he obviously adored. Then, there was *Angela,* evil husband stealer.

The right thing to do was to break up with him.

It would be a noble gesture of triplet solidarity.

It would be a sisterly sacrifice.

It would be like going on a hunger strike.

"Charlie, ask your sister why I can't see you anymore. Ask her why she doesn't look for wedding rings before she starts flirting and breaking *my* sister's heart."

Ah, but Charlie.

Charlie, Charlie, Charlie.

The night before they'd had their own special Christmas Eve dinner on Charlie's balcony. They cooked it together. "You've just got this mental block about cooking," said Charlie. "Anybody can cook." And it turned out when she was a little bit drunk and there was a good CD playing, so she was sort of dancing while she was cooking, with a wineglass in one hand and a wooden spoon in the other, well, she was in fact a *spectacular* cook! It was a wonderful discovery.

He gave her perfume and a book for Christmas.

The Kettle girls were allergic to perfume, but she bravely dabbed it on her wrist and only sneezed eleven times in a row, spluttering in between each sneeze things like, "Hay fev-er!" "Gosh!" "Must!" "Be!" "Pollen!" "In!" "The!" "Air!"

When she finally stopped sneezing, she examined the book. "I've been wanting to read this!" she said, which wasn't a complete lie as she had wanted to read it, before she did read it, a few months ago.

"Actually," said Charlie, tugging on his ear, which was what he did when he felt a bit awkward or shy. (She already knew that about him. She already adored that about him.) "I don't know anything about it. I just bought it because the picture of the girl on the front cover reminded me of you. I don't know why."

The girl on the front cover looked like a whimsical princess, and there was something about her expression that secretly reminded Gemma a little of herself too. It was her best self. The self she would be on a tropical island, on a perfect day, wearing a floaty dress and possibly a straw hat. A day when she didn't sneeze or drink too much and nobody got offended or had to rush off and everybody got everybody else's jokes. A day when Gemma had no memories except the good ones. A day when everything was funny and fascinating just the way it should be.

It delighted her that Charlie could recognize *that* self.

Wasn't there some rule that said you had to marry that sort of man—fast?

She walked downstairs in her swimsuit and found Maddie, still naked and in her floaties, banging away on her xylophone. She was sitting on the sofa next to Nana, who was sloshing her bare feet around in a bucket of water.

"Oh good, Gemma!" said Nana. "I was just thinking. If I die in this heat, make sure they don't have the funeral next Wednesday. That's bingo day at the club. Everybody would be put out. Tell them to have it on Thursday."

"You're not going to die."

Nana looked offended. "How would you know, Miss Smarty-pants?"

"Why don't you come swimming with Maddie and me?"

"Because I don't want to, thank you very much."

Maddie tossed aside her xylophone with a clatter and threw her arms around Gemma's leg. "Swim!" At least someone was in a good mood.

Lyn and Michael's swimming pool was magnificent, a curving turquoise shell with glittering views that made you feel like you were swimming in the harbor.

"Gem! Look!" demanded Maddie. She leaned forward with her bottom sticking out behind her in imitation of a grown-up's dive, her head squashed between upstretched arms. Then she launched herself into the pool, landing splat on her tummy. Her floaties kept her bobbing on the surface.

Gemma dived in next to her and swam along the bottom of the pool, feeling the voluptuous relief of immersion in a silent, cold, chlorinated world.

But it wasn't as if she were in love with Charlie or even in a relationship yet.

They didn't have nicknames, private jokes, photos of happier times, or joint friends who would be shocked and sad. No forthcoming social events. No joint purchases. It would be painless and clean. Just one sharp slice of the knife: "Charlie, I'm sure you understand. You're Italian after all. Family comes first."

"Look, Gem! Look!"

Maddie waded up the stairs and out of the pool, water dripping, and stood on the edge of the pool with her arms held high. She looked like a slippery little seal.

"Ooooh!" applauded Gemma as Maddie did a star jump into the pool and bobbed back up to the surface, gasping and choking, her hair flat across her face. She seemed to be under the impression that other people swam only for the pleasure of seeing her perform various awe-inspiring tricks.

"Maybe you could try and shut your mouth next time," suggested Gemma. "You'll swallow less water."

Maddie patted the surface of the water with flat palms, so that drops of water flew in her eyes, and gave a loud chuckle, to indicate she was being funny now.

"Ha!" cried Gemma, splashing herself in an equally hilarious manner, while she thought about what Cat had said in Lyn's office: "She'll break up with him eventually, anyway."

She wasn't joking or being sarcastic. She said it as if it were a fact. She thought it was inevitable. Of course, the two of them had been teasing her for years about her growing accumulation of ex-boyfriends. Lyn had even given her a book called *Ten Stupid Things Women Do to Mess Up Their Lives* and helpfully indicated with a Post-it note the chapter on the stupid thing she believed Gemma was doing. But still, Gemma had thought, rather idiotically she now realized, that they were as surprised as she was each time she broke up with another boyfriend.

Perhaps they already knew what Gemma secretly feared, that she wasn't actually capable of genuine, serious love. Sure, she was capable of an infatuation, like the one she was currently experiencing with Charlie, but they were right, it probably wouldn't last.

For weeks, sometimes months, she adored her men—and then

one day, without warning, it hit her. Not only was she over the infatuation, she actively *disliked* the guy. She remembered sitting on a beach with the plumber who liked country music.

"Where's the bottle opener?" he said, frowning and scrabbling through their basket.

And that was it. I don't like you, she thought, and it was like an icy cold breeze whistling around her bones.

Some people lacked hand-eye coordination. Some people were tone-deaf.

Gemma lacked the ability to stay in love with somebody.

"Gem! Look!"

"Ooooh!"

They sat down to eat Christmas lunch at the long table on Lyn and Michael's balcony. The table was set beautifully with tasteful Christmas decorations, the harbor glinted beside them, and the sun reflected rainbows in the crystal of the glasses.

It seemed to Gemma that the setting called for another, more functional, better-dressed family—especially today, when everybody had red faces and there was a discernible bubbling of hysteria just below the surface.

There were loud pops and insults as people pulled at their Christmas crackers far too aggressively. Cat and Dan nearly wrenched each other's arms off. People began to read out the jokes inside their paper crowns in loud sarcastic voices. Nobody listened except for Michael, who genuinely found them funny, and Nana Kettle, who kept missing the punch lines. "Eh? What did the elephant say?"

Maxine and Frank sat next to each other, which was a disconcerting sight. In fact, Gemma couldn't remember the last time she'd seem them sitting together. They seemed to be overcompensating by being excessively animated and polite to each other.

Kara was tipsy.

Maddie sat in her high chair, singing a loud toneless song to herself. She had to tilt her head up because her green paper crown was too big for her and had fallen down over her nose.

Gemma herself had slipped into full-on giggly, girlish Gemma. She could hear herself talking nonstop. Chatter. Chatter. Ha, ha, ha. Shut up, she thought, shut up for God's sake, but it seemed she was trapped in her own inane party personality.

As food began to circulate around the table, Lyn and Maxine both hovered just slightly above their seats, ignoring their own empty plates, hands poised like frenzied conductors, ready to pounce triumphantly on any unmet requirement.

"Nana, have some salad dressing!" ordered Lyn.

"Cat, pass your father the turkey!" called out Maxine.

It was a mystery to Gemma why they cared so much. Nobody was hungry. It was too hot.

"More wine anybody?" asked Frank.

"Yes, please, just a little drop, thank you, Frank," slurred Kara in a fake elegant tone and dissolved into hysterical giggles, slumping across the table.

"Would someone take her glass away?" implored Michael.

Maxine said, "I warned you hours ago she was drinking too much."

"A little drop won't hurt her." Frank leaned over with the wine bottle.

Lyn snapped, "Dad! She's fifteen!"

"Well, you three could sure put away the booze when you were fifteen."

"You see, I've always had an interest in lepers," Nana Kettle told Dan.

"I beg your pardon?" Dan looked dazed. His paper crown was leaving a stain of red across his forehead.

"Lepers!" chimed in Gemma. "Nana has always had an interest in lepers. It means your present is probably a donation on your behalf to the Leper Foundation. That's what she gave Michael last year. Don't you remember, Dan? We couldn't stop laughing."

"Gemma! Now you've ruined the surprise!" said Nana Kettle crossly. "Goodness me! Don't listen to her, Michael."

"I'm Dan."

"I know perfectly well who you are, Dan, for goodness' sake."

Nana Kettle turned to Gemma."I told that new young man of yours you were a butterfingers! Did you hear me?"

"I did hear you, Nana."

"I think he agreed with me. He seemed a very sensible fellow, don't you think, Dan?"

Dan's hands clenched tight around his knife and fork. "Very sensible."

"His sister was a pretty girl," observed Nana Kettle. *"Very* pretty girl. All that lovely dark hair. Don't you think, Gemma?"

Silently Gemma shrieked, *Shut up, Nana!* I will have to break up with him, she thought, I will. Her eyes were drawn irresistibly to Cat.

"She was gorgeous, Nana." Cat's face was hard. "Absolutely gorgeous. Don't you think, Dan?"

"Oh, Christ." Dan put down his knife and fork and dropped his head in his hands.

"Headache, dear?" asked Nana sympathetically.

There was a noise down the end of the table. Frank stood up and carefully tapped his fork against his glass.

He grinned self-consciously, boyishly, as everyone turned to face him. "I've got an announcement to make. It's going to come as a bit of a surprise."

"Good news, I hope," said Michael with a hint of desperation. His purple crown was balanced precariously on his springy new haircut.

"Oh very good, Mike, mate. Very good."

Gemma was barely listening to her father. She was wondering whether Dan really was having an affair with Angela, and if he was, then what? The thought of lugging around a secret of that magnitude made her feel ill. She was in the middle of giving Dan a private, powerful death stare to convey, "If you are having an affair, I know you are and you'd better stop," when her father's words penetrated her consciousness.

"Maxine and I are dating again."

Maxine and I are dating again.

Nobody said a word. From the house, the saccharine sounds of Michael's Christmas CD became audible. Sleigh bells rang and somebody dreamed of a white Christmas.

Kara hiccuped.

"You're *dating*." Cat leaned forward to look down the length of the table at Frank and Maxine.

"We've been seeing each other socially for quite some time now of course," said Maxine in a voice that sounded bizarrely too young for her, like one she'd put on to imitate what *a very rude young girl* had said to her in the supermarket. "And a few months ago we began a—well, I guess you could call it, a relationship."

"I think I'm going to be sick." Cat pushed away her plate.

"We didn't want to tell you earlier, until we knew for sure." Frank placed a hearty, proprietary hand on Maxine's shoulder. Maxine looked up at him, her face flushed with girlish color.

"Sure of what?" asked Lyn faintly.

"Well. Sure that we were in love. Again, of course."

"I *am* going to be sick," said Cat.

"Excuse me," Lyn stood up. "Excuse me for a minute." She threw down her napkin and walked off the veranda, pulling on the glass sliding door unnecessarily hard.

"Goodness me, you girls are crotchety today!" said Nana Kettle.

"But this is good news!" Frank put his wineglass down and leaned forward with his hands clutching the sides of the table, a perplexed frown creasing his forehead. "You're happy for us, aren't you, Gemma?"

"I'm very happy for you," said Gemma truthfully, but she had that slightly off-balance feeling she used to get when she was at school and Cat or Lyn gave a teacher a different answer from the one she would have given. No, she'd think. I'm sure that's not right. But how could we have got it wrong?

When their father first moved out of the house at Killara and into his new flat in the city, six-year-old Gemma wasn't particularly concerned.

In her mind it was somehow vaguely linked to his blown-off finger from Cracker Night. It was like when she or one of her sisters got sick. They had to move into the little room next to Mum and Dad's with the sofa that turned into a bed. That was so your nasty germs didn't float up your sisters' nostrils.

Probably Daddy had to sleep somewhere else for a little while because he didn't want to infect anybody with his horrible sick finger.

"But Mum and Dad sat us down in the lounge room and *told* us they were getting a divorce," said Cat and Lyn, years afterward, when she told them her childhood theory. "How could you forget that? It was awful. Mum was doing this weird twisting thing with her hands, and Dad kept bouncing up from his seat and walking around the room and then sitting back down again. We were so mad at them."

"I was probably thinking about something else at the time," said Gemma.

It had happened at intervals throughout her life: a piece of news of major social, political, or personal significance somehow slipped right past her.

When she was aged around ten, she asked her sisters, "What's an 'abba'?" They were staggered.

"Abba is a band!" cried Lyn. "A really famous, cool band!"

"Be careful what you say in front of people," advised a shaken Cat. "You'd better check with us before you say *anything*."

The first time Gemma registered the "divorce" word was the day they found out they were going on the fastest water slide in the world. The whole family was in the kitchen and Maxine was bent down by the oven, lifting up the corner of the foil to check on a yummy roast chicken. There had been a complicated incident involving Cat and a Barbie doll, and Gemma was just about to launch into a detailed account when Frank announced, "Lyn's staying here with Mum for the holiday."

Gemma took one look at the secretive expression on Lyn's face and instantly grasped the situation. A similar event had occurred at school just the other day when she went to buy an Icy Pole at the tuck shop. When she came back, Gemma's best friend, Rosie, had recruited Melinda as her new best friend. In the space of two minutes alliances had shifted!

Quite obviously, Mum wanted Lyn to be her best friend! She always did have a noticeable preference for Lyn. It was because she tucked in the corners so tidily when she made the bed and didn't drop stuff. Now they were going to have their very own little holiday together. They'd probably start whispering and giggling together at the dinner table. It would be awful.

The only solution was to get Mum and Lyn to come on holidays too. Surely Mum didn't want to miss going on the fastest water slide in the world!

But no. No, that couldn't happen; that was a typical laughable Gemma idea because Mum and Dad were getting a "divorce"—an ugly-tasting word, very similar to "zucchini."

And that was when one of Gemma's worst secret fears came thumping to the surface.

Cat and Lyn had recently decided to inform Gemma that she was adopted. They were a little surprised she hadn't worked it out for herself.

"If you were really our sister you'd look like us," said Cat with rock-solid logic. "Triplets are meant to all look the same."

"We still love you like a real sister," said Lyn kindly. "It's not your fault. But you have to do what we say."

"No, Gemma, you're not adopted, for heaven's sake," said

Maxine as Gemma cried into her lap. "Your sisters are liars—they take after their father."

But she was never really quite convinced, and when she heard that ugly "divorce" word in the kitchen that day, the enormity of what was about to happen stunned her. It was like that movie *The Parent Trap* they'd seen at Nana's place, where the divorced parents each took one little blond girl. There was no little redheaded girl in the movie.

Clearly, Mum was going to take Lyn, and Dad was going to take Cat. Neither of them would want Gemma because she was adopted.

What would happen to her? Where would she live? What would she eat for dinner? She didn't know how to cook a chicken! She didn't even know how to *buy* a chicken. What did you say? One chicken, please? What if they laughed at her? How much did a chicken cost anyway? She only had $3.00 saved up. That would probably buy her only, say, ten chickens. After that, she would be so hungry!

Six-year-old Gemma felt dizzy as she struggled not to collapse under the weight of everything she didn't know. Her parents and sisters receded into the distance. She was a tiny penciled dot on a huge white sheet of paper. There was only her and she reached only as far as the tips of her fingers and the tips of her toes and beyond that there was nothing.

She didn't even notice Barbie's head roll out of her unclenched hand and onto the floor.

Diving like Dolphins

It drives me bananas the way women tiptoe into the surf, flinching each time another body part gets wet. Look at 'em. Flapping their hands, scrunching up their faces. It takes them three hours to get their hair wet. And when there's more than one of them, it's even worse. Squealing and bleating and backing up and inching forward and backing up again. I ask you, what is the bloody point?

When I was about fifteen, the age when I was just starting to worry if a girl would ever deign to sleep with me, I saw these three girls sun-baking down at Freshwater Beach. They were probably about eighteen, and they were gorgeous. Legs up to their armpits. Athletic-looking. I was giving them the surreptitious once-over from behind my reflective Miami Vice shades, when all of a sudden the three of them jumped up and ran down into the surf. They got to about their knees in the water and then they dived under at exactly the same moment. That's what got me. Their synchronicity. It was bloody sexy for some reason. Three bodies suspended in midair, like dolphins.

If only those girls knew how many nights they spent with me and a box of Kleenex under the duvet. Ah, the fun we shared that year. I was fair, of course. All three of them got the treatment.

Anyway, I always swore I'd marry a woman who ran straight into the ocean, like they did.

I didn't of course. Would you bloody look at her? Get in, woman! Stop being such a girl!

CHAPTER 12

"Hello, you," said Charlie. "Happy Boxing Day."

He held his front door open with his foot and placed his hands on her cheeks to kiss her.

"Mmm." Every time Gemma kissed Charlie, she accidentally said "Mmm" as if she'd just taken her first mouthful of an unexpectedly delightful dessert.

Was it physically possible to break up with someone who tasted like that?

"I've been *very* domestic this morning," she said when he finally let her go and pulled her inside. "I've made us a proper picnic—and I've put it all in my backpack so I can sling it jauntily over my shoulders."

She spun in a circle to show him, faintly aware that she was deliberately being cute and charming.

The plan was to ride up on Charlie's bike to watch the start of the Sydney to Hobart.

The other plan, Lyn's plan, was for Gemma to ascertain whether Dan was having an affair with Angela. "Just find out what's going on," said Lyn. "But don't break it off. She's got no right to ask that."

Charlie stood back and surveyed her.

"I'm overwhelmed by your jauntiness. I'm also overwhelmed by the fact that you think you're coming on the bike wearing those shorts."

Gemma looked down at her bare legs. "Oh."

"Sorry. Not prepared to risk those very sexy legs."

She lifted one leg and pointed her sneakered toe like a ballet dancer. "We're vain about our legs. We got them from Mum."

"We?" Charlie raised an eyebrow. "Is this like the royal we?"

"My sisters."

"To be honest I'm only interested in *your* legs—not your sisters'."

"Speaking of sisters—"

His tone changed. "Let's not."

"Our worlds collide."

"Yes."

"This is a bit awkward." Gemma clutched the straps of her jaunty backpack.

"Oh well. Let's talk about something less awkward."

"Cat wants me to break up with you."

Charlie became very still.

"Cat was the one who stormed off? She's Dan's wife?"

"Yes."

"Do *you* want to break up? Because don't just use this—this thing—as an excuse. If you want to finish it, finish it."

"No. I don't want to finish it. It's nice. I like your eyelashes."

His shoulders relaxed. "Good." He smiled. "I like your legs."

"Is Angela having an affair with Dan?"

Charlie scrunched up his face in comical pain. "I really don't want to do this conversation. Can't we just go have a nice picnic and forget about our siblings?"

"We really have to do it." A pleasing touch of Lyn-type authority.

He sighed. "We didn't talk about it much because to be honest I didn't want to hear. Even though it was obvious something *very* strange was going on in that kitchen. But yes, she did have something going with him. I don't know how many times they saw each other. But he definitely ended it when his wife, your sister, got pregnant."

His wife. Cat was someone's wife who got pregnant. Gemma could see Cat sitting on the bathroom floor, looking up at her, pretending so hard not to care about the results of the pregnancy test—and visibly trembling. She was shaking all over, and she didn't even seem aware of it. And now Dan had put her in a situation where she was described as *the wife who got pregnant.*

That slimy scoundrel.

"She swears that it's definitely over," continued Charlie. "I believe her. She doesn't want to break up a marriage."

Gemma didn't say anything. She was busy punching Dan in the stomach.

"I thought about giving her a Chinese Burn," offered Charlie.

"Humph."

"If it makes you feel better, she's really upset about the whole thing."

"She's upset!"

"Jeez." Charlie held up his palms in surrender. "I know. Look, the real offender here is Dan the Man. I didn't like him the moment I saw him."

"Didn't you?" asked Gemma, momentarily diverted.

"Nope. Arrogant prick."

"Are you absolutely positive it's over?"

"Positive."

"Absolutely positive?"

"Absolutely. Look. It doesn't need to come between us, does it?"

"No."

Jesus, Mary—and Cat—willing.

"Because I think we could be good." He wound his fingers around the straps of her backpack and jiggled her back and forth.

"Do you?" There was that melting-caramel feeling again.

"Oooh yeah. I think we could really go places . . . Like North Head, for example. Like right now."

"Let's go then."

"Oh." Charlie stopped as he went to pick up the two helmets from the hallway. "One thing I wanted to ask you."

"Yes?"

"Angie said she remembers seeing the three of you outside her flat. You're not planning on stalking her, are you?"

Gemma felt the tips of her ears become mildly warm. "That was a one-off."

"Good. Because she's still my little sister. Even if she does stupid things."

"Well. Yes." A spark of embarrassed resentment.

She wore a pair of Charlie's jeans for the ride up to North Head. At each set of lights he put one hand back and caressed her leg. She squeezed her thighs around his hips and the top of her helmet clunked romantically against his. At North Head they found a space among the crowds for their blanket and cheered as the ocean became a frothy highway of busily zigzagging yachts, their sails blossoming in the breeze.

"Doesn't get better than this, does it?" said a man sitting next to them.

"Well, it could do," began Gemma thoughtfully.

"No, mate, it doesn't," interrupted Charlie, and he put his hand across her mouth, like an elder brother. She'd always dreamed—somewhat incestuously—of a lovely, protective, bossy older brother.

Once the boats had disappeared off the horizon, they went for a snorkel on Shelley Beach. It was a glimmery, hazy hot day and the water was dappled green. They saw darting shoals of tiny, iridescent fish and sleepy cod slithering mysteriously in and out of rocky hiding places. The rhythmic kick of Charlie's flippers created clouds of translucent bubbles and Gemma thought, At this particular moment, I am entirely happy. She felt his hand on her shoulder and lifted her head and trod water. He pulled his snorkel from his mouth and pointed downward, his animated face squashed by his mask, like a ten-year-old. "Giant *stingray!*" Then he shoved his snorkel back into his mouth and dived down deep to see it. Gemma followed him and swallowed a gigantic mouthful of salt water when she saw the size of the alien creature flapping its way along the sandy bottom.

Afterward, when they were making banana smoothies in the cool of Charlie's kitchen, she said, "Have you always lived in Australia?"

"Apart from when I was twenty—I lived in Italy for nearly a year, with my mum's family." He scooped ice cream into the blender. "They come from a little village in the mountains on the east coast of Italy. I'll take you there one day. My aunties will try and feed you up and my cousins will try and feel you up. Ha."

He was always doing that—talking as if they had a future.

Gemma watched him press the button on his blender. She licked her lips and tasted salt.

"You know what's funny about you?" she said suddenly. "It's like you're always on holiday. You're like a tourist. A happy one."

(When Charlie got dressed, he sort of *jumped* into his jeans or shorts. She didn't tell him that. She didn't want him to get self-conscious about it, or stop it.)

"That's because I'm with you. That's the effect you have on me."

"No it's not. I bet you're always like that. I bet you were born like that. One of those fat, gurgly little babies. Baby Charlie!"

"I hate to disappoint you, but I wasn't even called Charlie. My real name is *Carluccio*. It was my friend Paul who started calling me Charlie. Have I told you about him?"

Something about the expression on his face made Gemma think, Uh-oh, he's about to *share*. It was lovely of course, but she had a terrible habit of laughing in the wrong places when boyfriends got profound.

She tried to look meaningful. "No. Tell me."

Charlie handed her a tall frothy glass.

"He lived across the road from me. I don't even remember meeting him, he was just always there. We did everything together. You know the sort of adventures kids have together. Going places on our bikes. Finding stuff. Building stuff. Anyway. When we were fifteen, Paul died."

"Oh!" Gemma just managed to stop herself from dropping her smoothie. "Oh dear!"

"He died of an asthma attack in the middle of the night. His mum found him, with his inhaler still in hand. Teenage boys don't handle grief very well. The day of his funeral I punched a hole in my bedroom wall. My knuckles bled. My dad plastered it up and gave me a little pat on the shoulder."

"Poor, poor Charlie." She could just imagine his shattered, boyish face.

"It's O.K., no need for violins. Drink your smoothie, please. The thing about Paul was that he was always so enthusiastic about things. I was the laid-back one, the one who was hard to impress. He was always saying, Oh man, that's so cool! He'd see a blue-tongued lizard and he'd be down on his hands and knees with his eyes bulging just like the Crocodile Hunter and I'd be like Yeah, yeah', but secretly just as excited. When he was gone, I really missed that. So, one day, I decided, I'd *pretend* to be like Paul. When I saw a good movie or caught a great wave, I'd say to myself, Oh man, Charlie, that's so cool! It was like I was wearing one of Paul's old shirts. At first I was faking it, just to feel better. But then I wasn't faking it anymore. It was like a habit. So, blame Paul. He gave me my name and my personality."

"Lovely name. Lovely personality."

Charlie drained his glass and peered at the bottom as if he was trying to find something.

"What about your fiancé who died?" he asked, without looking at her. "That must have been pretty bad."

"Yes, it must have been," said Gemma, imagining how Charlie must be imagining her, young, in love, devastated. "I mean, yes, it was."

"And nobody else has managed to get a ring on your finger since him. Is that because nobody can live up to his standards?"

"Nobody can live up to *my* standards."

"Oh I see. And it's always you who does the breaking up?"

"Yes. I can't seem to break that six-month mark."

"I see." Charlie nodded his head wisely and pretended to peer at her over invisible glasses, while judicially stroking an invisible beard. *"Very* interesting. Why don't we move into my office and discuss this."

He took her by the hand and led her out to his living room. She lay down flat on the couch, only to find that her psychiatrist was lying on top of her, explaining that he had diagnosed her condition and was ready to administer treatment. Yes, it *was* considered rather unorthodox in certain circles, but he could assure her it was highly effective.

She just needed to lie very still.

"Say something in Italian to me."

"Io non vado via."

"What's it mean?"

"It means I'm going to break the six-month mark."

To: Gemma; Cat
From: Lyn
Subject: The Parents
Do you two want to get together some time to discuss the above? Maybe brunch at Bronte? Michael's mother has got Maddie all day Wed. if you're free.
I am blown away by this. L.

To: Lyn; Gemma
From: Cat
Subject: The Parents
Fine with me. I'll come straight from the joys of marriage counseling.

The parents' little love fest is completely nauseating.
Gemma—have you dumped the locksmith yet?

To: Lyn; Cat
From: Gemma
Subject: The Parents
He's not the LOCKSMITH—he's CHARLIE—and I said I would
THINK about it and that's what I'm still doing.
P.S. Wednesday is fine with me for brunch. I think it's NICE that
Mum and Dad are dating. What's wrong with you two??

Before the day Marcus went flying across Military Road, Gemma
had been living with him in his very expensive, very tidy Potts
Point flat for close to two years. It never felt like home. She just
slept at Marcus's place every night of the week.

Cat and Lyn came to stay with her the night before the
funeral.

Lyn was tanned gold from her interrupted holiday in Europe,
with jet-lagged circles under her eyes. She'd been gone for nearly
a year and her hair was longer and she was wearing an entire out-
fit Gemma had never seen before. Even her shoes were different.

"I love those shoes! Are they Italian?" asked Gemma.

"Don't even think about it," said Lyn automatically, and then
she looked stricken and said, "Or you can borrow them if you
want." Gemma said, "O.K. I will" and clomped around the flat in
Lyn's shoes and waited for her to say, "Walk properly! You're doing
your weird walk, you're going to ruin them!" but Lyn just smiled in
a strained, interested way and Gemma thought, My God, how long
are they going to keep this up for?

It made Gemma feel queasy, how nice they were being to her.
They were both speaking in strangely proper voices and every
now and then she'd catch them staring at her, almost as if they
were frightened.

Perhaps she was behaving oddly for someone with a dead

fiancé. She probably was, because she felt very odd. Extremely odd.

It was his *absence* that confused her. How could a tall, strong, definite man like Marcus just not be there anymore? She kept pushing the idea around in her head, trying to make sense of it. Marcus is dead. Marcus is dead. I will never see him again. Marcus is gone. Gone forever. A giant hand had reached down into her world and ripped out a large shred of her reality. It gave her vertigo.

Gemma's only other experience with death had been Nana Leonard but she'd been such a frail, unassuming presence. There was no gaping hole left when she died, she just gently slipped away, leaving the world pretty much as it had been. But Marcus? Marcus was big, booming, and *definite.* That's what she loved about him. You would never say to Marcus, "Are you sure?" because it would be a stupid question. Marcus had opinions and plans and a car and furniture. Marcus had a strong libido and strong political views. He could do one hundred push-ups without breaking a sweat.

Marcus must be very angry about not being there anymore.

"Yeah, mate, I don't *think* so." That's what he said on the phone when he disagreed with somebody. He wouldn't agree with dying. "Yeah, mate, I don't *think* so," he'd be saying at the Pearly Gates. "Let me speak to the manager. We'll straighten this out."

If Marcus wasn't there, how could Gemma still be there?

She looked down at her own feet in Lyn's Italian shoes and felt very, very weird.

"I feel weird," she said.

"Well, you would," said Cat.

"It's perfectly normal," said Lyn.

And they both looked petrified.

Gemma watched her sisters pinching their bottom lips in exactly the same way and realized she couldn't possibly confess to them the dreadful, blasphemous thought that had come into her head just before she went running across the road to see if Marcus was O.K. It would distress them. Even if they said, "Oh no, that doesn't mean anything! Don't worry about it! It was probably just the shock!" Gemma would know they were lying.

They would think of her differently forever. She had been hoping they could somehow make it right—but they couldn't. Of course they couldn't.

She put her hands up to her face, and now finally she was behaving properly. Both her sisters sprang to her side.

"Would you like a cup of tea?" asked Lyn, smoothing a lock of Gemma's hair behind her ear, like she was a little child. "And bun? More bun?"

"No, thank you."

Cat patted her arm nervously. "Would you like to get drunk?"

"Yes please. Or no. I know. High."

"Sorry?"

"Marcus has got some dope. It's in the cupboard above the stove."

So that's how they spent the night before Marcus's funeral.

Lyn rolled a beautiful neat joint and they sat cross-legged on his clean creamy carpet and passed it around, without saying a word. Gemma felt a satisfying rush of nothingness filling and expanding her brain.

"No wedding now," she observed finally, as she passed the joint to Lyn.

Lyn narrowed her eyes as she inhaled and the tip of the joint burned brightly. "That's right. No wedding."

Gemma said, "You won't get to wear your bridesmaid dresses."

"No," agreed Lyn, coughing a bit as she passed the joint to Cat.

"You hated your dresses, didn't you?"

They sat with very upright backs and exchanged solemn looks.

"Yes, we did hate them," Cat said slowly. "We really did."

And that's when they all started to giggle, wildly, rapturously, rocking back and forth with tears of hysteria running down their faces. Gemma watched Cat drop a piece of ash on Marcus's pristine carpet and imagined his face twisting with rage. She got onto her hands and knees and still sobbing with laughter, she crawled over to the piece of ash and used the tip of her finger to rub it hard against the cream wool.

"You're making it worse," said Lyn.

"I know." She rubbed her finger back and forth, harder and harder, smearing the black smudge across the carpet.

She never told anybody the thought that came into her head, the moment after Marcus collided with the concrete, while she was waiting for someone to tell her what to do, before she started running.

She didn't think it so much, as hear it, with bell-like clarity, as if a sober person had walked into a drunken, noisy party, snapped off the music, and made an announcement in the sudden, stunned silence.

She recognized her own voice. Four clear, cool, precise words:

"I hope he's dead."

CHAPTER 13

Between the ages of two and three, the Kettle triplets began to babble to each other in their own secret, unintelligible dialect, switching effortlessly to English whenever they needed to communicate with a grown-up.

Years later, Maxine discovered this was a relatively common phenomenon among multiples, known as "twin talk" or more impressively—idioglossia. (At the time, all she really cared about was that they weren't attempting to drown, suffocate, or bludgeon one another.)

Gradually, they talked less and less in their secret language and eventually it was erased from their memories, vanished like the lost language of an ancient tribe.

Psychic connections between twins and triplets are another well-documented and exciting phenomenon. In this area, however, the Kettle girls have always lagged. The idea, after all, is to *feel* your sibling's pain, not laugh uproariously at it. Elvis, before he went onstage, was able to feel the presence of his dead twin brother, Jesse. Yet nine-year-old Gemma, immersed in her new Enid Blyton book, couldn't even sense the stealthy presence of her very much alive sisters stealing a bag of mixed lollies from right next to her hand.

When they were eleven, Cat became obsessed with the idea of telepathic communication. Many hours were spent on complex experiments. Unfortunately, they all failed, due to the appalling incompetence of her sisters, who could neither send nor receive a coherent message.

No, the Kettle girls share no psychic connections. (A lot of the time they don't even understand each other in ordinary verbal, sitting-across-the-table conversation.)

And so:

At nineteen, Lyn's chin slams into her steering wheel in a car accident caused by a very drunk driver on the Spit Bridge. Gemma feels nothing, not the tiniest twinge, as she dances seductively in a dark, smoky club on Oxford Street, a frangipani in her ear, a cigarette between her fingers. And Cat doesn't even pause for breath in screaming at her computer, which keeps crashing while she tries to finish an overdue uni assignment.

At twenty-two, Marcus whispers vicious threats into Gemma's ear, and Cat senses nothing as she breathlessly wrestles with Dan while just outside the door his flat mate laughs heartily at *Hey, Hey It's Saturday*. And Lyn is far away in another time zone and another season and doesn't look up from suspiciously reading the label on a can of deodorant in a London chemist.

And at thirty-three, Cat rocks back and forth, back and forth, as her abdomen knots and locks and she silently screams, Stop it, stop it, stop it. Lyn feels nothing but pleasure as she watches Maddie's awestruck face illuminated by the colors of fireworks thundering across the sky. And Gemma feels nothing but Charlie's tongue and taste as she kisses him in the hallway of some friend of a friend's New Year's Eve party.

No, neither of them feels a thing until the first day of the New Year when Dan calls to say, "Cat's lost the baby."

CHAPTER 14

"Tell them I don't want to see anybody," Cat told Dan. Gemma, Lyn, and Maxine all agreed that was understandable and a good idea but obviously it didn't apply to *them,* and so they all arrived separately within fifteen minutes, running up the flat stairs, striding inside, breathless and flushed. When they saw Cat, they stopped and crumpled as if they thought just by coming they could fix things and seeing her made them realize there was nothing to be done and nothing to be said.

They squashed themselves shoulder to shoulder around Cat's little round kitchen table to drink cups of tea and eat fat pieces of iced walnut bun with lots of butter—Kettle family comfort food. Cat ate hers ravenously. It was what they ate when Pop Kettle died and when Marcus died a few months later.

The difference was that everybody knew Pop and Marcus. Nobody knew Cat's baby. Her baby didn't have the dignity of a name, or even a gender.

It was just a nothing. Cat had loved a nothing. How foolish of her.

"We'll try again," said Dan solemnly and determinedly at the hospital, as if the baby was a goal they'd just missed kicking and if they really put their minds to it they'd get it next time. As if babies were interchangeable.

"I wanted *this* baby," said Cat, and the nurse and Dan nodded their heads patiently and kindly, as if she were delirious.

"Darling! It was Mother Nature's way of telling you that something wasn't right with the poor little mite," said Nana Kettle on the phone. "At least you weren't far along." Cat said through a clenched jaw, "I have to go now, Nana."

Mother Nature can go fuck herself, she thought. It was my baby, not hers.

Cat stuffed bun into her mouth and looked at Lyn standing up to pour everybody's tea.

The heartbreakingly perfect curve of Maddie's cheek.

The ugly little ball of bloody tissue that was Cat's baby.

They took it away, with bland efficient medical faces, like it was something disgusting, like something from a science fiction movie that had been removed from Cat's body and now had to be quickly removed from everybody's sight, as a matter of good taste.

Nobody cooed in wonder over Cat's baby. Cat's hands trembled at the injustice. Only she knew how beautiful her baby would have been.

She had always suspected that deep within her, there was a secret seam of ugliness, of unseemliness, of something *wrong* that was the mirror of Lyn's right. And now her poor little innocent baby had been contaminated by her wrongness.

"Where's Maddie?" she asked.

"Michael," Lyn answered quickly, leaning over to pour Cat's tea. "You're not going back to work tomorrow. You'll have some time off?"

"Dunno."

Gemma gulped at her tea, her eyes anxiously on Cat.

Cat said to her, "You're doing that slurping thing."

"Sorry."

Sometimes Gemma got a particular expression on her face—a quivering pathetic puppy look—that aroused in Cat a powerful urge to kick or slap or verbally crush her. Then she felt racked with guilt. Then she felt angrier still.

I am not a nice person, she thought. I never have been. "You're an *evil, nasty* little girl, Catriona Kettle," Sister Elizabeth Mary informed her one day in the primary-school playground, the black band of her veil squeezed around puffy, red-veined cheeks. Cat felt an uplifting rush of wild courage, like she was about to run off the edge of the highest diving board at the swimming pool. "Well, you're an evil *fat* nun!" Sister Elizabeth grabbed her by the upper arm and slapped the back of her legs. Slap, slap, slap. Veil flying. Hefty shoulder heaving. Kids stopped to stare in sick fascination. Lyn and Gemma came running from opposite sides of the playground. "Oh!" moaned Gemma in sympathetic synchrony with each slap, "Oh!" until Sister couldn't stand it anymore and stomped off, after pointing a silent, quavering finger of warning at each of the three Kettle girls.

"You should certainly *not* go back to work tomorrow, Cat," said Maxine. "Don't be ridiculous. You need your rest. Dan can call work for you, can't you, Dan?"

Dan had his mouth full of bun. "Yeah," he said thickly, putting his hand over his mouth. "Course."

He'd been so gentle and loving last night—as if she were very ill, or as if she'd experienced some painful injury. He played the role of understanding, supportive husband to perfection—so handsome, so caring! But he was playing it wrong. Cat wanted him angry and irrational. She wanted him scornful and aggressive with the doctor: Wait a minute, this is our child, how the hell did this happen? But no, he was all understanding masculine nods as the doctor talked, two logical, reasonable men discussing such a— sadly!—common occurrence.

"I might leave you all for a bit, if that's O.K. with you, Cat?" Dan stood up and took his mug over to the sink.

"Fine." Cat looked down at her plate. "Whatever."

"Where are you going?" asked Gemma.

"Just out, got a few things to do." Dan kissed Cat on top of her head. "Are you O.K., babe?"

"I'm fine. I'm perfectly fine."

Had there been a sharp edge to Gemma's tone? There was something uncharacteristic about her asking Dan where he was going. Cat looked at Gemma, who was sitting cross-legged on her chair, twisting a long lock of hair around her finger. Did she know something? Had she got more sordid details from the locksmith about the one-night stand that Cat didn't know about? Did Cat even care? It all seemed irrelevant and childish now. She didn't even care if Gemma kept going out with the brother. What did it matter? When it came down to it, what did anything really matter?

"Gemma," she said.

"Yes?" Gemma nearly dropped her slice of bun in her eagerness to be accommodating. She picked up the milk hopefully. "Milk?"

"Just forget what I said on Christmas Day. You know. About Charlie. I should never have said that. I was upset."

There. Now she had redeemed herself for wanting to kick her.

"Oh. Well. That's O.K. I mean, who knows? You know, my relationships never seem to last longer than a few months these days. So probably we will break up but it's all going well at the moment, so if you—"

"Gemma?"

"Yes?"

"Shut up. You're babbling."

"Sorry."

Gemma's face closed down, and she picked up her teacup and slurped. "Sorry," she said again.

Oh God. Cat breathed deeply. Now she was back to feeling evil again. She would have been a bad mother anyway. A sarcastic, harping, carping mother.

"Did Nana Kettle call you?" asked Lyn.

"Yes." With enormous effort Cat managed to make her voice

sound like a normal person's. "She told me Mother Nature knew best."

Maxine gave a derisive snort. "Rubbish. Did she tell you that God needed another rose in his garden, too?"

"No."

"That's what she said to me when I lost my baby."

Lyn put down her teacup quickly. "I didn't know you ever had a miscarriage, Mum!"

"Well, I did."

"When?" Lyn obviously thought she should have been approached first for authorization.

"You girls were only three." Maxine stood up and refilled the kettle at the sink, her back to them. Her daughters took the opportunity to exchange raised eyebrows and surprised mouths. "You all knew I was pregnant. You used to put your little faces up to my stomach and pat me and chatter away to the baby."

She turned back around to face them, the kettle in her hand. "Actually, I remember you were the most interested, Cat. You used to sit there on the lounge whispering into my stomach for ages. It was the only time I could get a cuddle from you."

"We could have had a little sister or brother," said Gemma in wonder.

"It was an accident, of course," said Maxine. "At first I was hor-rified. I even thought about an abortion, which would have had your father at confession every week for a year. But then I got used to the idea. I guess the hormones kicked in. And I thought, imagine, just *one* baby. I could do everything right, with one baby. Of course, it was stupid thinking. You three were toddlers. It wasn't like I had any spare time."

Lyn said, "I can't believe we didn't know this, Mum."

"Yes, well, I lost the baby at thirteen weeks." Maxine flicked the switch on the kettle. "There was no reason to upset you. I just stopped talking about the baby—and you all seemed to forget. You were only babies yourselves, of course. So."

Cat looked at her mother, in her stylish Country Road slacks and blouse. Thin, brisk, and elegant. Short red hair, cut, colored, and styled at the hairdresser every three weeks. She would have been only twenty-four when she had her miscarriage, just a girl, a kid. It occurred to Cat to wonder if she would have liked Maxine if they'd been at school together. Maxine Leonard with her long swishing red hair, her long, long legs, and short, short miniskirts. "Your mum," Nana Leonard used to say, "was a little bit *wild,*" and they all stared, thrilled, at the old photos. Really, Nana? Mum? Our mum?

She probably would have been friends with her. Cat's friends were always the bad girls.

"Were you upset?" she asked. (Could this be the most personal question she'd ever asked her mother?) "Were you upset about losing the baby?"

"Yes, of course. Very. And your father—well. It wasn't a very good time in my life. I remember I used to cry when I was hanging out the washing." Maxine smiled and looked embarrassed. "I don't know why. Maybe it was the only chance I got to think."

"Ah." A sob of involuntary grief rose in Cat's chest. She took a deep breath and tried to stop it. If she gave in to it, she might fall to her knees and start wailing and keening like a complete lunatic.

Maxine came up behind her and put a tentative hand against her shoulder.

"Darling, you're perfectly entitled to grieve for your baby."

Cat turned in her chair and for a fraction of a second pressed her face against her mother's stomach.

She stood up. "Back in a sec."

"Don't, Lyn," she heard Maxine say. "Let her be."

She walked into the bathroom and turned on both taps at full blast and sat down on the edge of the bath and cried. For the baby she didn't know and for the memory she didn't have of a girl standing at the clothesline in a suburban backyard, a plastic clothes peg in her mouth and tears running down her face.

She'd bet she didn't stop pegging those clothes for even a second.

The sun on her face woke her. They'd forgotten to close the blinds last night. "Good morning, sweetie." Cat kept her eyes closed and reached down to touch her stomach.

Then she remembered and misery flattened her body, pressing her against her bed.

This was worse than Dan sleeping with Angela.

This was worse than finding out about Lyn.

This was worse than anything.

She was overreacting. She was being selfish. Women had miscarriages all the time. They didn't make such a fuss. They just got on with it.

And far worse things happened to people. Far, far worse.

Little children died. Sweet-faced little children were raped and murdered.

You saw parents on television whose children had died. Cat could never stand to look at their white faces and pleading bloodshot eyes. They looked like they weren't human anymore, like they had evolved into some other species. "Change the channel," she always told Dan. "Change it."

How dare she *change the channel* to escape from their horror and then lie here feeling desolate over an everyday, run-of-the-mill, happens to one-in-every-three-women miscarriage?

She turned over and squashed her face into her pillow, hard, until her nose hurt.

It was the second day of January.

She thought of all the hundreds of days ahead of her and felt exhausted. It was impossible to think of getting through a year. Day after day after day. Getting up to go to work. Shower, breakfast, blow-drying hair. Driving the car through rush hour. Accelerate. Brake. Accelerate. Walking through the labyrinth of cubicles at work. "Morning!" "Hi!" "Good morning!" "How are you today?"

Meetings. Phone calls. Lunch. More meetings. Tap, tap, tap on the computer. E-mails. Coffee. Driving home. Gym. Dinner. TV. Bills. Housework. Nights out with friends. Ha, ha, ha, chat, chat, chat. What was the point in any of it?

And *trying again.* Sex at the right time of the month. Carefully counting the days until her period came. What if she took another year to get pregnant? And what if she miscarried again? There was a woman at work who had *seven* miscarriages before she gave up.

Seven.

Cat couldn't do it. She knew she couldn't do it.

She felt Dan's thigh against hers, and the thought of having sex with him seemed bizarre. Slightly foolish even. All that grunting and groaning and ooooh and aaaaahing and we start up here, and now we move down there, and I do this and you do that and there goes you, and there goes me.

What a bore.

She rolled back over and looked at the ceiling. Her hands felt the little buttons on the mattress beneath the sheet.

She didn't even like him that much.

Actually, she didn't particularly like anybody.

The alarm began to beep, and Dan's arm shot out automatically to hit the snooze button.

I'm just going to stay here, she thought. I'm just going to lie still like this, all day, every day. Maybe forever.

"So! How about I treat you to a real nice dinner in some classy restaurant? Just you and me. How would you like that? That'd be fun, eh? Put a smile on your dial?"

"No thanks, Dad. But thank you."

"Lunch, then. That'd be better, eh? Smack-up lunch?"

"No. Maybe some other time."

"Or with your mother? All three of us? That would be something different, eh? Ha!"

"Yes, that would be different. Ha. But no. I'm really tired, Dad. I might go now."

"Oh. Well, O.K. Maybe another time. You call me when you're feeling a bit better. Bye, love."

Cat let her arm flop and the phone thud onto the carpet beside the bed.

She yawned hugely and thought about lifting her head to look at the clock, but it seemed like too much effort for too little return. It didn't matter. She wasn't getting up. It was her third day in bed and already it felt like she'd lived this way forever. Huge chunks of time vanishing in deep, dark, druglike sleep that dragged her down like quicksand. When she woke up, she was exhausted, her eyes gritty, her mouth bitter.

She curled up on her side and rearranged the pillows.

Her father had sounded like a used-car salesman on the phone. He always put on that fake, fiercely happy voice when things were going wrong, as if he could sort of bulldoze you into being happy again.

Dad was better in the good times.

A memory appeared so clearly in Cat's head that she could smell it. It was the smell of cold, crisp Saturday mornings and net-ball. The sickly sweet Impulse deodorant all three of them used to wear, the wedges of orange that Mum brought along in a Tupper-ware container. They were always running late and the car was filled with tension and Maxine drove so *slowly* and then they'd pull into the netball courts—and there was Dad.

They wouldn't have seen him all week and there he was wait-ing for them, lifting a casual hand in greeting. He'd be talking away to the other parents and Cat would crunch across the gravel in her sneakers and squash her head under his arm and he'd hug her to him.

He loved watching them play netball. He loved the fact that the Kettle girls were famous in the Turramurra District Netball Club. A-grade players. And lethal, all three of them. "Even the dippy redhead turns into a hard-faced bitch as soon as the whistle blows," people said admiringly. "It's just their long legs. They're just *tall,*" said the jealous short girls.

Cat was goal defense, Lyn was goal attack, and Gemma was center. The three of them had the court covered, with the wings and keepers all but irrelevant. It was the one time in their lives where the roles were divided up evenly, neatly, fairly—equally distinct but equally important.

"Good play, girls!" Frank would call out from the sidelines. Not embarrassingly enthusiastic like some parents. Just cool and smooth. A little thumbs-up signal. He wore chunky woolen sweaters and jeans and looked warm and comfortable, like a dad in an aftershave commercial.

And where was Maxine? On the other side of the court, sitting very straight on a fold-out chair, her elegant shoes in neat parallel lines. Her white face pinched and set. Cold weather made her ears ache, and she was not the sort of woman to wear a warm hat: not like Kerry's mum, Mrs. Dalmeny, who wore a bright red tea cozy of a beanie and danced joyfully up and down the sidelines, calling out, "Oh, well *done,* Turramurra, well done!"

Cat hated her mother then. Hated her so much she could hardly bear to look at her. She hated the discreet little clap, clap, clap of Maxine's gloved hands when *either* team scored a goal. She hated the way she spoke to the other parents, so stiffly and carefully. Her manners were so good they were like a put-down.

Most of all, Cat hated the way her mother talked to her father.

"Max, how are you?" Frank would say, his eyes hidden by designer sunglasses, his tone as warm and sexy as his chunky sweater. "Looking as gorgeous as ever, I see!"

"I'm perfectly well, thank you, Frank," Maxine would respond with an unflattering flare of her nostrils. Frank's teeth would flash with humor and he'd say, "Hmmm, I think it might be a bit *warmer* on that side of the court."

"Why does she have to be a bitch to him?" Cat would say afterward to Lyn, and Lyn would say, "Well, why does he have to be so sleazy?" and then they'd have an enormous fight.

Twenty years later Cat lay in a sweaty tangle of sheets and thought, What if the three of them had been just plain mediocre netball players—or even bad, D-grade, fumbling-for-the-ball bad? Would Dad have still been there every week, smiling in his sunglasses?

Maybe not.

No, not maybe at all.

He wouldn't have come.

Well, so what? Dad liked winning. So did Cat. She could understand that.

But Mum would still have been there. Shivering and sourfaced in her little fold-out chair, peeling off the lid on the Tupperware container full of carefully cut oranges.

That particular thought was somehow too irritating to deal with right now.

Once more Cat let herself submerge into deep, murky sleep.

"Cat. Babe. Maybe . . . Maybe you'd feel better if you got up and had a shower."

Cat heard the sound of the blind being opened and sensed evening light filling the bedroom. She didn't open her eyes. "I'm too tired."

"Yeah. But I just think maybe you wouldn't feel so tired if you got up. We could have some dinner."

"I'm not hungry."

"Right."

A tiny "I give up" twist on the word "right."

Cat opened her eyes and rolled over to look at Dan. He had turned around toward the wardrobe and was taking off his work clothes.

She looked at the perfect muscled V-shape of his back as he

shrugged himself into a T-shirt, pulling it down in that casual, don't-care boy-way.

Once upon a time—was it that long ago?—watching Dan put on a T-shirt used to make her feel meltingly aroused.

Now, she felt . . . nothing.

"Do you remember when we first started going out and I thought I was pregnant that time?"

Dan turned around from the wardrobe. "Yeah."

"I would have had an abortion."

"Well. We were pretty young."

"I wouldn't have thought twice about it."

Dan sat down on the bed next to her. "O.K., and so?"

"And so I'm a hypocrite."

"We were like, I don't know, eighteen. We had our careers to think about."

"We were twenty-four. We wanted to go backpacking around Europe."

"Well. Whatever. We were too young. Anyway, it's irrelevant. You weren't pregnant. So what does it matter?"

He reached out to touch her leg, and she moved away on the bed. "It just matters."

"Right."

"It didn't suit me to have a baby then so I would have got rid of it. I was even a bit proud of how O.K. I was about it—as if having an abortion was making some sort of feminist statement. My body, my choice, and all that crap. Deep down I probably thought having an abortion made me *cool*. And now . . . so, I'm a hypocrite."

"Christ, Cat, this is the most ridiculous conversation. *It never happened.*"

"Anyway, I probably aborted this baby."

Dan exhaled. "What are you talking about?"

"The night of your work Christmas party. I drank a whole bottle of champagne in the Botanical Gardens. I would have been pregnant then. God knows what damage I did."

"Oh, Cat. I'm sure—"

"Before that I was being so careful whenever I thought there was a chance I could be pregnant. But I was a bit distracted by your little one-night stand with the slut."

He stood up abruptly from the bed. "O.K. I get it. It's my fault. Your miscarriage is my fault."

Cat pulled herself up into a sitting position. It was good to be fighting. It made her feel awake. *"My* miscarriage? Isn't it *our* miscarriage? Wasn't it our baby?"

"You're twisting my words."

"I just think it's really interesting that you said *your* miscarriage."

"Christ. I can't talk to you when you're like this. I hate it when you do this."

"When I do *this*? What's this?"

"When you fight for the sake of it. You get off on it. I can't stand it."

Cat was silent. There was something unfamiliar about Dan's voice.

His anger was cold, when it was meant to be hot. Their fights weren't biting and contemptuous. They were violent and passionate.

They looked at each other in silence. Cat found herself touching her hair and thinking about how she must look after three days in bed.

What was she doing thinking about how she *looked*? This was her husband. She wasn't meant to think about how she looked when she was fighting with him. She was meant to be too busy yelling.

"I know this is really hard for you," said Dan in his new cold, calm voice. "I know. I'm upset too. I really wanted a baby. I really wanted this baby."

"Why are you talking like that?" asked Cat, really wanting to know.

His face changed, as if she'd attacked him.

"Oh, forget it. I can't talk to you. I'm going to make dinner."

He headed for the door and then suddenly turned back, and she felt almost relieved as his face contorted with anger.

"Oh. And one thing. She's not a slut. Stop calling her that." He closed the door hard behind him.

Cat found herself breathing hard.

She's not a slut.

You used present tense, Dan.

Present tense.

And why are you *defending* her?

The thought of Dan feeling protective toward that girl gave her such a violent, unexpected thrust of pain that she almost whimpered in surprise.

"Where are you going?" Gemma had asked him the other day, as if she had a right to know. Gemma never talked liked that. Sharply. Looking straight at Dan, with a touch of accusation. Most of the time Gemma didn't even notice people leave the room. Dan always said Gemma had the attention span of a goldfish.

And then there was Christmas Day. "Danny!" Angela had said and there was pleasure and surprise in her voice. Was that the right reaction for someone you slept with once and never heard from again? Someone who went slinking shamefaced off in the night, without even bothering to say, "I'll call"?

She's not a slut. Don't call her that.

Cat lifted and dropped the sheet over her legs.

So.

So.

So.

So, she wasn't having a baby.

So, it seemed there was a very real possibility that her husband was having an affair with a gorgeous brunette with very large breasts.

So the gorgeous brunette had a brother who just happened to be dating Cat's sister.

And Cat's divorced parents were having sex, instead of politely despising each other, like nice, normal divorced parents.

And sick leave didn't last forever.

And as far as she knew Rob Spencer was still alive and breathing clichés and spite.

And there was no point in any of it. No point at all.

Cat got out of bed and walked with wobbly legs to the dressing table mirror.

Ugly. So ugly.

She bared her teeth in a mockery of a smile and spoke out loud.

"Well, Happy New Year, Cat. Happy fucking New Year."

"Why don't you just say *sorry* to Daddy?" For days after Frank moved out, six-year-old Cat followed her mother relentlessly around the house, questioning and nagging, her fists clenched with frustration. It was like pushing and pushing against a gigantic rock that wouldn't budge—and you really, really needed it to budge so you could open the door to where everything was good again.

She didn't care what Mum and Dad said when they had their little talk in the living room. All that stuff about how they still loved them and it wasn't anybody's fault and these things happened and everything would be just the same except that Mum and Dad would live in separate houses. Cat knew there was no question about what had really happened. It was her mother's fault.

Dad was the one always laughing and making really funny jokes and coming up with really fun ideas. Mum was the one always cross and cranky, ruining everything. "No, Frank, they haven't got sunscreen on yet!" "No, Frank, they can't have ice cream five minutes before dinner!" "No, Frank, we can't take them to a movie on a school night!"

"Oh school, schmool! Relax, Max, babe. Why can't you just relax for a minute?"

"Yeah, relax, Mum! Relax!" chanted her daughters.

That's why Daddy had moved out. He couldn't stand it any longer. It was no fun living in this house. If Cat was a grown-up, she might have moved out herself.

All Mum had to do was say sorry for being such a misery-head.

Cat followed her mother as she lugged a basketful of laundry into the living room and upended it on the sofa.

"You always tell us," Cat said shrewdly, "to say sorry when we're fighting." Her mother began sorting the clean clothes into neat piles across the top of the sofa, one for Lyn, Cat, Gemma, Mum—and none for Dad.

"Your father and I are not fighting." Mum lifted up a T-shirt of Gemma's and frowned. "How in the world does she get these marks on her clothes? What does she do?"

"Dunno," said Cat, bored by this topic. "I just think you should say sorry. Even if you're not really."

"We're not fighting, Cat."

Cat groaned with frustration and slapped both her hands to her head. "Muu*uum*! You're driving me crazy!"

"I know just how you feel," answered her mother and when Cat tried to change tactics and be nice by saying, "Mum, I think you should just *relax* a bit," it was like she'd pushed a button. A button right in the middle of her mother's forehead that turned her into wild, crazy, lunatic Mum.

"*Catriona Kettle!*" Her mother threw down a clump of clothing forcefully and her face went a familiar bright red, causing Cat to immediately begin strategic escape maneuvers. "If you don't leave the room this instant, I'm going to get my wooden spoon and smack you so hard that, that . . . you won't know what's hit you!"

Cat didn't bother to point out what an amazingly stupid thing this was to say because she was already running. "I hate you, I hate you, I hate you," she muttered under her breath. "Hate, hate, hate!"

A few days later their father took them to see his new flat in the city.

It was on the twenty-third floor of a very tall building. Through his windows you could see the Harbour Bridge and the Opera House and little ferries chugging frothy white trails across the flat blue water.

"So what do you think, girls?" Dad asked, spreading his arms wide and turning around and around in circles.

"It's very, very pretty, Daddy," said Gemma, running happily through each room and stopping to caress different things. "I like it a lot!"

"I'd like a house with a window like this." Lyn pressed her nose thoughtfully against the glass. "That's what I'm going to have when I grow up. How much does this cost, Dad? Quite a lot?"

They were both so *stupid*. Didn't they see? Everything in Dad's new house gave Cat a bad feeling in her stomach. Everything he had—his own fridge, his own TV, his own sofa—proved that he didn't want *their* TV or fridge or sofa. And that meant he wasn't coming back and this was what it would be like forever and ever.

"I think it's a really dumb place to live." Cat sat down on the very edge of her father's new sofa and crossed her arms tight. "It's all small and squashy and stupid."

"*Small* and *squashy* and *stupid!?*" Frank opened his eyes very wide and let his mouth drop in shock. "Now would a house be small and squashy if you had a room to swing a cat? But where could I find a cat to test it out? Hmmmm. Let me think."

Cat kept her arms folded tight and compressed her lips, but when Dad was being funny it was like the very tip of a feather dancing ticklishly across your cheeks.

She was already laughing when her father grabbed her under the arms. "Wait a minute! Here's a cat. A really big grumpy one!" and swung her wildly around the room.

There was no point being mad with Dad. It was all Mum's fault. She would just stay mad with her, until Daddy came back home.

• • •

"You're up." Dan was at the door, car keys in his hand.

"Yes."

"That's good."

"Yes."

Cat stood in her dressing gown with her hair wet from the shower and her limbs heavy and doughy. She imagined her arms falling straight to the floor like stretched-out plasticine.

Someone should mold her into a nice, neat smooth ball and start again.

He said, "I was just going to Coles. I thought maybe a nice steak for dinner."

Dan always thought maybe a nice steak for dinner.

"Oh. Good."

"You want a steak too?"

"Sure." The thought of steak made her want to gag.

"O.K. I won't be long." He opened the door.

"Dan?"

"Yeah?"

Do you still love me? Why were you talking in that cold, hard voice? Do you still love me? Do you still love me? Do you still love me?

"We need more tea."

"O.K." He closed the door.

She would ask him when he came back. She would match his cold tone. "Is something going on with that girl?" and there would be no undignified catch in her voice.

She sat down at the kitchen table and placed her hands flat in front of her and bent her head till she was close enough to examine the tiny pores and wrinkles on the joints of her fingers. Her hands looked elderly in close-up.

Thirty-three.

At the age of thirty-three, she thought she'd be a proper grown-up doing whatever she pleased, with a snazzy car that she could drive wherever she wanted and everything—all the confusing parts of life—worked out and checked off. In fact, all she had was the not especially snazzy car. She had more worked out when she was twelve. If only bossy, know-it-all twelve-year-old Cat Kettle were still around to tell her what to do.

There was a messy pile of bills sitting on the kitchen table from today's mail. Bills bored Dan. He threw them down in disgust when he saw one, leaving them half sticking out of their envelopes for Cat to worry about.

She pulled the sheaf of papers toward her.

The bills would keep on coming, no matter what else was happening in your life and that was good because it gave you a purpose. You worked so you could pay them. You rested on the weekends and generated more bills. Then you went back to work to pay for them. That was the reason for getting up tomorrow. That was the meaning of life.

Electricity. Credit cards. Mobile phone.

Dan's mobile phone bill.

She picked it up almost eagerly, a sick sense of satisfaction, a refreshing injection of adrenaline. Twelve-year-old Cat Kettle always wanted to be a spy.

The paper quivered in her hand. She didn't want to find something bad, but she almost did. For the sheer satisfaction of solving a tricky problem. For the pleasure of the "gotcha!"

Many of the phone numbers she recognized. Home. Work. Her own mobile.

Of course, there were a lot she didn't recognize. And why should she? This was stupid. Silly. She was smiling mockingly at herself as she scanned the page and then, there it was:

25 Dec. 11:53 P.M. 0443 461 555 25.42

A twenty-five minute call to someone late on Christmas Day.

Cat had gone straight to bed as soon as they got home from

Lyn's place. On the way home in the car they were O.K. They'd talked, calmly, without fighting, about the day's events. Angela turning up in Lyn's kitchen. Frank and Maxine getting back together. They'd even managed to laugh—Dan a touch warily, Cat a touch hysterically—about how horrible it had all been. Nana with the lepers. Michael clicking his fingers to his awful Christmas music CD. Kara finally collapsing face-first on the tabletop.

Of course, that was when she was still carrying her baby like a magical talisman.

"Next year," she'd said to Dan as she sighed with the comfort of cool sheets and a pillow. "We could have a Kettle-free Christmas. We could go away somewhere. Just us and the baby."

"That sounds like a perfect Christmas," he'd said. "I'll come to bed soon. I'm going to walk off some of Lyn's cooking."

He'd kissed her on the forehead like a child, and Cat fell immediately into a dreamless sleep.

And then he'd spoken to someone for nearly half an hour, till past midnight.

It could be anybody of course. It could be a friend. It could be Sean, for example. It was probably Sean.

Although his conversations with Sean were always short and to the point. They weren't chatters, Sean and Dan. Yeah, mate. No, mate. See you at three then.

Maybe they had long, meaningful, sharing-their-feelings conversations when Cat wasn't around.

She looked back through the bill for other calls to the same number.

It appeared eight times in December. Most of them long conversations. Many of them very late at night.

On the first of December, there was an hour-long call at eleven o'clock in the morning.

That was the day after Cat found out she was pregnant. It was when she would have been at Lyn's place, looking after Maddie.

She's pregnant. I can't leave her now.

No. It would be Sean. It would be a work friend. It could even be Dan's sister, Melanie. Melanie. Of course it was Mel. Of course.

Cat stood up, walked to the phone, and dialed the number, and found she was breathing in exactly the same way as when she forced herself to sprint up that killer hill by the park. Frantic little gulps for air.

The phone rang once, twice, three times. Cat wondered if she was having a heart attack.

It switched to voicemail.

A bubbly girl's voice spoke clearly and sweetly into Cat's ear, in the tone of a special friend who is so sorry she's missed you: "Hi! This is Angela. Leave me a message!"

She hung up, hard.

Gotcha.

Scrape and twist of the key in the lock. He walks into the kitchen with plastic bags of shopping hanging from his wrists.

She waits till he dumps them on the bench. Then she stands in front of him and puts her hands flat against his chest and automatically he links his hands behind the small of her back, because this is the way they stand. This is what they do. Her hands here and his hands there.

She looks at him. Full in the face. Right in the eyes.

He looks at her.

And there it is. She wonders how she missed it and for how long.

He's already gone. He's already looking back at her, politely, coolly, a little sadly, from some other place far off in the future.

He's gone.

Just like her baby.

Heads or Tails, Susi?

Do I have a problem with gambling? No! I've got a problem with winning! Ha! That's a joke I heard once. I don't know if I told it right, though. It's not really that funny.

So, you want to know about the first time I gambled. Yeah, I remember. It was Anzac Day and I was sixteen. I was down at the Newport Arms. You know, it's the one day of the year you're allowed to play two-up until midnight. It's legislated! Only in Oz, eh?

It's a good atmosphere in the pubs on Anzac Day. A lot of old codgers. And you've got this big, excited circle of people standing around a guy in the middle, who tosses the coins. He's normally a bit of a performer. He uses a special little wooden stick and the coins go spinning up into the sky and everybody looks up and watches them come down. The way it works is everybody bets with one another. You just hold up your money in the air and call out ten on heads, or whatever.

It was the first 2-Up game I'd ever seen, so I was watching for a while, seeing how it worked. I was mostly watching these girls, 'cos they were pretty easy on the eye. They were there with their grandpa, I think, they called him Pop. He was wearing one of them old-fashioned hats. He called them all "Susi" for some reason. They were all four putting away the beer. Jeez, were they into the game! They bet on every toss and they'd be yelling out, just like the men, "Head 'em up!" or "Tail 'em up!"

When one of them won, their grandfather would do a little old-fashioned dance with them. Like a waltz. Just a couple of little steps whirling them around. And then they'd be back, holding up their cash, yelling and laughing, giving each other high fives.

So finally I got up the guts to have a go. Bet five bucks on tails and won. I was hooked. Mate, I loved it. I can still see those coins flipping and turning in the moonlight and those three girls jumping up and down and hugging their grandpa.

Oh, yeah, I was hooked. Big time.

CHAPTER 15

The first time it happened, she was driving out of the Chatswood Shopping Center parking lot.

Maddie was in the back, silently strapped into her car seat, her thumb in her mouth, one finger locked around her nose. Lyn could see her accusing eyes in the rearview mirror. They weren't talking to each other after a particularly horrible experience in the bookstore.

Maddie had spotted a copy of her favorite bedtime book in the children's section and grabbed it triumphantly off the shelf.

"Mine!"

"No, Maddie, it's not yours. Yours is at home. Put it back."

Maddie looked up at Lyn as if she were nuts. She shook the book vigorously at her, eyes blazing righteously. "No! *Mine!*"

Lyn felt quietly browsing customers around her lifting their eyes and tilting their heads in an interested way.

"Shhhh!" She put a finger to her lips. "Put it *back.*"

But Maddie wasn't having any of it. She stomped her feet like a demented tap dancer and hugged the book tight to her stomach, hollering, "No, shh! Mummy, mine, mine, *mine!*"

A woman walked into the same aisle as Lyn and smiled sympathetically.

"Ah. The terrible twos, is it? I've got that to look forward to!" She was pushing a stroller with a cherubic blond baby, who observed Maddie with surprised round eyes.

"Actually," said Lyn. "She's not even two yet. She's starting early."

"Ah. Advanced for her age," the woman said nicely.

"You could say that," began Lyn. *"No,* Maddie!"

She leaped forward too late. The angelic baby had reached out a hand as if to grab *Good Night, Little Bear* and Maddie had responded with swift, efficient retribution, using the book to swipe the child across the face.

The baby dissolved, as if her feelings had been hurt for the first time ever. One shocked chubby hand went up to the bright red mark on her cheek. Her blue eyes swam with fat tears.

Lyn looked at the rather satisfied expression on her own daughter's face and died of shame.

There was nothing worse, Lyn and Michael had always agreed, than seeing a parent slap a child in anger. Maddie would not be smacked. There would be no violence in their household.

Violence begets violence.

She believed it absolutely.

And now she grabbed Maddie and smacked her hard. She smacked her very hard and very angrily, and Maddie's startled cry reverberated around the bookstore like a child abuse victim.

"It's O.K.," said the nice woman, picking up her nice child. She had the same round blue eyes as her baby.

"I'm so, so sorry. She's never done that before."

And I've never done that before, either.

"It's O.K. Really." The woman rocked her baby to her shoulder. She had to raise her voice to be heard over Maddie's ear-splitting wail. "Kids!"

Maddie backed herself up against the bookshelf and doubled over, crying with luxurious, hysterical abandon, only stopping to take a breath of air to help her reach a new level of volume.

People around them were now openly looking, some of them craning their heads over bookshelves to see. They stared blank-faced, their mouths slightly slack, like people in an audience.

"I'll have to get her out of here. I'm so sorry."

"It's fine," smiled the woman, jiggling her child on her hip. My God, she was *freakishly* nice.

Lyn picked up Maddie, who continued to scream relentlessly, arching her body and throwing back her head so it caught Lyn painfully on the chin. With her arms pinned tightly around her daughter's violently wriggling body, she walked rapidly out of the shop. The mother-with-screaming-child walk of shame.

"Excuse me, madam!" A pounding of footsteps behind her.

"Yes?" Lyn looked up. Maddie's legs continued to kick.

"Um." It was a very tall teenager with a "How can I help you?" smiley badge pinned to his blue denim shirt. He looked apologetic about his height, as if he didn't quite know how he'd got all the way up there. He locked big knuckles awkwardly. "Only, I think maybe you haven't paid for those books."

Maddie was still clutching *Good Night, Little Bear* and Lyn herself was holding a copy of *Coping with Miscarriage* as well as, humiliatingly, *Taming the Toddler: A Survival Guide for Parents.*

Well, why not? The sort of woman who hit her children would also do the occasional spot of shoplifting.

She marched back to the cash register, trying to smile ironically and humorously. If she had had someone with her, Michael or one of her sisters, then it *would* be funny. If she had both her sisters it would be pure slapstick. It would make their day.

But she was on her own and so she could only imagine it being funny.

"Wasn't that Lyn Kettle?" she heard someone say as she paid for the books, including a second copy of *Good Night, Little Bear,* and stuffed change into her purse. "You know. The Brekkie Bus woman."

Oh, funny. What a riot.

Maddie's sobbing had subsided into piteous little hiccups by the time they got back to the car.

"Mummy's very sorry she got cross," Lyn told her as she buckled her into the seat. "But you must never, never hit little babies like that."

Maddie stuck her thumb in her mouth and blinked, as if she was well aware of the lack of logic in Lyn's argument and it wasn't worth a response.

Her eyelashes were still wet from crying.

Guilt came to rest directly at the center of Lyn's forehead. She imagined the nice woman describing the incident to her undoubtedly nice friends, while all their nice children frolicked quietly and shared their toys. "I mean it's *obvious* where the child learned to behave like that."

She turned on the "tranquility sounds" CD she'd bought as part of achieving her New Year's resolution: *Reduce stress in measurable, tangible ways, both professional and personal, by no later than 1 March.*

The warbles and chirps of happy little birds filled her car, a waterfall gurgled, a single bell chimed.

Oh, Jesus. It was unbearable. She switched it off and reversed her car.

Where was the "exit" sign? Why did they make it so difficult to get out of shopping center parking lots? You'd done your shopping—they weren't going to get any more money out of you. What was their objective here?

She couldn't give Cat that miscarriage book. She'd sneer at her. Make some contemptuous remark. Make her feel like an idiot. The other day when she asked, "Who's got Maddie?" her eyes were so hard and hate-filled, Lyn had felt herself flinch.

Dan. Something wasn't right there. It didn't matter what Gemma said, he was still seeing that girl. She could see it in his face. He looked right through them all. The Kettles didn't matter to him anymore.

Around and around she went. The "exit" signs disappeared completely to be replaced by cheerful "more parking this way" arrows.

Gemma looping her hair around her finger. They all laughed at Gemma but—well, was she *normal?* At school she was the smartest of the three of them. "Gemma is extremely bright," Sister Mary told Maxine, who had looked quite baffled. "Gemma?" And now Gemma seemed to be frittering away her entire life like a sunny Saturday morning.

NO EXIT. STOP. GO BACK.

This had to be a joke. There was no way to get out of this shopping center. Was there a hidden camera somewhere with some manic presenter about to jump out and shove a microphone in her face? Because it wasn't funny. "That wasn't funny," she'd say.

She backed up and started driving again. Around and around.

Frank and Maxine on Christmas Day. That shiny, smug expression on Dad's face. Mum all sweetly girly and stupid, stupid, stupid.

EXIT THIS WAY. O.K., fine. If you so say so. She swung the wheel.

Bloody, bloody hell. She'd forgotten cockroach spray. Maxine had suggested a promisingly murderous-sounding brand called "Lure & Kill." This morning one had scuttled evilly across the pure white expanse of her fridge door.

NO ENTRY.

Fuuuuck!

She slammed on the brake.

And that's when it happened.

She forgot how to breathe.

One second she was breathing like a normal person, the next she was making strange choking sounds, crazily gasping for air, her hands clammy and cold against the steering wheel, her heart hammering impossibly fast.

My God, I'm having a heart attack. Maddie. Car. Have to stop.

With stupidly shaking hands she turned off the car engine.

Pop Kettle died of a heart attack. Dropped dead in the backyard giving Ken from next door a tip on the doggies.

Now Lyn was going to drop dead in Chatswood Shopping Center. It would be in the papers. Women across Australia would all secretly ask, What sort of irresponsible mother drops dead with a toddler in the backseat?

Unadulterated panic pumped through her body. Her chest heaved, and her hands fluttered uselessly in the air.

She couldn't breathe.

Droplets of moisture slid down her back.

Why couldn't she breathe?

And just when she thought, O.K. this is it, this is the end, somehow, someway, she began to breathe again.

The relief was ecstasy. Of course she could breathe. Her heartbeat slowed more and more until it was almost back to its normal quiet, unobtrusive rhythm.

Limp with relief, she turned around to check Maddie. She was deeply, soundly asleep, her thumb still in her mouth, her head lolling trustfully against the side of her car seat.

Lyn turned back on the ignition and adjusted the rearview mirror to look at herself. Her face looked back at her perfectly calmly, her lipstick was still perfect.

She pushed the mirror back into position and drove straight out of the parking lot.

When Michael arrived home that night, Maddie went rocketing into his arms and wrapped her arms around his neck.

"Daddy!" She gave his head an extra happy, pleased-with-him pat.

"Hello, my precious."

"She hasn't exactly been precious today." Lyn kept chopping garlic and tilted her cheek to be kissed.

"Hello, my other precious. I thought I said I'd cook tonight."

"I'm just doing a quick stir-fry."

"You wanted to get your accounts done today."

"This won't take me long."

"I did say."

The unspoken accusation—Lyn-the-Martyr. She'd been hearing it all her life. If she just gave people a chance, they would get around to doing things. If she would just relax, chill out, loosen up.

"Feet, Daddy!"

Michael balanced Maddie's bare feet on top of his own black business shoes and, holding on to her hands, he began to walk around the kitchen with exaggerated lifted knees.

"So what did our Ms. Madeline get up to today?"

"There was a little baby in the bookshop who reached out for Maddie's book. So she backhanded her with it."

"Ah."

"So I smacked her."

"Ah."

Lyn turned around from the chopping board to look at him. He was grinning down at Maddie, who was dimpling up at him, her eyes shining. With their curly black hair, they looked like a perfect Daddy and daughter in a movie. Lyn had a sudden memory of Cat standing on Frank's shoes in exactly the same way, except Frank was whirling her around the room in a crazy, dizzy waltz and Cat was pink-faced and shrieking, "Faster, Daddy, faster!" while Maxine yelled, "Slower, Frank, slower!"

Relax, Mum, they used to tell her. Poor Mum.

"I smacked her quite hard."

"I expect she deserved it. You know what this proves?"

"What?" Lyn had gone back to the chopping board. So much for shared parenting values.

"It's time for us to *breed* again! She's ready for a sister or brother."

Lyn snorted. "Right. So she can have someone to abuse on a daily basis."

"I mean it. She's the sort of kid who needs brothers and sisters. We did say we'd start trying this year. That was the five-year plan if you recall."

Lyn didn't answer.

Michael's tone turned teasing. "I'm sure you've got it written down somewhere."

Of course she had it written down. She'd planned to go off the Pill after her next period.

Lyn pushed the garlic into a neat little hill and poured oil into the wok. "Yes, well, obviously that's got to be put on hold now."

"What do you mean obviously?"

"Cat, of course."

"Oh, Cat, of *course.*"

"Imagine how she'd feel if I just happily announced I was having a baby."

"So how long do we put our life on hold for?"

"As long as necessary."

"That's ridiculous. What if Cat takes months to get pregnant again? Or has another miscarriage?"

"Don't say that."

She couldn't understand why this wasn't as black-and-white obvious to him as it was to her.

Lyn put the garlic into the hot oil and it sizzled and popped excitedly, while Michael lifted Maddie off his feet and allowed her to go running off on some mission.

"You're serious."

"I told you. The other day with Gemma and Mum, she was just, I don't know. When we were sitting there eating bun, she had exactly the same sort of surprised hurt expression on her face that she got when Mum and Dad sat us down in the living room and told us they were getting a divorce. I've never forgotten it. Her little face just crumpled."

"Well, your little face probably crumpled too."

"I don't know if it did or not. That's just my memory of it. Cat's face."

"So. Do you think Cat would do the same for you if the situations were reversed?"

"Yep."

"I bet she bloody well wouldn't."

"I bet she bloody well would."

Kara appeared in the kitchen. "Yum, it smells good in here. I'm *starved* to *death*!"

Lyn's eyes met Michael's in shared surprise at this unexpected cheeriness.

"Shall I set the table?"

Michael's mouth dropped.

"Thanks," said Lyn, trying for the nonfussy, not-too-enthusiastic tone that Cat seemed to use so effectively with Kara.

"No problemo."

She opened a cupboard door and began pulling down plates.

Michael gestured wildly and silently at Lyn. "Drugs?" he mouthed frantically, doing something peculiar to his forearm that was presumably meant to be his imitation of somebody injecting a vein.

Lyn rolled her eyes.

Kara closed the cupboard door. "What are you *doing,* Dad?"

"Oh! Just—you know!"

"You are such an idiot."

Michael looked relieved and nodded agreeably.

"Mummy!" Maddie toddled back into the kitchen, an expression of perplexed delight on her face. "Look!"

She held up two copies of *Good Night, Little Bear.*

Lyn said, "Fancy that!" and Maddie plunked down onto her bottom with both books in front of her, her head turning back and forth, as she flipped each page, intent on solving this mystery. The smell of frying garlic filled the kitchen and Michael chomped on a piece of capsicum and the ghost of his childhood dimple dented his cheek as he happily poured too much soy sauce into the stir-fry. Kara rattled efficiently through the drawer for knives and forks and her bare shoulders were young and tanned with skinny white lines from her swimsuit. And for just a moment, in spite of all the reasons not to feel happy (like the sinister bruise of worry over today's parking lot incident), Lyn experienced an unexpectedly lovely unfurling of happiness.

It didn't last, of course.

Michael became overexcited by Kara's sunshiny mood and asked too many offensive questions, like, "So! What have you been up to?" causing her to slump with disgust and ask if she could please eat her dinner in peace and quiet in front of the TV.

After dinner, Maddie had a sudden revelation that her nightly bath was actually a physically painful experience, tantamount to torture. At Michael's insistence, Lyn finally succumbed to the ferocity of her tantrum and let her go to bed dirty, which went against all of her deepest-held beliefs about personal hygiene and good discipline.

And when the house was finally quiet and Michael and Lyn were settled around the dining room table with coffee and Tim Tams and their respective laptops, Lyn started to tell Michael about what happened in the parking lot and found she couldn't find the right words.

She could have found the right words if it had happened to someone else. In fact, she'd be the first one offering a diagnosis. "You weren't having a heart attack, silly!" she'd say and then she'd tell them that they almost certainly had a—and she'd use the words with such calmly knowledgeable, pseudo-psychologist, women's-magazine authority—panic attack. Yes, a panic attack, which was really nothing to worry about. Oh, she'd be so enthusiastically sympathetic, so know-it-all, typical Lyn. She'd explain how she'd read all about these "attacks" and they were really quite common and there were techniques you could learn to deal with them.

But they weren't meant to happen to *her*. Other, more fragile people were meant to have panic attacks. People in need of looking after. O.K., if she was being completely honest—slightly *silly* people.

Not Lyn.

An event occurred. You flicked through your mental filing case of potential emotional responses and you *chose* the appropriate response. That was emotional intelligence, that was personal development, that was Lyn's specialty. So why was she suddenly having a panic attack over not finding an exit and forgetting to buy cockroach spray?

Maybe it *was* something medical.

Maybe she should talk to a doctor about it.

The problem was that the very thought of talking about it out loud, to Michael or even more so to a doctor, seemed to cause a perceptible quickening of her heart. She imagined trying to describe that horrible pain across her chest and involuntarily pressed her hand to her collarbone. God, it had been awful.

If she told Michael about it, he'd insist that she see a doctor. He would react with immediate, loving, husbandly concern. "Let's rule out the physical reasons first," he'd say. And then he'd go on and on about reducing stress in her life and delegating more and not taking on so much and hiring more staff and getting more sleep and a cleaner—and it would make her feel really, really stressed.

That was the problem with a perfect husband. A lesser man might laugh and say something like, "Well, you're a bit of a head case, aren't you!" and that was exactly the sort of unsupportive reaction she needed.

A little contempt might make it dwindle away. It would be like laughing at the scary bits in a horror movie.

She looked at Michael and thought about saying, "I'm going to tell you something and I want you to be *un*supportive, O.K.?" He was sitting back in his chair, munching his biscuit and double-clicking in that casually authoritative way he had with computers, as if the laptop was an extension of his own body. Computers and other electrical equipment seemed to shrink when Michael was around, becoming malleable and obedient in his large hands. It was a pity he couldn't do the same with every problem. Tap a few keys, frown in an interested way. "Mmmm, let's give this a go, then," and hey presto, confidence about the functionality of your personality rebooted and restored.

She would tell him another day.

Or perhaps she wouldn't tell him at all.

She went back to the twenty-three unanswered e-mails that had just filled her computer screen. She could see the words "problem," "urgent," and "help!" featuring heavily in the subject headings.

"You're not still worrying," Michael looked over at her, "about Maddie missing her bath."

"I'm not that anal."

"She's testing her boundaries."

"Yes, and finding they can be knocked over with ease."

"The solution is a sibling."

"Pffff. She's got too many Kettle chromosomes. Anyway, of course we're going to have another baby one day. Just not right now."

"For some reason I have a problem with Cat's life having such a major impact on my life."

"Well, that *is* life. People impact on each other. *Siblings* impact on each other."

"Not mine."

"Yours are weird."

"Oh, please. From the mouth of a Kettle. Now that's the kettle calling the pot black." Michael chuckled contentedly at his own wit.

"Oh, very good, yes, good one, darling."

Lyn applauded lavishly with one hand on the tabletop while using the other one to continue scrolling through her e-mail. She hadn't really been concentrating on the conversation due to a distractingly intriguing e-mail that had just arrived from an address she didn't recognize.

Hi Lyn,
Well, it has been a long time, hasn't it? Too long. I think about you a lot and the other day I happened to see an article about a business called the "Gourmet Brekkie Bus." There was your face smiling back at me. I couldn't believe it. It seems to me that I might have played a small part in the success of . . .

With a pleasant buzz of anticipation—could it be?—she was scrolling to the end of the e-mail to see if the sender was who she thought when the phone rang.

"Hello?" Lyn snatched up the portable phone from the table in front of her and kept looking at her computer screen.

There was silence for a second, a muffled sound, and then, "Lyn."

It was Cat. Her voice was wrong.

Lyn stood up, pressing her hand against her other ear.

"What's the matter? What is it?"

"Well. One thing is that I've had an accident."

"A car accident? Are you O.K.?"

"Oh! Yes, I'm O.K. Although one little problem. The thing is . . . The thing is I'm probably over the limit. I had maybe four glasses. Five glasses. Maybe one was a glass of water? Yes, rehydrate, like Gemma says. But. Yes. Too many glasses. And this guy's wife, this stupid, stupid *bitch,* she wants to call the police. I said it's not necessary, we can just exchange details. But she's such a fucking . . . I think they're calling now."

"Where are you?" Lyn was running toward her bedroom as she spoke.

"Me? Oh, I'm on the Pacific Highway. Down the road from the Greenwood."

"What are you wearing?"

"What?"

"Cat—what—are—you—wearing?" She unzipped her shorts and wriggled out of them. Michael had followed her into the bedroom, carrying his chocolate biscuit.

"Jeans and a T-shirt. But look I have to tell you—"

"What color T-shirt?"

"Black. Lyn. What I'm calling to tell you . . . I need to tell you that Dan is leaving me. Yes. For that girl. He loves her. He doesn't love me."

"I'm coming now. Just stay where you are. Don't talk to anybody."

She hung up, threw the phone on the bed, and pulled jeans and a black T-shirt from her wardrobe.

"What's going on?" Michael absentmindedly stuffed the rest of his biscuit in his mouth.

"Cat's been in an accident. I'm going there."

"O.K., and why are you changing your clothes?"

"She's over the limit. She thinks the police are coming."

"So . . . ?" Suddenly he understood. "Oh, Lyn, don't be so stupid. You can't get her out of this."

She finished zipping up her jeans and pulled the elastic from her hair and ran her fingers through it, I-don't-care-what-you-think Cat-style.

"Probably not. It's worth a try."

"No, it's not worth a try. You're being ridiculous."

His paternal, pompous tone was really irritating her. She ignored him and grabbed the car keys from the dressing table.

"I'll come with you," he said. "I'll tell Kara."

"No." He would slow her down. She was running for the door to the garage. "No. Better stay here."

"Don't you drive too fast! Lyn, are you listening to me? You drive *carefully,* for Christ's sake! You promise me? Promise me!"

The fear and frustration in his voice made her stop for a second and look at him calmly. "I promise. Don't worry."

"You three girls," he called after her, as she ran down the stairs, her car keys held out in front of her like a sword, ready to push the button to deactivate the alarm, "You are so bloody, bloody . . . !"

"I know," she called back, comfortingly. "I know."

She prayed he didn't hear the screech of tires as she accelerated out of the garage.

According to family folklore, swapping identities was a game Cat first played when they were just two years old and she was caught by her parents in the act of creating her own crayon Picasso on the living room wall.

Maxine and Frank exploded as one, "Naughty girl, Cat!"

Cat turned her head, red crayon artistically in hand, and realized from the identical expressions of horror on her parents' faces that she had committed a terrible crime.

"Me Lyn," she said craftily. "Not Cat."

And for just a split second they both believed it was Lyn, until Frank lifted her up by the strap of her overalls for a closer look at Cat's evil little sparky face.

When they were in primary school, the two of them regularly swapped classes, just for the sheer pleasure of conning their teachers. Lyn found it strangely exhilarating being naughty Cat Kettle, talking to the bad boys up at the back of the classroom and not listening to the teacher. In fact, she found it so easy and natural being Cat that when they went back to their own classrooms, she sometimes wondered if now she was just pretending to be Lyn. (And if she was pretending to be Lyn, she wondered, was there another Lyn—the real Lyn—deep down inside?)

When they turned sixteen the Kettle girls made the pleasing discovery that boys liked them, quite a lot. One night, Cat accidentally agreed to go out with two different boys on the same night. She only realized at the very last possible minute when one boy arrived to pick her up. The other boy was due to meet her at the movies in twenty minutes' time.

It was a thrilling mix-up, with Cat dramatically clapping her hand to her mouth, her eyes wide with the wonderful horror of it. They all fell about smothering whoops of laughter in Cat's bedroom, while the poor boy made strained conversation with Maxine. The only solution was for Lyn to go meet the other boy, Jason, at the movies.

Lyn went off to the movies feeling pleasantly frightened, like she was on a covert mission to save the world. It was only when she saw Jason leaning against a wall outside Hoyts, chewing nervously on the tickets that he'd already bought, his face lighting up when he saw her, that she suddenly felt awful.

"Hi, Cat," said Jason.

"Hi, Jason," said Lyn, and remembered not to apologize for being late.

It all went well in the beginning. They saw *Terminator* and Lyn avoided giveaway girly gasps, instead grunting with satisfaction at the most violent bits. At one stage she did worry she might have overdone it—she was laughing raucously at Arnie pulling out his eyeball, when she noticed that Jason had turned his head to look at her. But when she said, "What?" he grinned and pretended a piece of popcorn was his eyeball and ate it, so that was O.K., although revolting.

It wasn't until afterward, when they were standing outside the movies, that everything went horribly wrong.

Suddenly, without warning, he leaned forward and kissed her, slithering his tongue weirdly along her gums. It was horrible, disgusting, mortifying. It was like being at the dentist with your mouth forced agape and unexpected violations with strange instruments and excessive saliva buildup.

When he'd finally finished with her mouth and Lyn was feeling an urgent desire to gargle and spit, he stood back, narrowed his eyes, and said, "Are you Lyn? Are you Cat's sister Lyn?"

She tried to explain, but he was squaring his shoulders and squinting his eyes with cold contempt, just like the Terminator. "You Kettle girls are bitches, prick teasers," he said. "And *you*, you can't kiss." Then he delivered his final, devastating blow: "'Cos you're frigid!"

Lyn went home on her own, disgraced, humiliated, and . . . frigid.

She told Cat and Gemma that they'd been caught, but she never told them about the absolute confirmation of her worst secret fears. All she said was, "I will never, ever do that again."

She was too late.

The flashing blue lights were visible from a block away, illuminating the little group of people, policemen, cars, and tow trucks in ghastly turquoise, like a stage set for a play.

As she pulled over, her own headlights shone a spotlight on the sickening, crumpled, caved-in side of Cat's precious car. It was a proper accident. The idiot could have killed herself.

The reality of it was shocking. Now she wished she'd let Michael come with her.

She parked her car and walked toward the circle of people. Cat was in the center, all eyes upon her as she blew into a little white tube held by a policeman who looked like a teenage boy.

As Lyn approached she heard him say in a somber tone, "I'm afraid your reading is well over the limit."

"Oh well." Cat kicked at the ground.

A woman said to the man standing next to her, "I told you she was drunk!"

"Good for you, Laura." The man shoved his hands into his jeans and frowned.

Lyn fought the desire to say saying something crushing to Laura-the-bitch and walked straight up to the policeman.

"Hello, I'm Lyn Kettle," she said, in her bright but stern working-day voice. "I'm her sister."

The policeman looked at her and seemed to drop his own working-day tone. "Gee, you can really tell you're sisters! People must get you mixed up all the time."

"Yes, ha! They do sometimes." Lyn smoothed down her hair uneasily and hoped he wasn't trained to pick up guilty body language. "Um. What happens now?"

The policeman switched back to his somber voice of authority. "Well, your sister will have to come down to the station with us. I'm afraid she's likely to be charged with negligent driving and driving under the influence."

Cat looked around her vaguely, as if all this had nothing to do with her.

Lyn reached over and touched her on the arm. "Are you O.K.?"

Cat raised her hands in a sort of hopeless gesture. "Oh. Never better."

Her hands were bare, Lyn noticed. No wedding ring.

CHAPTER 16

"So she's going to have to go to court!"

"Yes."

"With a judge?"

"A magistrate, I think."

"Will we get to go and watch?"

"Oh, for God's sake."

Gemma had often observed a strange phenomenon in her conversations with Lyn. The more serious Lyn's tone, the more lighthearted Gemma became. It was like they were on a seesaw with Gemma flying high on the childish axis "Wheeee!" while Lyn banged down heavily onto solid, grown-up ground.

If Gemma started to become more serious, would Lyn start to lighten up—or did the seesaw go in only one direction?

"Gemma. She's going to have a criminal record."

"Oh." Actually Gemma thought there was something rather thrilling about having a criminal record (did Cat have a *mug shot*?) but that was not the sort of thing you said out loud, especially to Lyn. "How terrible."

"Yes. But anyway. There's more. She and Dan are separating. He's leaving her for Angela."

"No!" There was nothing funny about that at all. "But how can he do this now, of all times? She only lost the baby a few days ago!"

"Apparently, he was going to wait awhile to tell her, but then Cat found something on a telephone bill. I don't really know the full story."

"But what if she hadn't lost the baby?"

"He said he was going to stay and try and make it work."

"He makes me ill."

"Me too."

"And how is she?"

"I think she's suffering from depression. She just wants to sleep all the time. Listen, are you still seeing Charlie?"

"Yes. Why?"

"It's all a bit more complicated now, isn't it?"

"I guess so."

Charlie said firmly, "It's nothing to do with us."

"It's everything to do with both of us," said Gemma.

"It's nothing to do with us," he repeated. "I don't want it to have anything to do with us. I love you."

It was the first time he'd said it, and she didn't say it back. She said, "No, you don't!" and then he looked surprised and hurt and tugged at his ear.

You're getting me mixed up with someone else, she wanted to explain. Don't look at me so seriously. Don't look at me as if I'm having an impact on you. I don't have real relationships. I don't have a real job. I don't have a real home. The only part that's real about me is my sisters.

And if I'm not really real, then I can't really hurt you.

Marcus told Gemma he loved her for the first time on a warm October night. It was also the first night he called her a silly bitch.

They'd been going out for about six months, and Gemma, at nineteen, was still floating, spinning, bubbling with the delight of her first full-on proper, sophisticated, older (living on his own!), well-off, funny, smart boyfriend.

He was a *lawyer,* for heaven's sake! He knew about wine! He'd been to Europe *twice*!

She adored everything about him and he seemed (it was a miracle, really!) to adore everything about her.

This was the boyfriend she'd dreamed about when she was fifteen.

This was like, *it*!

They were going on a picnic. A romantic picnic by the harbor that he had organized and she was wearing a new dress that she was swirling for him and he was laughing at her swirling and then he told her he loved her.

He meant it. She could tell that he hadn't planned to say it. It had just come out of his mouth. It was an involuntary I love you, which meant it was the genuine article.

"I love you too!" she said and they smiled at each other foolishly and had a lingering, lovely kiss against his kitchen counter.

About twenty minutes later, they were ready to go out when they remembered the bottle opener. Marcus opened the top drawer and made a "tsk" sound. "It's not here."

"Oh," said Gemma, who was still feeling woozy and wonderful. "I put it away last night. Didn't I put it in that drawer there?"

"Clearly you didn't."

"Oh." She leaned over to look in the drawer and suddenly he slammed it shut, so she had to pull her hand back fast. He yelled so loudly that it was physical, like a blow to her chest, "For fuck's sake, Gemma, where did you put it? I've told you at least five fucking times where it goes!"

It was just so unexpected.

"Why," she asked, and it was a bit difficult to breathe, "are you yelling?"

The question enraged him. "I'm not," he yelled, "fucking yelling, you silly bitch!"

He slammed drawers open and shut with such force that she was backing out of the kitchen thinking, My God, he's gone crazy!

Then, "Why did you put it there?" and he lifted the bottle opener out of the wrong drawer and put it in the picnic basket and said in a perfectly normal voice, "Right, let's go!"

Her legs were shaking.

"Marcus?"

"Mmmm?" He carried the basket out of the kitchen, collecting his house keys from the table. "Yeah?" He smiled at her.

"You were just yelling at me like a complete maniac."

"No, I wasn't. I just got a bit irritated when I couldn't find the bottle opener. You've just got to put it in the right drawer. Now are we going on this picnic or not?"

"You called me a silly bitch."

"I did not. Come on now. You're not going to be one of those fragile, sensitive types, are you? I don't want to have to walk on eggshells. That used to drive me mad with Liz."

Liz was his ex-girlfriend, and, up until now, she had represented a very pleasing element in their relationship. "Oh, she couldn't have been that bad," Gemma would say happily whenever Marcus brought up one of Liz's faults. Liz had lived with Marcus for two years and was a bit of a loser. Attractive enough, but she didn't have Gemma's legs and she was a sulk, a prissy girl, always nagging. Not as smart as Gemma. Gemma didn't want to lose that enjoyable feeling of gentle superiority whenever Liz's name came up.

Plus, she knew she did have a tendency to be oversensitive. Her sisters had been telling her about this tendency all her life.

Perhaps she was overreacting. People got angry sometimes.

And so it began.

They went on the picnic and at first she was a little tense but then he made her laugh and she made him laugh and it was another wonderful night, in a string of wonderful nights. The next day when Cat said to her, "So how was your night with the big hunk?" she said, "He told me he loved me! *Involuntarily!*"

There was no need to ruin the lovely picture she could see reflected in her sisters' eyes by telling them a silly story about a bottle opener. So she pressed it down, brushed it away, crumpled it up.

And she would have forgotten all about it, if a few weeks later, it hadn't happened again.

This time there was sand on her feet when she got in his car. Well.

He loved his car—and he'd been under so much pressure at work and she should really have washed her feet more carefully.

Selfish. Stupid. Lazy. Did she just not care? Did she just not listen? He pushed her out of the car, and it was her own fault for being so clumsy that she dragged her foot along the gravel parking lot, ripping a chunk of skin off her big toe.

There was a family in the parking lot at the beach, two little boys with pink-zinked noses and foam surfboards under their arms and a mum with a flowery straw hat and a dad with a beach umbrella. The little boys stared, and the parents hurried them along, as Marcus roared and swore and thumped his fist against the car.

Afterward, she put her head back against the seat, closed her eyes, and felt grimy with a strangely compelling sort of shame.

Marcus was singing along to a song on the radio, tapping his fingers on the steering wheel. "Good day, hey?" he said, reaching over to pat her on the leg. "How's that toe of yours, you poor little thing. We'll have to get a Band-Aid on it."

Sometimes it happened every day for a week. Sometimes a whole month would pass without incident. It was never in front of anyone they knew. With their families and friends, he was charming and adoring, holding her hand, laughing affectionately at her jokes. It was a dirty little secret that they shared, like a perverse sexual habit. Imagine if they knew, Gemma would think, imagine if they ever saw, how shocked they would be, when they think we're normal and nice, just like them.

But it was fine. She could deal with it. All relationships had their problems after all. There was no need for her blood to turn to ice the moment she saw him pause, become still, the muscles in his back tensing.

He never hit her, after all. He would never do that. He only hurt her accidentally when she didn't get out of his way quickly enough.

She just had to work out an appropriate response for these little "episodes." Yelling back Cat-style? Calm, rational reasoning Lyn-style?

But both tactics only amplified his rage.

The only thing to do was to wait it out, to fold herself up inside, to pretend she was somewhere else. It was like ducking under a big wave when the surf was especially rough. You took a deep gulp and closed your eyes and dropped as far as you could beneath that raging wall of white water. While you were under it pushed you and shoved you as if it wanted to kill you. But it always passed. And when you broke the surface, gasping for air, sometimes it was so calmly-lapping-gentle you could hardly believe the wave ever existed in the first place.

It was fine. Their relationship was fine! They loved each other so much.

And she *was* forgetful and annoying and clumsy and selfish and hopeless and boring.

And it *was* highly unlikely that anyone else would put up with all of Gemma's faults. She was, after all, fundamentally irritating.

She started having very long, very hot showers, scrubbing hard at her skin. Other women, she noticed, were so much *cleaner* than her.

"Right," said Lyn. "Deep breaths."

The three of them were standing outside Cat and Dan's place, except that now, the moment they opened the door, it would only be Cat's place.

Dan had spent the morning moving his stuff out.

"I'm fine," said Cat. She went to put her key in the door, and Gemma caught Lyn's eyes as they both looked away from the clumsy tremor of her hands.

They walked in and stopped. Gemma's stomach turned as she saw the blank spots on the walls and the dusty grooves across the carpet where pieces of furniture had been pulled. She hadn't really believed he would do it.

Dan was such an automatic, everyday part of the Kettle family. It seemed like he had always been a part of their family dinners and birthdays, Christmas and Easter celebrations, making jokes, slouching on the sofa, complaining and teasing and giving his opinions, loudly, Kettle-style. Maxine told him off without formality. Frank opened the fridge door and tossed him beer bottles without looking. Dan knew all the family stories, he even starred in some of them, like "the time Frank tossed the beer bottle over his shoulder to Dan only Dan wasn't there" and "the day Cat bet Dan that he couldn't make a pavlova and he made the most stupendous pavlova of all time for that barbecue and Nana Kettle trod on it and the cream went up to her ankle!"

What would happen to those stories now? Would it be like they never happened? Would they have to rewrite all their histories as if Dan weren't there?

Gemma realized she was feeling somehow hurt by Dan, as if he'd left her too. And if she was feeling betrayed and shocked, then she couldn't even imagine the depth of Cat's feelings.

She had to say something.

"Oh dear," she said.

Lyn rolled her eyes and said, "You didn't tell me you were letting him take the fridge, Cat." She took out her mobile from her handbag. "I'll call Michael now and you can have that old one we've got in the garage."

"Thanks," said Cat vaguely. She was standing at the kitchen bench reading a handwritten note without picking it up. It was sitting next to a set of keys.

She pressed her fingertips gently against the piece of paper and then walked into the bedroom.

Gemma looked at Lyn, who was issuing bossy instructions to Michael. She gestured with her head for Gemma to follow Cat.

Gemma pulled faces at her. "What should I say?" she mouthed.

"Gemma's being pathetic," Lyn told Michael, and she pushed her firmly between the shoulder blades toward the bedroom.

Feeling slightly sick, Gemma allowed herself to be shoved.

The awful things that were happening to Cat made it seem like she was a different person—and that was wrong. She remembered Cat's and Lyn's scarily polite behavior when Marcus died. She must try to not to be polite to Cat. Sympathetic. But not at all polite.

Cat was standing with her hand on the mirrored door of the bedroom cupboard. "All his clothes are gone. Look."

"More room for you!" Gemma began to spread out Cat's coat hangers so that the empty half of the wardrobe disappeared. "Hey. I haven't seen that skirt before. Hmmm. That's very sexy." She held it up against herself and swiveled her hips. Cat sat down on the bed in front of her and lifted up the hem of the skirt.

"Good. I can wear it clubbing when I'm out on the prowl again."

"Yep. You'd pick up in no time."

"Give those twenty-year-olds a run for their money."

"For sure."

They looked at each other, and Cat smiled wryly.

"Actually, I don't have a great track record competing with the twenty-year-olds, do I?"

Gemma put the skirt back in the wardrobe and sat down next to her.

She put her arm around her. "You could get a hot young twenty-year-old yourself. They've got all that stamina."

"Yeah," Cat sighed. "The thought of some twenty-year-old pumping away at me makes me feel exhausted."

Gemma laughed. "He wouldn't last long. You'd get breaks in between pumping."

"You know what I found this morning?" asked Cat.

"What?"

"A *gray pubic hair.*"

"*No!* I didn't even know you went gray down there! Are you sure? Let's see it."

"Get lost!" Cat elbowed her. "I'm not letting you see my pubic hair, for God's sake."

"Well, your fridge is on the way. What's so funny?" Lyn stood at the bedroom door, half frowning and smiling.

Gemma said, "Lyn's probably got an identical one."

"An identical what?"

But Cat had looked up and seen something on the top shelf of the cupboard.

"Oh," she said. "Oh."

She stood up and pulled down some sort of soft toy, it looked like a little furry football.

Gemma and Lyn watched as she held it gently and her face dissolved like a child's.

She spoke as if she were telling them some very bad news that she'd only just received. "I'm never going to have a baby now."

"Of course you are," said Lyn firmly.

"No question," said Gemma.

But it took at least twenty minutes before they could get her to stop crying.

Later that night, after Lyn had gone home and Gemma and Cat were on to their third bottle of wine, Cat said, "What did you do with Marcus's engagement ring?"

"I gave it to a lady sitting on George Street."

"*What?*"

"She was singing 'Blowing in the Wind.' She had a beautiful voice. I took the ring off my finger and put it in her guitar case."

"It was worth ten thousand dollars!"

"Yes. Well, she was singing really nicely. And I've always liked that song."

"I'm going to pretend Dan is dead. Like Marcus."

"Oh. Good idea."

"But I'm not going to give my ring to some busker, for God's sake. What's wrong with you?"

"I don't concentrate. That's the problem with me."

Gemma's twenty-first birthday present from Marcus was a pair of ski gloves. Inside one of the gloves was a business-class ticket to Canada.

Her friends said, "Oh my God, Gemma, this guy is a *catch*!"

She'd been going out with him for eighteen months.

On their first day's skiing, Gemma felt elated. The snowy peaks of Whistler were outlined against a cloudless blue sky. There had been a huge snow dump the day before, and people everywhere were in good moods, calling out things like, "Magic! Pure magic!" as they tramped in their boots through crunchy new snow toward the lifts.

She felt clean. She felt like they were a normal couple.

And then she forgot to concentrate.

It was because she hadn't been skiing for a few years and she was overexcited, not thinking properly.

Skiing with Dad in the August school holiday was an annual event for the Kettle girls, an exuberant circle on Mum's kitchen calendar, a brightly wrapped package of seven gleaming days. Sun reflecting off your sisters' goggles. Exhilarated shouts. The rasp of skis sliding across ice on the early morning T-bars. Dad teaching you the fine art of pushing your way to the front of a lift queue without anybody noticing. Steaming hot chocolates with melting marshmallows and red, cold faces.

Skiing occupied a special place in Gemma's heart.

That's why she forgot she wasn't a carefree little girl anymore.

She forgot to be careful, she forgot to think about the consequences, and on their first run, she just skied straight to the bottom, without even looking to see what Marcus was doing.

It was fantastic. She stopped near the gondola, the scrape of her skis sending a shower of snow in the air, and turned around to squint into the sun, breathless and smiling, to look for Marcus.

As soon as she picked him out from the weaving colorful figures on the mountain, she knew. She punched the ends of her ski poles deep into the snow and waited. Stupid, stupid, stupid.

He waited till he was right next to her. She smiled at him, pretending they were still normal people but she didn't bother to say "Shhhh" when he started yelling.

She *should* have waited for him. She *was* fucking ungrateful. She *was* selfish and stupid. The problem with her was she *didn't* think.

When he finished, he shoved his poles in the snow and skied off, banging his shoulder painfully against hers, almost knocking her off balance. She watched him go and took a shaky breath. It would be all right. In a few minutes he would calm down.

"You O.K. there?"

It was a woman in a bright yellow ski suit, with a long plait of blond hair. She had an American accent.

Gemma smiled politely at her. "Yes, thank you."

The woman pushed back her goggles, revealing the fanatical skier's raccoon face: a distinct white silhouette around her eyes.

She said, "Sweetie. The only part that's your fault is that you stay with him."

Gemma flushed. Stupid, nosy woman. "Oh. Well, thank you very much," she said as if she were talking to a madwoman and she skied off to catch up with Marcus.

That same night Marcus proposed to her in the hotel restaurant. He went down on one knee and produced a diamond ring and all the other diners clapped and cheered and called out "Whoo whoo!" just like in a schmaltzy movie. Gemma followed the script perfectly.

She put one shocked feminine hand to her throat, said, "Yes, of course, yes!" and threw her arms around him.

Sometimes, she thought about leaving him—but she thought about it in an abstract way, the same way that you dream about living an entirely different life. Imagine if I were a princess. Imagine if I were a famous tennis player. Imagine if I weren't a triplet. Imagine if I were with someone other than Marcus.

Sometimes, just as she was falling asleep, he would whisper to her what he'd do to her if she ever tried to leave him. He whispered so softly it felt like she wasn't really hearing it, she was thinking it. She lay so rigid that her muscles ached the next day.

The church was packed for the funeral. His parents and brother were distraught. Person after person got up to tell poignant, funny stories about Marcus. Their voices cracked with grief. They ducked their heads, hid their faces.

Cat and Lyn stood on either side of Gemma. They stood so close she could feel the entire lengths of their bodies next to hers.

After the funeral, she resigned from her teaching job and moved in with Maxine for a while. Her mother behaved the way she did whenever they hurt themselves when they were little— extremely crossly. "How did you sleep?" she snapped each morning. "Drink this please!" She didn't hug her. She just handed her a carrot juice.

Gemma walked for hours and hours around the neighborhood streets. Her favorite time was twilight, when people began switching on lights, with their curtains still undrawn. You could see straight into the bright little cubes of their lives. It fascinated her. The minutiae of their existences. The potted plants on their windowsills. Their furniture. Their pictures. You could hear the sounds of their music, television sets, radios. You could smell their dinners cooking. People called out to one another. "What's this plastic bag in the fridge?" "What?" "This plastic bag!" "Oh, that." Once she stood still for five minutes, listening to the soothing sound of someone's shower running, imagining steam billowing, soap lathering.

She wanted to go into every house, curl up on their sofas, try out their bathtubs.

When she saw the notice asking for an experienced housesitter it was the first time she'd felt definite about something in years.

She became a drifter through other people's homes, other people's jobs, and other people's lives.

A year later she dated the second of the fourteen boyfriends.

He was a sweet-faced chartered accountant called Hamish. One day after they'd been going out for a few months, they went to the beach. "Wash the sand off your feet, will you?" asked Hamish mildly, before she got in the car.

On the way home, Gemma yawned and said, "You know, Hamish, I don't really think this is going anywhere, do you?"

Hamish was shocked. He hadn't seen it coming. He cried when they said good-bye, ducking his face against his shoulder to wipe away his tears on his sweetly uncool checked shirt.

Gemma felt terrible.

But somewhere deep inside of her she felt a tiny hard kernel of pleasure.

CHAPTER 17

It seemed to Cat that she'd been gathering momentum ever since the night of the spaghetti, slipping and sliding, grabbing frantically to save herself. The night of the mobile phone bill was when her fingers finally uncurled from the rockface and she went into freefall.

"You called her on Christmas Day."

He didn't look away, didn't look at the bill she was waving at him. "Yeah, I did. Cat, babe—"

"Please get that *gentle* expression off your face."

"O.K."

"Why did you pretend to be happy about the baby?"

"I didn't. I was."

"Don't patronize me. I don't want my feelings spared! I want the truth."

And like an idiot man he took her literally. He didn't spare her feelings; he beat them to a bloodied pulp.

The thing was, he'd been having doubts, *little* doubts, sort of niggling feelings for a long time. A year at least.

A year at least? Cat felt her whole world tilt.

He thought maybe it was normal after being married for so long. He just felt, you know, flat. Didn't she feel that way sometimes?

"I don't know," said Cat, because she didn't know anything anymore.

That night with Angela, even though he hated himself, he also *liked* himself. For the first time in ages. Angela made him feel good. Sometimes Cat treated him like such a moron.

"We've always been so competitive. Sean's mentioned it. How we were always making little digs at each other."

As if their marriage was something that happened a long time ago.

"Go on," said Cat. "It's all so fascinating."

She felt as if she'd committed a social gaffe of gigantic proportions. Had their relationship appeared bitchy and cruel to the world instead of sexy and fun? Had Dan been lying beside her each night, separated by an entirely different reality?

"Just go on," she repeated. He seemed too brightly defined under the kitchen lights.

That week after he told her about Angela was pretty rough. Cat wasn't talking to him, or else she was screaming at him, and he didn't get much sleep on the sofa bed. He was exhausted.

So, one day, without really thinking about it, he accidentally rang Angela.

Cat laughed—a contemptuous bark. "Are you telling me that this all happened because you were *tired*? Because I was giving you a hard time about your little fling, you decided to turn it into a bigger fling?"

"You're twisting my words again."

"I am not twisting your fucking words. I am trying to understand you!"

"It's complicated."

"So, while we were trotting off each week to fat Annie, you were having an affair?"

"It wasn't like an affair! Every time it happened I said, O.K. this is it, never again. It was like when we were giving up smoking. I just kept falling off the wagon."

Cat snorted and stored that one up for Lyn and Gemma. It

was like giving up smoking. It was on the tip of her tongue to say, You *are* a moron.

He said, "And then you got pregnant."

"Yep. Then I got pregnant." She remembered the joy like a crisp, clean scent.

"So then, it was easy. I broke it up. When we saw her at Lyn's place, I hadn't spoken to her in, well, days. I only rang her that night because I knew she'd be upset."

"And now I'm not pregnant anymore."

He looked at the floor.

"How very convenient for you." Fat, salty tears blocked her sinuses. "You must have been pleased."

"No." He moved as if to hug her, and she backed away.

"You're only here because you don't want to look like a bastard by leaving too soon after the miscarriage!"

"That's not true."

"Well, what do you want? Do you want me or her?"

He said, "I don't know what I want."

He was a child in the six-foot-body of a thirty-seven-year-old man.

"You *wimp*! You fucking *coward*!"

"Cat."

"If you don't love me anymore, then have the guts to say it."

"I do love you. I just think, maybe, I'm not *in* love you with anymore."

"And you think maybe you're in love with her."

"Yes."

It felt as if he'd just thrown a bucket of icy cold water at her. She blinked and tried to catch her breath.

"Leave."

"What?"

"I'm making it easy for you." She tugged her engagement ring and wedding ring over her knuckle and threw them across the room. "We're not married anymore. Go to your girlfriend's place."

"I don't—"

Suddenly she was filled with manic hatred for him. She couldn't bear the sight of him, his worried face, his reaching hands, and his slack, stupid mouth.

"Go! Just go! Go now!"

She screamed harder than she knew it was possible to scream and shoved him violently in the chest. "Get out!"

She was frightened and fascinated by the unrecognizable sound of her own voice. Cool, cynical Cat appeared on the sidelines of her consciousness to observe the whole performance with interest. Wow, I must really be upset. I must be mad with grief. Look at me!

"Cat. Calm down. Stop it. People are going to start calling the police."

He grabbed for her wrists, and she writhed away from him, bucking her body like a true mental patient.

"Go! Please, please just go!"

"Fine," he said, releasing her hands and lifting his own in surrender. "I don't know where I'm going, but I'm going."

But she could see little pinpoints of relief in his eyes. He left, slamming the door behind him.

Cat slid to the kitchen floor and wrapped her arms around her knees. She rocked back and forth, her eyes dry.

What are you doing Cat? Why are you rocking like that? Nobody's watching. Who are you trying to impress with the terrible depths of your pain?

"Oh shut up!" she said out loud to the empty kitchen.

She stood up, dressed, and drove herself to the pub. Her mind was a burning white-hot rectangle of nothing.

She sat at the bar and drank tequilas, one after the other, and didn't allow her mind to think one single thought.

It wasn't surprising that she got drunk.

She hadn't eaten all day.

She hadn't had a drink since the day with Gemma when she found out she was pregnant.

And five tequilas will do that to you.

At some point the world became blurry and confused, like a strangely edited MTV clip.

She was talking with the bartender about cricket scores.

She was tearing up her beer coaster into tiny little pieces.

She was telling a girl in the toilets about her miscarriage.

"OmiGod," the girl said to her mirrored reflection while she pursed her lips to apply her lipstick. "That is just so awesomely sad. A little fucking baby."

And then she was out in the parking lot and she was going somewhere, somewhere important, to fix things.

He doesn't love me anymore.

The crunch of metal. Her head snapping back.

"I think she's drunk. I think we should call the police."

Lights flashing red and turquoise.

Lyn suddenly, confusingly, right there in the middle of it all, in the same way that new people popped into your dreams, without actually arriving.

Sitting in the back of the policeman's car, watching the back of his neck. It was a boy's neck, slightly flushed, his hair cut in a very straight, scissored line. Another young boy pressed her black, inky fingertips one by one against official white stationery. He held her hand so respectfully, even though she was an evil, drink-driving, baby-killing criminal, that Cat started to cry.

And then arriving at Lyn's place and Michael meeting them at the door and being nice to her, his arm around her waist, helping her up the stairs to the spare bedroom.

"I love you, Michael," she told him.

"I love you too, Cat," he pushed her gently onto the bed.

"But I'm not at all physically attracted to you." She shook her head sadly.

"Well, that's quite O.K."

Kara materialized, carefully placing a glass of water and aspirin next to her bed.

She didn't know if she imagined the bit where Lyn kissed her forehead just before sleep finally, thankfully, closed her mind down.

The next afternoon, she didn't love anyone.

Lyn and Michael dropped her back home. They were like solicitous parents, twisting their heads to offer advice to Cat sitting slumped in the backseat. Cat felt hungover and immensely irritable. She also uncharitably suspected that Lyn and Michael were enjoying the drama.

"With your first offense, I'm sure you only lose your license for a year at the most. That won't be that bad," said Lyn.

Why was she using words like "first offense"? Did she think this was an episode of *Law and Order*?

"Don't forget you girls have appalling driving records," said Michael cheerily.

Oh, he was a *dork*.

The flat was empty, and Dan hadn't called.

She took a taxi to the smash repairs where her car had been towed and winced in empathy when she saw her beloved car parked sadly against a grotty paling fence, a violently scooped-out dent in one side. She felt exactly the same way.

"You need a courtesy car, love?" asked the manager, his head down as he filled in forms.

"Yeah," she said. What did it matter if she got caught for driving without a license? Dan didn't love her anymore. All the rules that mattered had already been broken.

There was a framed photo of a baby on his desk.

"Your baby?" asked Cat.

"Sure is!" The man stood up and grabbed a set of keys from a hook.

"I've got a little boy about the same age," said Cat.

"Oh yeah?"

"He's just started walking," she said, as they walked out of the office. "My little boy."

"Yeah?"

He took her to an aggressive-looking ute with a gigantic sign on the back: SAM'S SMASH REPAIRS, YOU SMASH 'EM, WE FIX 'EM.

"Hope you don't mind the free advertising," he said.

"No. Good slogan." Because mothers were nice like that, generous with their praise.

His face became animated. "You like it? I thought of it. Says it straight."

"It sure does."

She gave him a smiling little waggle of her fingers as she drove slowly out of the driveway, the mother of a little boy, the sort of woman who feels a little nervous driving a big wide truck. But when she pulled out onto the highway, and put her foot hard on the accelerator, she felt the evil tentacles of her true self spreading and multiplying.

The sort of woman with an impending court case.

The sort of woman with a dry hung-over mouth going home to no one.

The sort of woman who automatically looks for the next side street when she sees a police car in the distance.

She and Dan decided to separate.

Separate.

She practiced conversations in her head:

"How's Dan?"

"Oh, we've separated."

"My husband and I are separated."

Sep-a-rat-ed.

Four sad little syllables.

She went back to work seven days after her miscarriage, two days after Dan moved his things out of the flat.

It was the first time in her life that she had lived on her own. No sisters. No roommates. No boyfriend. No husband. Just her.

Cat the silent observer appeared to have moved in permanently. She felt herself watching everything she did, as if every move were significant.

Here I am waking up. This is the new quilt cover with big yellow sunflowers that Gemma gave me. Dan hasn't even seen it. And I'm tracing each petal with my fingertip.

Here I am eating Vegemite on multigrain toast, a single, professional woman, living on her own, preparing for another long day at the office.

"Good *morning*!" Her secretary, Barb, popped her head around the cubicle door. "How *are* you? Oh God, you look terrible."

This last sentence sounded to Cat like the most genuine thing Barb had ever said to her. She had long ago accepted that in spite of her excessively bubbly demeanor, Barb actually held Cat in the greatest contempt. It didn't matter because she was an excellent secretary.

"Are you sure you're well enough to be back?"

Nobody at work had known about the pregnancy.

"It was just a very bad flu."

Cat looked up from her computer and caught Barb's eyes rest momentarily on her ringless left hand.

"Well. Take it easy. Can I get you a cup of coffee?"

Barb had been Cat's secretary for two years, and this was the first time she'd ever offered to make her coffee. She was way, way above that.

Cat took a shaky breath. If *Barb* started being nice to her, she would fall apart.

"No thanks," she said shortly.

One night, Frank and Maxine turned up at the flat, their arms laden with a strange collection of offerings.

Multivitamins. Frozen casseroles in neatly labeled Tupperware containers. An indoor plant. An electric wok.

"Why are you bringing me a wok?" asked Cat.

"It's mine," said Frank. "Thought I'd try my hand at that orien-
tal stuff. But I never used it."

"I told him you had a gas stove," Maxine said irritably, but Cat
saw her pat him gently on the lower back as she bustled by, filling
up Cat's freezer.

"What, no bun?" asked Cat in mock surprise.

Maxine pulled out a white paper bag. "Yes, of course. Make
yourself useful, Frank. Put the jug on."

Cat watched them acting as if they'd been these types of parents all her life.

"So, how's the *relationship* going then?"

"Oh, your mother's always been the woman for me!" said
Frank.

"Bloody hell, Dad," Cat said. "You barely spoke to each other
for ten years."

He winked at her. "I still adored her from afar."

"Oh for heaven's sake!" said Maxine.

"You two," Cat reached for a piece of bun, "are very weird."

"Weird, eh?" said Frank.

They both smiled at her, as if they couldn't be more pleased to
be weird.

There were moments when she thought she might survive. And
there were other moments when she would catch herself thinking
about her life as if it was a party she couldn't wait to leave. If she
lived to say eighty, then she was nearly halfway there. Death was
the hot bath you promised yourself while you endured small talk
and uncomfortable shoes. You could stop pretending to have a
good time when you were dead.

One day at work, there was a mini-commotion outside Cat's office
door. She looked up to see a knot of cooing, rapturous women
and sheepishly grinning men.

Somebody called out, "Come see, Cat! It's Liam's baby!"

Cat carefully plastered a delighted smile across her face and walked out to join them. She liked Liam, and this was his first baby, a little girl born back in November. Liam was worth a little fake delight.

"Oh, she's beautiful, Liam," she said automatically, but then she actually looked at the baby, clinging like a little koala against Liam's chest, and she found herself saying, "Can I?" Without waiting for an answer she eased the baby out of his arms, responding to an overwhelming, physical desire.

"Someone's feeling clucky!" cried the women.

The warmth of the baby's body nestled against her own was an exquisite ache. The baby looked up at Cat pensively and suddenly smiled—a huge, gummy grin that sent the crowd wild.

"Oh! The little cutie!"

The noise frightened the baby, and she began to whimper.

Liam's wife, a short, flowery, feminine woman, the sort who made Cat feel like a giant, said, "Oh, dear, I think she wants her mummy."

She held up her arms with sweet authority, and Cat handed her back.

After they'd gone to visit another department, Cat sat back at her sterile computer screen and felt bereft.

Barb walked in with a pile of documents for her in-tray.

"Sweet baby," she commented. "Such a pity she inherited Mummy's ears," and she made flapping moves on either side of her head.

Cat smiled. She was becoming rather fond of Barb.

"It's nearly time for our 'health and beauty weekend,'" Lyn said one day, pulling out the certificate Cat had given her and Gemma for Christmas.

There was something incongruous to Cat about that piece of paper. It was a cheerful relic of her former existence, like those miraculously unharmed possessions people retrieved from the ashes of their fire-ravaged homes. Even her handwriting looked different: unguarded and confident. "You should organize a trip with the boys for that weekend," she remembered telling Dan, while she wrote the date on their wall calendar, never thinking that by January, everything would be different.

"You and Gemma go," said Cat. "I don't think I will."

"I think you will, young lady. We're not going without you."

It was easier not to argue, and when Lyn pulled into her driveway to pick her up, with Gemma sitting in the front seat wearing Maddie's *Little Princess* tiara in her hair, she felt a tiny gleam of happiness.

"Remember when we went away together up the coast after our last HSC exam?" said Gemma, twisting around in her seat to look at her. "How we all stuck our heads out the windows and screamed, even you, and you were driving! You want to do that again?"

"Not especially." Although she did remember how good it felt, with the air rushing wildly into her lungs.

"Do you want to wear Maddie's tiara?"

"Not especially."

"Do you want to play a game where I play the beginning of a song and you guess what it is for a prize?"

"O.K."

So, as they wound their way around the twisting mountain roads toward Katoomba and the air outside became cooler, Gemma played songs from an ancient mixed tape collection. After the first opening bars, Lyn and Cat shouted out the names of the songs, and Gemma awarded snake lollies as prizes.

"I'm predicting a draw with this one," she said, and before she'd even pressed play, Cat and Lyn yelled, *"Venus!"* Bananarama's "Venus" was their "oh-my-God-I-*love*-this-song!" from the year they turned eighteen. They used to dance to it on top of their beds, feeling almost unbearably erotic, until their mother came in and spoiled it, just by the expression on her face.

As soon as they walked into the resort and breathed in the heavily scented air, Cat's sinuses began to twitch, Lyn dropped her bag and said, "Oh dear," Gemma said, "What is it?" and then all three of them began to sneeze. And sneeze, sneeze, and sneeze.

Wet-haired women in white fluffy robes making their way through reception stopped to stare at the interesting sight of three tall women, sneezing uncontrollably. Tears of mirth streamed down Gemma's face, Lyn distributed tissues, and Cat walked up to reception and between sneezes said, "We need our money back."

The weekend was now an adventure, a story to tell. They were ecstatic with themselves when they found a house, perched on the side of a mountain, with four-poster beds in each room, and a truly amazing bathroom! It had a huge spa bath right next to a giant window that revealed the valley tumbling dramatically away beneath them, so that when you sat in the bath, it was like *flying on a magic carpet*. "That's what one of our visitors wrote in the guest book," explained their hostess proudly.

Gemma insisted they share a spa bath immediately, before it got dark and the view disappeared.

"It's like we're all back together in the womb!" she said when they were sitting in the bath, their backs up against the sides, legs crisscrossing in the middle, wineglasses in hand. "It was just like this, except without the sauvignon blanc. Or the bubbles."

"You do not remember being in the womb, Gemma," said Lyn.

"I do!" said Gemma airily. "We used to float around all day, having fun."

"Mum thinks we were fighting," commented Cat. "She read somewhere about twins actually thumping each other in the womb."

"Oh no," said Gemma. "I don't remember any fighting."

Lyn widened her eyes fractionally at Cat and lifted her hair away from her neck. Gemma held her nose and slowly slid down until her head disappeared beneath the noisily bubbling water.

Cat closed her eyes and felt the childlike, familiar comfort of her sisters' legs pressed casually against her own.

It might actually be rather nice to return to that shadowy time of preexistence, she thought, when there was nothing particularly pressing to do except the occasional somersault, no thoughts, just interesting sensations of light and sound, and no loneliness, because those other two versions of you, who had been there forever, were right there beside you, not going anywhere.

CHAPTER 18

All her life Cat had never had a problem falling asleep. Now she battled ferocious attacks of insomnia. Each night she lay in bed with her eyes firmly shut, her body carefully positioned for sleep, and felt like a fraud. Her body wasn't deceived. The mechanics of falling asleep had become mysterious to her.

Eventually she would give up, turn on the lamp, and read, for hours, till three, four o'clock in the morning. She never closed the book. One second she'd be reading a sentence, the next the alarm was beeping insistently and she was groggily opening her eyes, the book still open in her hand, the light from the lamp insipid in the morning sunshine.

One night, in the middle of the night, she was sitting propped up in bed, turning the pages of her novel without taking in a word.

She was thinking about how she and Dan had shared over a decade of *events*.

They were together, cooking steak at the pub barbecue, when they overheard somebody asking if it was true that Princess Diana had died.

They were part of the crazed crowd in the stadium on Bondi Beach, chanting "Aussie, Aussie, Aussie, oi, oi, oi!" when the women's beach volleyball team won Olympic gold.

There was the Tuesday night when Dan was watching the late news and she was cleaning her teeth. She heard him swear and then call out, "You'd better come look at this." She walked into the living room with her toothbrush still in her mouth and for the first time saw that plane make its unrelenting, cold-blooded flight across the skyline. They sat up until dawn, watching the twin towers crumble, over and over.

And then there were the personal events. The auction when they bought their unit. *"Sold!"* the auctioneer cried out, and they leaped to their feet, punching their fists in the air.

The scuba dive when they saw their first Weedy Sea Dragon, a fragile, mythical creature. Dan drew three big exclamation marks on his slate.

The trip to Europe. The wedding. The honeymoon. The trek in Nepal.

A million minuscule events. The pizza that never came. The Pictionary game where they slaughtered Lyn and Michael. The first time they used their breadmaker and the bread was so hard they kicked it around the kitchen like a football. The weird, druggy guy from next door who inexplicably said, "Bitchin' Barney!" whenever he met Dan at the garbage bins. How could she not be with someone who shared such a major chunk of her life?

Just six months ago they'd had a weekend away in a B&B in the Southern Highlands. It rained and they made up a stupid game called Strip Scrabble. She laughed so much her stomach hurt. Was he experiencing his "niggling doubts" *that* weekend?

Each time Cat looked the other way did his smile vanish and his face go blank, like a movie character letting the audience know what he was really thinking?

She slammed the book shut and looked over at his empty side of the bed. Was he sleeping peacefully next to Angela right now? Had they made love? Had they worked out positions for sleeping together? Did he complain about her hair tickling his nose? All that long, lovely black hair.

Oh God, this pain was unbearable, excruciating. Nobody could expect her to bear this.

She got out of bed and went around the flat swiching on lights. She stood under the shower and held her face up to the water. She turned on the television and flicked dully back and forth between channels. She stood in front of her open fridge, staring blankly at its contents. A basket of ironing killed off forty-five minutes.

By five A.M., she was dressed and ready for work.

She sat on the sofa with dry, burning eyes, her hands folded in her lap and her back straight, as if she were waiting for a job interview.

Dan was supposedly staying on Sean's floor until he got a new lease on a flat. He wouldn't be there every night, of course. Sometimes he'd stay with his girlfriend.

Girlfriend. A girlfriend sounded so much younger, sexier, and prettier than a wife.

Cat hadn't seen him now, or talked to him, for thirteen days. Thirteen days, where she hadn't known what he wore to work, what he ate for dinner, who pissed him off, what made him laugh on TV.

And that lack of knowledge about his life would just keep accumulating and expanding, pushing them further apart, a cold empty space between them.

Decisively, she stood up and went looking for the keys to the courtesy truck. She needed to know where Dan had spent the night. If he'd stayed at Sean's place, she would be able to make it through the day. If he'd stayed with Angela, well, at least she'd know.

It felt good to be outside, moving. The truck made her feel tough and capable. The streets were deserted, the streetlights still glowing.

At Sean's place in Leichhardt, she drove up and down the narrow street, peering hopefully at each parked car. Finally, she gave up with a sickly sort of calm. So he was with her. Right now, he was with her, in a bedroom Cat had never seen.

It was light by the time she turned into Angela's street in Lane Cove.

She remembered driving there that first time, filled with righteous hurt. Looking back, it seemed like she'd been luxuriating in her pain, safe in the knowledge that their marriage was a given, that Dan's love was a given.

Dan's car was parked outside Angela's block of units, parked with the assured confidence of a regular visitor. It looked like it belonged there.

Then she saw the car in front of Dan's. A blue VW. She remembered Charlie on Christmas Day. "Her Vee-dub conked out this morning."

She looked in the car window and Dan's long-sleeved blue top was lying on the passenger seat. It seemed she had an endless capacity to be hurt. The casual familiarity implied by that shirt was somehow more shocking than anything.

"Ange? Have you seen my shirt?"

"Your blue one? I think you left it in the car."

And was Cat in Dan's consciousness at all when he had these conversations with Angela? Of course not. Cat no longer existed, except as a problem to be solved, a memory to put behind him.

She was an ex-wife. Ex-wives were vindictive women with bitterly lined faces. Fine then, she'd act like one.

There was a Swiss Army pocketknife in Sam's smash repair truck. It slid back and forth in the center console each time she turned a corner. She got the knife from the car and unsnapped it. The morning sun caught the blade.

It was a beautiful Friday morning. The cicadas were already humming a promise of a hot summer's day and a weekend especially created for brand new-couples.

Tomorrow was Saturday, and she'd be waking up alone.

She squatted down besides Angela's car and plunged the tip of the knife into the black rubber of the tire.

Something unlocked in her mind. She tipped right over into blind fury.

She hated Dan. She hated Angela. She hated herself.

She hated the tires for resisting her. It was so typical: nothing ever went right for her! "Fuck you!" In a frenzy she ripped and slashed with all her strength, not moving on to the next tire until she was sure it was satisfactorily butchered.

After she finished Angela's tires, she moved on to Dan's, becoming efficient and deadly in her movements. And now it was for her baby. Her baby had been betrayed too. Her baby didn't have a chance to live and that was somebody's fault and she was going to *kill* them!

"Hey!"

The sound made her jump.

She looked up and saw Dan and Angela walking out of the glass doors of the block of units.

Dan's face changed as he got closer and recognized her.

"Cat?"

The knife was clenched hard in her hand as she stood up. Her chest was heaving, her face hot and sweaty.

It was a moment of profound humiliation.

On their faces she could see fear, pity, and a touch of revulsion.

And the worst of it was, this was an *event* happening to *them*. They were experiencing it together; they would talk about it later. It was the first in their collection of shared stories. "The time Dan's ex-wife slashed our tires."

Cat didn't say a word. She turned away from them, climbed into her truck, and drove off, without looking back.

Her hands on the steering wheel were filthy black.

What is happening to me?

She drove home to clean up. She had a nine o'clock meeting.

• • •

Gemma turned up at lunchtime.

She sat in Cat's office with that mystified expression she always got when she visited, as if she'd landed in a foreign country, instead of a normal, everyday workplace. It was an expression Cat found simultaneously charming and irritating.

She said, "I don't have time to go out for lunch."

"Oh, that's O.K., I'm not hungry." Gemma looked up from reading a memo in Cat's in-tray. "Goodness. It's all so serious here."

"Yeah. Deadly serious. We sell chocolates."

Gemma put down the memo. "Did you happen to slash a few tires before you came to work today?"

Cat was startled. She had just come back from a meeting where she had given a highly professional presentation. That knife-wielding maniac of this morning was somebody else entirely.

"How did you know? Oh. Stupid. The brother."

"So you did! Was it satisfying?"

"Not really." Cat scraped away a rim of black from her fingernail. "Did you come in just to ask me that?"

"They're thinking of taking out a restraining order against you."

Cat looked up and felt her neck becoming hot.

"A restraining order?"

"I know! It's exciting, as if they're scared of you! But still, I thought I should warn you with your court case next week. The prosecutor might mention it. Of course, your lawyer will object, and the judge will say, Sustained, the jury will disregard that! And the jury will all look thoughtful and your lawyer will say, This is a *travesty*, Your Honor! My client—"

"Oh shut *up*! It's not that sort of court case."

"I know. I was being funny."

"Not."

"No. Sorry. Really, I just wanted to tell you that, ah, I don't think you should go near them again."

"Thanks. Is that all? I've got work to do."

"That's all." Gemma stood up. "By the way, I've broken up with him."

"With Charlie," said Cat dully. She was thinking about how she must have looked that morning, holding a knife. "You didn't need to."

"It wasn't because of you."

"Oh."

"I nearly forgot!" Gemma picked up her bag and began fumbling through it. "I got you a present."

She pulled out a foam hammer with a ribbon tied around the handle.

"It's for stress relief." She banged it on the edge of Cat's desk and it made a sound like glass shattering. "I thought you could hit things with it when you got mad at Dan."

Cat made a sound that was halfway between a laugh and a sob. "I should have had it this morning."

"You can even hit people with it. See!" Gemma hit herself on the arm with the hammer. "Doesn't hurt! Do you want to hit me and pretend I'm Dan?"

"That's O.K."

"Or Angela?"

"Cat, could I have a word?" Graham Hollingdale poked his head in the office, just as Gemma furiously smashed the hammer against her own forehead, crying, "Take that, Angela!"

He looked alarmed. "Oh, excuse me! I'll come back."

Gemma rubbed her forehead. "Actually, it does hurt a bit."

To: Cat
From: Lyn
Subject: Dinner
Hi
How are you? Do you want to come to dinner tonight?
Love, Lyn

P.S. Gemma told me about this morning. She said Dan saw you driving off in some truck. Just wondering how that could be when you DON'T HAVE A LICENSE? Are you mad?

To: Lyn
From: Cat
Subject: Dinner
Can't come to dinner, thanks. Just promised the CEO I'd go to a boring-as-hell work function.
P.S. Yes, I am mad. Possibly certifiable.

Saturday morning welcomed Cat with a thumping headache, dry mouth, and furry tongue.

Why did she keep doing this to herself?

She lay still, fingertips to her temples, her eyes closed as she tried to remember the night before.

"Hello there."

Her eyes flew open.

Sweet Jesus, don't let this be true.

Snuggled up next to her, with the pillow making wings on either side of his pealike balding head, was her CEO Graham Hollingdale.

She just managed to stop herself from screaming.

"How are you feeling?" She watched in horror as he wriggled himself up and the sheet slipped to reveal a not unattractive naked chest. Graham Hollingdale, naked, in her bedroom. She'd never seen him without a tie before! He was way, *way* out of context.

She closed her eyes.

"Ah. Not that great," she mumbled.

The sordid details of last night tumbled back into her head. She'd gone with him to the Confectionery Manufacturer's Association Annual Meeting. They had endured astoundingly boring speeches, and afterward he'd suggested a drink. After the second drink she told him she was separated. After the third she had the startling revelation that Graham was a rather distinguished, handsome man. After the fourth she was suggestively suggesting they share a cab back to her place and feeling pleasantly promiscuous, as if she were the slutty one from *Sex and the City*.

You fool, Cat. You stupid, stupid fool.

She was giving up alcohol forever.

"Would you like me to get you a cup of tea?" asked Graham. Was that his hand on her leg? Or, surely not, something else?

"No, thank you."

She fought back welling hysteria and opened her eyes to confirm her state of undress. Her shirt was still buttoned decorously but her skirt had vanished. Underwear appeared to be intact.

"It's O.K. We only fooled around a little." His tone was avuncular and cozy.

Oh, yuck, yuck, yuck! She remembered it all. She'd kissed him! Worse, she'd kissed him *enthusiastically.*

She'd had a clumsy heavy-petting session with Graham Hollingdale, of all people! She'd have to get a new bed.

How utterly disgusting. How utterly humiliating.

She looked at her boss, lying on Dan's side of the bed, his hands crossed comfortably behind his head, and felt ill.

How much lower could her life sink? Self-disgust filled her mouth. Dirty-gray, sordid misery wrapped itself around her.

"I thought you were married," she said coldly.

He smiled. "Oh, that's O.K. I'm poly."

"You're who?" Was he trying to say that he was really a woman trapped in a man's body?

"Poly. Polyamorous. It means 'many loves.' If you're poly, you believe in having committed relationships with more than one person. My wife and I are both poly."

"So, you're swingers." Cat began to shift unobtrusively as far away as possible to the other side of the bed. Thank God no bodily fluids had been exchanged.

"Ha! Everybody thinks that!" Graham sat up with enthusiasm, a finger held in the air. She wished he could show this much enthusiasm for her marketing plans. "Not at all! Swinging is just about sex. Polyamory is about sharing your love with more than one person. It's about romance!"

"This is romance?"

"Not yet, Catriona. Not yet. My wife will always be my primary partner, but I would be honored if you would consider a poly relationship with me as a secondary partner."

Cat stared at him.

"I've always felt we've had real chemistry."

She was flabbergasted. "Really?"

"Really." Graham beamed. "I could commit to you fully, on Wednesdays. Wednesdays would be just for us."

This was becoming surreal.

"Graham. Last night, was ah—great. But I don't think I'm a *poly* sort of person. I have this thing about monogamy. Just ask my husband. My ex-husband."

"Oh, *monogamy.*" Graham looked slightly disgusted by the word. "Polyamory is so much more enriching. I can give you a Web site address."

"And Wednesdays aren't good for me." Laughing would be a big mistake.

"Oh well! I can look at my schedule!"

"Actually, Graham, can I ask you a big favor?"

"Of course." He looked at her expectantly.

"Do you think you could leave now?"

Venus on the Dance Floor

Christ! Get it off! I hate this song! "Venus"!

It reminds me of this time I went to a nightclub in the city. I was with a group of mates and we were watching these three girls dance.

They weren't bad, so I think, I'll have a go. Worth a go. So I boogie on up to 'em, feeling like a complete loser, like you do. One of 'em smiled at me and I'm thinking I'm in like Flynn. And then this bloody song starts and I became invisible! They went right off, laughing, screaming, and doing these really over-the-top sexy dances. No way could you break into that little circle. All they could see was one another. So I had to slink on back like a total dickhead. My mates never let me forget it. For years afterward, whenever I walked into the pub, they'd be singing lines from that song.

Never tried to pick up a girl on a dance floor ever again. Scarred me for life, mate. I'm not kidding ya.

CHAPTER 19

I am doing nothing wrong, thought Lyn. She sat at her desk listening to the distant, singsong sound of her computer dialing up its Internet connection.

She wasn't hurting Michael. The only person who could conceivably think that was, well, Michael. She knew he'd be hurt. If the situation were reversed, she'd be hurt.

But it was nothing. The whole thing was nothing.

It wasn't as if she hadn't told him straightaway about the "blast from the past" e-mail from her ex-boyfriend Hank. She'd even printed off a copy and coyly presented it to him. Michael had been obligingly macho in his response.

"Hmmm. 'Fond memories of our time in Spain.' This guy better watch himself!"

Hank's erotic appearances in her dreams weren't the problem. After all, more often than not, Michael also featured, looking on with benign approval. (In one he cheerfully mopped the kitchen floor and said "shift your feet" while Hank did interesting things to her up against the fridge.)

Everyone knew that sexual fantasies were perfectly acceptable. Healthy. Even necessary!

Michael probably had them about Sandra Sully on Channel

10. Lyn often caught him smiling fondly back at the television while he watched the late news.

So the fantasies weren't a problem. (In fact, their sex life had picked up recently. What did it matter if the credit went to Hank and Sandra?)

And the problem wasn't that she and Hank were now e-mailing quite regularly. Hank was happily married. He wrote in rather dull detail about his wife and his two little boys. There was even talk of him coming to Sydney for business.

The betrayal was simply this:

She had just written an e-mail to Hank about her "little problem."

Her secret little problem with parking lots.

It had happened twice more since the first time with Maddie. Once she was in an underground parking lot in the city, running late for a meeting. The next time she was doing the grocery shopping. Both times had been equally horrific. Both times she had been convinced, no, this time, I'm *really* going to die.

Now, hilariously, she was avoiding parking lots—pretending that it suited her to walk an extra two blocks with a stroller and a laptop. She even found herself looking the other way when she drove *past* one. Oh, what's that interesting billboard over there? she would think, swiftly turning her head, as if she could put one over on her sensible, sane self.

Nana Leonard, Maxine's fragile, wispy mother, had been a nervous woman, or as Frank so delicately put it, "off her bloody rocker." She became breathless and dizzy in shopping centers, and the older she got, the less and less she ventured out of her home. Nobody ever used the word "agoraphobia," but it was there in the room with them, a silent, hulking presence, whenever they had a conversation about Nana. "She said she wouldn't come to afternoon tea after all," Maxine would say tersely. "Tummy bug."

By Lyn's calculations, when Nana died, she hadn't left her house in two years.

Mental illnesses were hereditary. What if Lyn had been the one marked at birth to end up "off her rocker"? The one the wicked fairy godmother had cursed, *This one shall be the nut case!*

She had to nip it in the bud!

And so, there were numerous, logical, justifiable reasons why she had chosen to share her little problem with an ex-boyfriend—someone she barely knew—out of all the people in her life.

For starters, Hank was American. Americans were more open about this sort of thing. They *liked* chatting about deeply embarrassing emotions. They loved weird phobias! There was no such thing as an Aussie Oprah.

Then there was Hank's profession: He published self-help and self-development books. He spoke a language that most of the people in Lyn's life found cringe-worthy. He could provide articles and facts and stats and lists of instructions.

Finally, there was the fact that Hank didn't really know her. He didn't know, for example, that Lyn was meant to be the sensible one, the calm one.

"There's this special tranquillity about you," Michael had said once, and she'd treasured that remark, especially when he followed it up with, "which is most definitely missing in your mad sisters!"

Hank didn't know that Lyn had no right to feel anxious when everyone knew her life was so wonderful, while Cat's was falling to pieces and Gemma couldn't seem to make one.

It made perfect sense to tell someone on the other side of the world, someone who wouldn't tease or guffaw or say with disappointment, "But that's not like *you*, Lyn!"

"You haven't published a book on parkinglotaphobia by any chance, have you?" she had written to Hank, trying to sound wry and self-deprecating, not panicky and weird.

She put her elbows on her desk, rested her head in the palms of her hands, and watched the little blue stripe zip across her computer screen.

"Lyn! Have you seen my mobile?" called out Michael.

She picked up the phone on her desk and dialed Michael's mobile number.

"Don't worry, honey!" There was a banging of feet. "I think I hear it ringing!"

"I have to say, these *tubby* creatures set my teeth on edge," commented Maxine, as she helped Lyn decorate a giant, Teletubby-shaped birthday cake the night before Maddie's second birthday.

"Gemma said she had nightmares after she watched Maddie's latest video." Lyn formed a licorice stick into a smile and pressed it down on the bright yellow icing. "She was being attacked by feral Teletubbies."

"That child says the strangest things." Maxine frowned distractedly at the garishly colored photo in the recipe book.

"That child is thirty-three."

"Humph."

Lyn opened a packet of M&M's and observed her mother. She was leaning forward and a lock of red hair had escaped from behind her ear.

"I think I know what they've been up to," Michael had whispered when Frank and Maxine came breezing into the house that evening, both of them looking giggly and pink.

"Are you growing your hair, Mum?" asked Lyn suddenly, suspiciously.

Maxine pushed her hair back behind her ear. "Just a little."

"For Dad?"

"Don't be silly."

Oh, sure. Dad wanted his long-haired sixties babe back.

She changed the subject. "You know Cat's not coming tomorrow? She hasn't seen Maddie now for weeks, months even. I understand, but—"

"But you don't."

"No, I don't at all! Her own niece's birthday party. I told her that Maddie has been asking for her!"

That was the part she found inconceivable. It broke her heart to see Maddie's head pop up hopefully when the doorbell rang. "My Cat?"

"A miscarriage and a marriage breakup in the space of a few weeks is a lot to handle. She adores Maddie. You know that."

"I know." Lyn scratched irritably at her neck and wondered if she was coming down with the flu. Her whole body felt like it had been rubbed with sandpaper.

"Cat seems to think she's lost her chance of having children," said Maxine. "I think it genuinely hurts her to see Maddie."

"She's being overdramatic," said Lyn. "She's young enough to meet someone new and still have children. What's she going to do? Avoid Maddie for the rest of her life?"

Maxine raised her eyebrows. "Lyn. She deserves a little slack right now."

Lyn dotted M&M's around the Teletubby's head and thought, Well, I've been giving Cat slack her whole life. Just because you've suddenly turned into Doris Day.

She wondered whether her mother would disapprove if she knew she was trying to get pregnant again. Michael had convinced her that three months after Cat's miscarriage was a long enough waiting period.

She'd agreed but with conflicting emotions. Besides feeling guilty about Cat, she sometimes wondered if she really did want another baby. How could her already overcrammed life cope?

Then she remembered the wonder of a wrinkly, wise little face, miniature fingernails, that exquisite clean-baby smell. And *then* she remembered cracked nipples, bleary-eyed 3-A.M. feeds, and the earsplitting scream of a baby who has been fed, changed, and burped and should therefore have no *reason* to cry.

Oh, it was all so simple for Michael!

Maxine said, "Apparently Gemma and Cat are thinking of moving in together."

Lyn looked up sharply. "How incredibly stupid. They'll kill each other."

"That's what I said. But Cat wants to buy Dan out of the flat and Gemma could help her pay the mortgage. At least it would be more permanent than this house-sitting nonsense."

"She likes house-sitting," said Lyn, even though she'd said exactly the same thing herself before. "Gemma doesn't have any money. I don't see why she has to help pay off Cat's mortgage."

"Maybe if she has to pay rent she'll be forced into taking on a proper full-time job. A career, for heaven's sake," said Maxine.

Lyn found herself passionately in favor of Gemma's bohemian lifestyle. "Gemma doesn't want a career!"

"Gemma doesn't need a career." Frank strolled into the kitchen and scraped a finger around the icing bowl. He and Michael had been giving Maddie a bath, and his short-sleeved shirt was drenched. "She's making a mozza from this online trading stuff."

"Really?" Lyn didn't believe it. Gemma was always trying to impress Frank with outlandish stories.

"She does it all by intuition. Says it's like roulette."

"Ridiculous!" said Lyn and Maxine simultaneously.

"Did you two get into the bath with her?" asked Lyn as Michael appeared looking even wetter than Frank. Even his hair was wet.

"She kept throwing things at us," he explained. "It was worth it because it put her in a good mood. I only had to listen to her read me *Good Night, Little Bear* twice."

Maddie had recently decided to take on responsibility for reading bedtime stories. She flipped the pages, babbling in perfect imitation of the excited up-and-down rhythms of her parents' reading voices, sneaking little glances at them to make sure they were enjoying the story.

"Are you talking about Gemma's shares?" asked Michael. "Because from what she's said to me, I think her intuition is based on some pretty astute reading of the financial pages."

Lyn and her parents stared at him in disbelief. That seemed even less likely.

"Gemma only pretends to be a ditz," Michael told them. He looked at the cake and with his arms held close to his side and his hands splayed began to totter around saying in a squeaky voice, "Oooh, yummy!"

"What on earth is he doing?" asked Maxine.

"He's being a Teletubby," said Lyn. Frank, who had never seen the Teletubbies but didn't like to miss an opportunity to be stupid, began to totter around in a similar fashion, while Maxine giggled.

Watching them, Lyn scratched viciously at something invisible on her arm and wondered if her parents had only pretended to hate each other for all those years.

"I must be such a bitch," Lyn said later that night, after her parents had left and she and Michael were packing the dishwasher. "I can't bear the fact that my parents are happy, and I'm sick of feeling sorry for Cat."

"You're a very sweet bitch," said Michael. He stuck his thumbs and fingers out like a rap singer and waved his arms around, "Yo mah bitch."

Lyn smiled and had a sudden memory of Cat and Dan dancing together at Michael's fortieth. They were laughing their heads off while they parodied rap moves, but they were actually pretty good, their bodies loose and rhythmic.

"Actually, I do feel sorry for Cat," she said, removing the dishwasher powder from Michael's hands before he overfilled it. "Sometimes, it makes me want to cry."

"O.K., I think I'm having trouble following this conversation."

The day of Cat's court case was when Lyn's sympathy had first begun to fray around the edges.

Frank, Maxine, Nana Kettle, Lyn, and Gemma all came to give their support. The atmosphere, Lyn felt, was inappropriately festive.

Cat could have killed herself that night. She could have killed someone else. Drunk drivers killed people, for heaven's sake!

Frank was especially cheery, bouncing around, hugging Cat to him, and telling her he'd arrange the breakout when she got sent to jail.

"Managed to get away from work, did you, Dad?" asked Lyn. "That's nice."

Very nice. He'd missed Lyn's university graduation and Maddie's christening because he couldn't take time off work but Cat's drink-driving charge—oh well, that was a special event.

"Quite a crowd here," said Cat's solicitor as she shook hands with each of them outside the courthouse.

"It's a nice day out for us all!" beamed Nana Kettle.

"They're giving her a penalty, Gwen," said Maxine. "Not an award."

"Maxine, I'm not senile!" snapped Nana. She gestured at her multicolored Sydney Olympic Games Volunteers shirt. "That's why I'm wearing this. So that the judge will see that Cat comes from a real community-minded family!"

She gave the solicitor a cunning look. "Smart thinking, eh?"

The solicitor blinked. "Yes, indeed."

As if to prove her point, a man passing by saw the familiar uniform and called out, "Good one, love!" and gave her a thumbs-up signal. Nana smiled graciously and waved one hand at him like the queen.

In fact, Nana had done about five minutes volunteering before she tripped and twisted her ankle. She spent the next two weeks enjoying the events on TV. Her ankle was fine by the time of the Volunteers' Tickertape Parade. She marched through showers of colored paper with her head high, giving her regal wave to the cheering crowds.

"Cat's a good girl really," Nana told the solicitor. "Although she does like a little drink now and then."

Gemma looked at Lyn and began to laugh with her usual abandon.

"Her sisters are *terribly* upset," confided Nana.

Gemma made a strangled sound.

Cat didn't say anything. She was wearing sunglasses and looked pale and bad-tempered and not at all repentant.

The Kettle family squeezed into a row of seats at the front of the room. Lyn wondered if she should warn them not to applaud. Frank and Maxine held hands like teenagers at the movies. Nana complained loudly about the uncomfortable seats. Gemma, who was sitting next to Lyn, twisted back and forth, checking out the audience.

"What are you doing?" asked Lyn.

"Just seeing if there are any cute criminals."

"What happened to Charlie?"

"Long gone."

"Because of Cat?"

"Of course because of Cat."

"That's a bit sad."

Gemma swung back around. "Well, you're the one who *said* I should break up with him. The day Dan moved his things out."

"If it wasn't going anywhere!"

"Well, I guess it wasn't going anywhere." She was dismissive. Lyn took out her Palm Pilot and began scrolling through her day's diary entries. Gemma looked at it and scrunched up her nose.

"What?"

"Nothing."

Lyn sighed. "It's not pretentious. It's practical."

"Whatever."

They had to sit through six dull cases before it was Cat's turn, and by then the Kettle family was starting to fidget and whisper.

The magistrate herself seemed bored and businesslike. She

frowned deeply as she flipped through the evidence of Cat's driving records. "Fifteen speeding offenses in the last five years," she remarked.

Maxine coughed meaningfully. Gemma elbowed Lyn, and they both dropped their heads, sharing Cat's guilt.

The magistrate's face remained bland as the solicitor presented affidavits to prove Cat had been overwrought due to her miscarriage and the breakdown of her marriage.

"My client regrets her actions. They were the result of severe and unusual stress."

"We all suffer stress," the magistrate commented irritably, but she sentenced Cat to only a six-month license suspension and a thousand-dollar fine.

"The best you could have hoped for," the solicitor said afterward.

"Six months will fly by!" agreed Frank. "Lyn and Gemma can give you lifts!"

Lyn gritted her teeth. "Or you can just pretend you've still got a license and keep driving."

Everybody turned on her.

"What a silly thing to say, Lyn!"

"That wouldn't be a good idea," The solicitor spoke without irony. "The risk is too high."

Lyn groaned and suppressed a childish desire to tattle, Ask her about the truck she's been driving!

"I was joking," she said.

Cat pulled her to one side as they all walked toward their cars.

"I've given back the truck to the smash repairers. So don't get all fucking sanctimonious."

Lyn felt her pulse accelerate in response to Cat's contemptuous tone. It was like turning the dial on her gas stove. This is my biological fight or flight response, she reminded herself. Breathe! Cat was the only person who could make her feel this angry. It was like every fight they'd ever had over the past thirty years was all part of the one endless argument. At any moment, without notice, it could be started again, hurtling them straight into the middle of irrational, out-of-control, name-calling fury.

"Do you know how hard it was for me to get here today?" she said furiously.

"You came because you wanted to gloat, and now you're disappointed because you think nobody took it seriously enough."

The colossal injustice of the first accusation, combined with the element of truth in her second, made Lyn want to pick up her briefcase and slam it into Cat's face.

"That night, I was going to take the blame for you! I was going to try and get you out of it!"

Cat wasn't listening. "I'm not an idiot. Do you think I don't know I could have killed somebody? I know it! I think about it!"

"Well, good," said Lyn nastily. "Because it's true." Suddenly Lyn felt her fury slide away, leaving her weak with remorse. "O.K. then. Well. Want to go for a run this weekend? Do the Coogee to Bondi?"

"Oh *sure*! I'd love to!" Cat hammed it up, and they grinned at the absurdity of themselves. "Could I trouble you for a lift?"

Lyn rolled her eyes. "Of course."

It was always like that. They never said sorry. They just threw down their still-loaded weapons, ready for next time.

The weather chose to be kind for Maddie's birthday. The air was crisp, the sun warm, and it was a pleasure to look at the sky. A birthday picnic at Clontarf Beach would be just right.

Maddie, thankfully, had woken up as sweet and sunny as the weather, but Lyn's cold had gotten considerably worse. She dosed herself up on aspirin and felt wooly-headed, muffled from the world.

They were just about to leave the house when the phone rang.

"It's for you, Lyn," called Michael.

She called back, "Take a message! We have to get going!"

A couple of minutes later he came down into the kitchen and picked up the giant picnic basket to take out to the car.

"Who was it?" asked Lyn. She was squatting down, retying the laces on Maddie's shoes. Maddie's hands rested gently on her head.

"It was Hank."

She looked at the bright red laces on Maddie's shoes and felt as caught out as if she'd been unfaithful to him.

"Did he leave a message?"

"Yes. He said he got your e-mail about your panic attacks and to hang in there, because you're not alone, and he's got lots of really helpful information he's putting together for you."

Lyn finished tying up Maddie's shoelaces and stood up, swinging her onto her hip. "O.K. Look. It's nothing."

"It's *something.*" He was agitated, bouncing up and down on the balls of his feet, swinging the picnic basket. "You're telling some bloody ex-boyfriend your problems. Some strange guy I've never met telling me about my wife's problems!"

Lyn put a hand on his forearm and deliberately allowed a fragile note to creep into her voice. "I've got a cold. I'm really feeling terrible. Can we please talk about it after the party?"

He immediately, as she knew he would, lifted Maddie out of her arms and said without malice, "Of course."

Oh, Georgina, no wonder you cried when I stole him.

With her head heavy against the passenger car seat and the Teletubby birthday cake safely on her lap, Lyn let her eyelids sink and wondered if she'd make it through the day.

Maddie kicked and chattered in her car seat between Kara and one of her more likable best friends, Gina. The girls were taking turns playing Around and Around the Garden, like a teddy bear tracing a circle on Maddie's palm, causing her to chortle with rising anticipation until they tickled her tummy and she completely dissolved.

Every time she laughed, everyone in the car laughed.

As they pulled up at a set of lights on the Spit Road, there was a loud bip of a horn.

Michael looked out his window and said, "Look who made it after all."

Lyn leaned forward and saw Cat in the passenger seat of Gemma's car. They were both waving extravagantly. Cat wound down her window and held out a bunch of brightly colored balloons.

Watching their lips move excitedly and silently reminded Lyn of some moment in her life when she had understood something, for the first time. Something sad and inevitable. Her blocked sinuses and muffled head wouldn't let her pin down the memory.

The lights changed and Gemma's car sped off down toward the blue-green glitter of the harbor, the balloons still bobbing merrily out of Cat's window.

Maddie went wild when they arrived at Clontarf and saw Gemma and Cat already unpacking picnic things and tying balloons to a tree.

"Mummy! Look! Cat! Gem!"

"This O.K.?" called out Cat.

Lyn waved an approving hand, and Maddie went running drunkenly across the grass to be scooped up by Cat and spun around.

Kara and Gina didn't offer to carry anything from the car. They also went straight to Cat, both of them pulling out sheets of paper from their knapsacks. Lyn craned her neck to watch as the three of them bent their heads over the papers, the two girls laughing and pointing. She wished Kara could be as relaxed and natural with her.

"What do you think those three are talking about?" she asked Michael, as she slammed shut the boot.

"Homework?"

"In your dreams."

The birthday picnic was well under way when Lyn got a call on her mobile from her play-group friend, Kate. They weren't coming because her little boy, Jack, had just come down with chicken pox.

"Maddie probably has it too," said Kate. "Nicole's kid was the culprit; she would have been contagious at Julie's lunch. Anyway, good to get it crossed off! Some parents have 'pox parties' to pass it around."

"I had Maddie immunized."

"Oh, I see. Well, I looked into it obviously but—"

A child roared in the background, so Lyn was spared the sweetly veiled criticism she knew she was about to receive. She felt far too woozy for it.

"You know, *you* missed out on chicken pox, Lyn." Maxine looked up from her foldout chair, where she was delicately balancing a paper plate on her knees. "Gemma and Cat caught it when they went on that Christmas holiday with their father."

"Oh, don't remind their father," said Frank. "What a nightmare."

Now she remembered that memory. It was the day Cat and Gemma drove off in Frank's car for the water-slide holiday. They were both up on their knees in the backseat, their faces pressed against the back window, shouting things to her that she couldn't hear.

Different things will happen to us, six-year-old Lyn had realized and felt a little sad and shocked but also almost immediately accepting. It was logical. It made sense. There was nothing you could do about it.

"We probably infected about a thousand kids on that water slide," said Cat.

"Oh shit," said Lyn. She was thinking about Julie's lunch and how Nicole's runny-nosed little girl had wrapped her arms around Lyn's knees.

Everyone looked at her.

"I think I've got chicken pox."

Gemma patted her shoulder in a motherly fashion. "Nooo, you've just got a little cold!"

Lyn pushed back her cardigan sleeve to look at her wrist where she'd been scratching. There was a tiny little red sore. "I think this is the start of the spots."

Michael dropped his bread roll onto his plate.

"But what if you're pregnant? Is it dangerous?"

"Pregnant?" said Cat. She was sitting cross-legged on the picnic rug, a bottle of beer in her hand. "Are you trying to have another baby?"

Lyn watched Cat and Gemma exchange loaded looks and closed her eyes. How many more people would she upset today? Suddenly she felt unbearably ill. She opened her eyes again.

"Where's Maddie?"

Nobody took any notice of her question.

"So do you think you *are* pregnant?" asked Cat.

"Where is Maddie?"

She got to her knees on the rug and looked around wildly, fear clenching her heart.

"She's right there with Kara and her friend." Maxine looked closely at Lyn. "Darling, I don't think you *are* well. Feel her forehead, Gemma."

Lyn saw that Maddie was in fact only a few feet away, sitting on Kara's lap.

She collapsed back down on the blanket and looked mutely at her family.

Gemma put her hand against her forehead and announced, "She's burning up!"

"Right," Michael stood up. "We're getting you home."

"You're not to worry about Maddie," ordered Maxine.

Gemma said, "We'll sing her '"Happy Birthday."'"

And before she knew it, Michael and Frank were on either side of her, practically carrying her off to the car.

"I'm not paralyzed," she protested.

But her legs did feel strangely wobbly and her head was spinning and it was rather nice to be carried off, away from all those plates of food that needed handing around, candles that needed lighting, and Cat's hard, closed-up face.

CHAPTER 20

Lyn Woke Up the next day to find an army of weeping, seeping spots had ravaged every part of her body. They crouched on her scalp, lurked in her pubic hair, huddled at the roof of her mouth.

"This is like a joke," she croaked, as she lay in bed and lifted up her nightie to look with sick fascination at the vile rash of dots marching purposefully across her stomach. "This shouldn't be allowed."

She couldn't remember ever feeling more ill.

Michael took time off work, and Maddie was packed off to Maxine's house.

"I'll be fine," she told Michael pathetically. "Don't use your holiday time."

"For once in your life, will you just shut up and let me look after you! Now, I've rung the doctor about complications for pregnancy."

She interrupted him: "My period came this morning, along with the spots."

"Good. You're my only baby to look after."

Over the following days he did so much research on the Internet he became a chicken pox guru, nodding with rather annoying professional pleasure as each new symptom presented itself.

When the spots started to itch, he was ready with cotton wool, a refrigerated bottle of calamine lotion, and damp cloths.

"Hmmm, this is rather erotic," he said, as she lay facedown on the bed and he dabbed at the blisters on her bottom.

"I'm hideous," she moaned into her pillow.

"Now I need to cut those nails," he said, rolling her over. "So you don't scratch yourself and end up with scars."

"That's for children, you big idiot. I'm a grown-up."

The concentration on his face as he manipulated the nail scissors reminded her of Pop Kettle painting Nana's nails. She had to look away and blink.

One afternoon she woke up from a sleep with a raging throat, to find a carefully quartered orange sitting on a saucer next to her bed, together with a jug of iced water, a pile of magazines, and three brand-new paperback novels.

"You're wasted in I.T.," she told him. "You should have been a nurse."

"I'm only interested in *your* spots."

New ones kept materializing, including a five-cent-piece-sized monstrosity on the end of her nose.

"Oh, *gross!*" said Kara, delivering a cup of tea from Michael one morning. I'm glad I had chicken pox when I was a baby! That one on your nose—man!"

Lyn laughed, put her hand to her face, and started to cry.

"Oh, no!" Kara was beside herself. She put down the cup of tea and crawled onto the bed next to her. "I'm such a bitch! And it's not *that* bad."

"I'm only crying because I'm sick and emotional. It's O.K."

Kara slung an arm around her. "Poor Lyn."

Lyn sobbed harder. "Oh! When you were a little girl you used to hug me all the time. Remember your Crafty Case?"

Kara patted her kindly on the shoulder but obviously thought the disease had spread to her brain. "Daaad!" she shrieked. "I think we need you up here! Like, *now!*"

Kara came in after school that same afternoon, carrying a plastic bag from Kmart and a *Women's Weekly* magazine.

She showed Lyn a picture in the magazine of a mobile with silver stars and moons, hanging in a child's bedroom. "I thought we could make this together for Maddie," she said. "To take your mind off, you know, how bad you look. I've bought all the stuff we need."

"You lovely girl." Lyn pulled cardboard, glitter, glue, and crayons out of the bag. "But what's this?"

It was a new black bra with a label promising "fuller, firmer, more beautiful breasts" and a picture of a woman demonstrating two magnificent examples.

"That's a get-well present for you," said Kara, elaborately avoiding Lyn's eyes, as if she needed to be tactful. "It's your size. I checked in the laundry basket."

"Well, thank you!" said Lyn. Teenagers really were perplexing. "Thank you so much."

"Yeah, O.K."

An hour or so later, when the bed was covered with cardboard shapes, Lyn asked, as casually as she could manage, "What were you and Gina talking about with Cat the other day? Was it an assignment?"

"Ha," said Kara. She was cutting out a star, and Lyn noticed that when she was concentrating she still stuck out the tip of her tongue just like when she was a little girl. She wanted to say, *There you are! I've missed you!*

"It's just these e-mails Cat sends me and my friends. She started last Christmas."

"Oh." Trust Cat not to even mention it. "E-mails about what?"

"Stuff."

"What sort of stuff?"

"You know, stuff. It started out just for me after Christmas, when I got depressed about something. But then I showed it to a couple of friends and then everybody started wanting copies.

Girls have started e-mailing her questions and things. It's like a newsletter now. She does it every week. It's cool. She cracks you up."

Lyn pushed her luck. "I don't suppose I could see it?"

Kara sighed and put down her scissors. She looked at Lyn with stern benevolence. "It's sort of private, you know. But you can look at the last one for like *ten* seconds, if you really want."

She went off to her bedroom and came back with a sheet of paper that she held in front of Lyn's eyes while she counted out loud, "One elephant, two elephant, three elephant . . ."

Lyn just had time to read the headings:

The problem with diets
The problem with boyfriends like Mark
The Donna/Sarah/Michelle dilemma
Handling Alison's mum
Ideas for cheering up Emma (& anyone else suffering from Emma-type symptoms)
ANSWER FOR MISS X: No, that does not sound like herpes!

". . . *Ten* elephant!" Kara snatched the paper away.

"Thank you," said Lyn humbly, praying that Kara wasn't Miss X. "You know, you can always ask me things too. About—stuff."

Kara groaned and rolled her eyes. "The whole *point* is that it's stuff you would never in a million years ask your parents. And even though you're not my real mum, you sort of are."

You sort of are. Lyn picked up the tube of gold glitter and poured a little pile into her palm. She looked back up at Kara and smiled.

"Oh no," said Kara with disgust. "Please tell me you're not going to cry again!"

The next day she felt well enough to sit for a while on the balcony. She lifted her spotty face up to the sun as Michael pushed a cushion behind the small of her back.

"I spoke to Georgina yesterday," he said. "She rabbited on about changing her next weekend with Kara, but I think the real purpose of her call was to tell me she's doing a tandem skydive."

"Why would she want to tell you that?"

"When we were together she was always frightened of doing anything physical, or even sporty. I think she's implying I made her like that. Or I was holding her back. I don't know."

"What an idiot."

"It happens, though, doesn't it? When you're in a relationship you get stuck playing out your different parts. With me, she was the princess. Now she wants to say, See, there's *more* to me than you thought!"

"We're not stuck playing different parts."

"Of course we are. You're Wonder Woman and I'm—who am I? I'm Donald Duck. No. I'm Goofy."

The tiny thread of bitterness in his voice dismayed her. She stretched out her fingers and battled a mad desire to itch and itch and itch until her skin lay in bloody shreds at her feet.

"You're not Goofy!" she cried, and her itchiness made her sound frenzied.

Michael looked amused. "Thank you, honey."

She burst out with it: "O.K.! I've been having these ridiculous panic attacks in parking lots and I'm frightened I'm turning loony like Nana Leonard and I know I should have told you and, oh my God, my God, I want to *scratch*!"

That afternoon, while Lyn slept, dosed-up on aspirin and slathered in cold calamine, Michael did a Google search and downloaded every word ever written about panic attacks and parking lots.

Four days after the picnic, Lyn felt strong enough to withstand a visit from her sisters.

They came bearing get-well cards, a creamy bun, and a bombshell.

"What did you just say?" spluttered Lyn.

"I said I'm four months pregnant," answered Gemma.

"And—but—*four* months?"

"Yep. Freaky, hey? I had no idea until about a week ago."

Lyn didn't know why she was so stunned. Gemma wasn't exactly the Virgin Mary, and if anyone was likely to accidentally fall pregnant it would be her.

But pregnancy and Gemma just didn't go.

"The father? Was it Charlie?"

"Well, yes."

"How did he react?"

"He hasn't reacted. I'm not telling him. I haven't spoken to him since January."

"Obviously you have to tell him."

"No, she does not," Cat put down the teapot unnecessarily hard. "Obviously."

"That's the other thing," said Gemma. "Cat's going to adopt the baby."

"Adopt it?" repeated Lyn dumbly.

"It makes sense. I don't want a baby. Cat does. We've formed a synergistic partnership."

"I knew you wouldn't approve," Cat said aggressively.

"I haven't said anything!" Lyn put a finger to the healing scab on her nose. "I'm just trying to take it all in."

But Cat was right. She didn't approve at all.

Maxine dropped off Maddie later that afternoon.

She was fizzing. "You've heard about their appalling little plan?"

"Yes." Lyn rocked Maddie's compact little body to her. "Oh, I've missed you! Has she been good?"

"Not in the least."

"Ooh, Mummy fall?" Maddie sympathetically pointed at Lyn's face. "Whoops-a-daisy!"

Maxine tapped her nails rapidly on the coffee table. "When

you were little, whichever toy you picked up, Cat wanted it. Didn't matter what it was, the moment you wanted it, *she* wanted it. She'd be throwing a tantrum, screaming like a banshee—and what would Gemma be doing?"

"What?"

"Giving Cat her own doll or teddy bear or whatever! I said to her, Gemma, a baby is *not* a toy! It's not something you just hand over to your sister because she hasn't got one! She just giggled in that ridiculous way of hers. I mean *really*, the child is *deranged*! Ever since that dreadful Marcus got himself killed she's been quite odd!"

"What does Dad say?"

"Oh, Frank is no help. He's always been far too soft on Cat. I'm surprised we've only been in court with her once. We had our first argument about it."

"Your *first* argument?!" said Lyn.

Maxine stopped tapping and smiled. "First one this time around."

The Twist

I remember I was in a record shop once and I saw a woman shopping with her grown-up daughters.

The girls were probably in their early twenties. The mother was one of those grim North Shore types, sensible shoes, pursed mouth.

Anyway, the record shop starts playing some rock 'n' roll music and one of the girls says, "This is your era, Mum!" and she starts dancing the twist. The woman says, very firmly, "That's not right, this is how you do the twist!" And she actually starts dancing right there in the record shop and blow me down if she's not damned good!

It was obviously out of character for her. You could see her daughters' jaws drop. But then they start dancing with her! All three of them—laughing, swiveling their hips, imitating their mother.

It was rather lovely. Then the song stopped and they stopped and that was it.

I went home that night and asked my kids if they'd like to see me do the twist, but they just said, "Oh please don't, Mum."

CHAPTER 21

The breakup With Charlie happened fast, without warning, just like every time.

It was a Tuesday morning, and Gemma woke up feeling vaguely queasy and out-of-sorts. (She thought it was probably the sardines on toast she'd eaten the night before. She certainly didn't relate it to that day six weeks earlier when she stood in Charlie's bathroom, watching a tiny yellow ball rolling rapidly around and around the bathroom sink, as if it were on a spinning roulette wheel, until it vanished down the murky black tunnel of the drain. "Oops," she'd said. *Oops. I just got a new destiny.* But she hadn't even considered the possibility of pregnancy. After all, she'd *intended* to put the Pill in her mouth, and besides which, it was minuscule! It was only months afterward, sitting in the doctor's office, that she remembered and was impressed by the power of that little yellow ball.)

She and Charlie hadn't stayed together the night before, so she should have been pleased to have him drop by unexpectedly. Up until now, each new sight of him standing in a doorway had filled her with fresh pleasure. But today, for the first time, their hello kiss was a little perfunctory, a little rushed. He looked too businesslike and distracted. Plus, he was getting over a cold and his nostrils were pink and flaky.

He didn't smell as delicious as he normally did. Actually, nothing that morning smelled very nice.

Gemma was in her dressing gown, her hair wet from the shower. She had an 8:30 start at a job walking around North Sydney railway station excitedly handing out free "energy" drinks. Eight-thirty was too early to be excitable. People would pretend not to see her. The thought of the gritty morning odors of North Sydney station was making her feel ill.

"Angela just called me," he said. "Your sister slashed her tires."

"Good for her," said Gemma. It was a stupid thing to say. She didn't even mean it.

"Gemma! She can't go around just destroying people's property. She's got to get herself together. People break up. It happens."

Yes, thought Gemma. It happens.

It was the first time she'd ever heard him angry, and there was a pedantic, schoolteacherish tone to his voice that Gemma didn't like. People's property—really! Men were so precious about cars, as if they were people.

"Anyway," Charlie had his motorbike helmet under his arm, and he was rapping the top of it with his knuckle, "Ange is upset about it obviously and she's thinking about taking a restraining order out against your sister. I just thought I should tell you. Maybe you could talk to her. Explain, you know, she can't do this sort of thing."

"That's ridiculous. That's just going over the top! Restraining orders are for big, violent ex-husbands with guns."

"She had a knife. Their tires were mutilated."

"That doesn't mean she's going to start mutilating *people*!"

Charlie compressed his lips and puffed out his cheeks, drawing his eyebrows together.

And there it was. That feeling. The icy breeze whistling through her bones, except this time it was combined with nausea clutching at her stomach.

"I don't think we should see each other anymore."

His hand holding the motorbike helmet dropped by his side.

"Are you serious? Don't say things like that if you're not serious."

"I am serious."

"Gemma, don't. Come on. This is silly. This is nothing."

"It's not about Cat."

"So what is it about?"

"I don't know. I'm sorry." She pulled out the old, well-worn favorite. "It's me. Not you."

"What? You've been thinking about this?"

"Yes."

"Oh."

She looked at his face, and it was like watching something close down—shutters pulled, curtains drawn, doors slammed shut. A polite, immobile, stranger's face emerged. It wasn't Charlie anymore. It was just some guy she didn't know, who didn't know her, who didn't particularly want to know her.

Two minutes later he was gone. She sat at the Penthursts' kitchen table and looked at a photo on the fridge door of Don and Mary all dressed up at their daughter's wedding, smiling and squinting into the sun.

She listened to his bike roar off down the street. A trajectory of sound that ended in silence.

And that was that.

So he didn't make the six-month mark, after all.

The weeks that followed were an odd time. She missed him, but in a dreamy, nostalgic, inevitable way, as if it had been a holiday romance, where neither of them had ever seriously considered a future together.

Her stomach problem kept coming and going. She lost her appetite and took a lot of afternoon naps, lying on the big four-poster bed, listening to the wails of the crows. "Aaah" they cried dolefully to one another.

"Aaah," said Gemma to the ceiling.

"I had no choice, did I?" she said to the Violets.

No, they answered silently. No choice at all.

The day before Gemma found out her tummy bug was actually a baby, she and Cat spoke on the phone about Maddie's birthday.

"But you can't just not go!" said Gemma.

"I've implemented a new policy," said Cat. "No more children's birthdays. Saturday was my last one for all time."

"Who was the child?

"Emma Herbert's daughter. They had a jumping castle."

"Emma from school? Well, that explains it. She was always a bitch. She probably gave birth to a bitch."

"I was the only childless one there. Also the only single one."

"So? Why didn't you just play on the jumping castle?"

"So, I am sick to death of holding other people's babies and smiling at other people's babies and hearing about other people's bloody babies!"

Gemma herself thought there was nothing nicer than other people's babies. It was especially pleasing the way you got to hand them straight back when they started doing anything complicated, like crying.

"O.K. But you will have your own children one day."

"I'm thirty-*three*," said Cat, as if it were someone's fault.

"Yes, I do know that, actually. Well, you could meet someone new. Or you could get back together with Dan. Or you could pop by your local sperm bank."

"I'm thinking about it!" said Cat in an ominous, "that'll show 'em" tone that made Gemma think of Cat as a little girl, a darkly frowning little girl plotting lavish schemes of revenge against nuns and schoolteachers.

"Apparently cloning technology is really advancing. You could get a little Cat Clone."

"I've already got a clone thanks very much."

"Yes and she's not going to be happy when she hears you're not going to Maddie's party."

"I can't have a baby," Gemma told the doctor.

She had never thought that *her* body would do anything so serious, so definite, so permanent.

"Four months is a little late to be considering a termination."

"Oh no. I can't have an abortion!"

"Well, then."

"But I can't have a baby."

The doctor lifted her hands in a "What do you want me to do about it?" gesture.

Gemma looked down at her own hands. They were shaking, just like Cat's did that day in the bathroom when they found out she was pregnant. She thought about that bag with the bright red elephants that Lyn always carried around. It was full of *stuff* for Maddie. In her room there was more stuff. Important, technical-looking, necessary stuff that kept her alive.

"I read once about some teenagers who had a baby," Gemma said. "They gave their baby breakfast cereal and it died."

"Too much salt," said the doctor.

"But I could do that!" cried Gemma. "I could *easily* do that! How would you know?"

"You wouldn't do that. There is plenty of information available. Plenty of support. There are clinic centers for new mothers. Mothers' groups."

I don't even have the right stuff for myself, thought Gemma. I don't have a fridge. I don't have a job. I don't have a boyfriend. I don't concentrate!

"Yes." Gemma stood up. There were a lot of people in the waiting room. "Thank you."

The doctor looked up at her. "Adoption is always an alternative, if your circumstances really are such that you can't have a baby."

"My circumstances really are such," said Gemma. I don't *have* any circumstances!

"I can give you some information."

"Actually, that's O.K.," she said, because she already knew who would be adopting her baby.

"Don't be so stupid!" said Cat, who seemed a little doubtful that Gemma was pregnant at all. She kept asking if she was quite sure, as if Gemma might have misheard the doctor's diagnosis. "I can't adopt your baby. You'll be fine. Everybody will help you. Mum. Lyn. Me. You'll be fine. It's just the shock. Every new mother feels nervous."

She was adamant. Gemma pleaded and cajoled, to no avail.

It was only when Gemma put her elbows on the table, her head in her hands, and began to cry that Cat finally said, "O.K., O.K., I'll think about it!"

She brought her a cup of tea and sat there looking at her doubtfully, carefully. "You seriously don't want to be a mother? You seriously don't want this baby?"

There was a wrench of longing in her voice.

"Seriously," said Gemma. "Really! And you would make a wonderful mother. And we're triplets! The baby is practically yours anyway."

"But you're not just suggesting this to make *me* happy, are you?"

"No. I can't have a baby and I don't want to have an abortion."

She didn't, because already she adored the baby. Cat's little boy or girl, another little niece or nephew. Of course she adored it.

Everything was going to be O.K.

It was a win-win.

Lyn wouldn't stop talking about Charlie.

"You only met him once," said Gemma. "I don't know why you care so much."

"I just think he's the sort of guy who would want to know he was having a baby."

"You're just saying that because he saved Maddie's feet from the glass. As if that demonstrated his paternal instincts!"

"I'm saying it because you have a moral obligation to tell him!"

"What if he wants to be involved with the baby? That won't work. Cat won't want that."

"I thought you cared about Charlie."

"I don't want to talk about it anymore."

Much to Maddie's amusement, Lyn picked up a cushion from the lounge, held it to her face, and head-butted it.

Gemma tried not to think about Charlie during the day, but it felt like she spent every night with him.

Her dreams became garishly colored horror films. They were very vivid, very long, and they all featured Charlie.

Dream-Charlie was not a nice man.

One night he stabbed her, right in the stomach, with the end of a ski pole. Gemma looked down and saw bright splatters of her own blood blossoming on freshly fallen snow. "Here it is!" Charlie plunged his hands into her stomach and triumphantly dragged out a baby. The baby was Maddie, in her blue denim overalls and covered in entrails and bloody mush. She grinned at Gemma and held out her palm for Around and Around the Garden. "Fucking nice, Gemma!" yelled Charlie. "You knew we were going snorkeling!" and he skied off with Maddie on his hip. Gemma tried to run after him but her legs were buried in the snow and she couldn't move. "Lyn's going to be really mad at you!" cried Cat, whooshing past on skis. Maxine came stalking across the snow in her high heels. "Retrace your steps, Gemma. Where did you last see Maddie? Think!"

With a tremendous effort, she wrenched herself out of the dream, and her eyelids fluttered open.

Was that a giant splotch of spreading blood on the sheets?

Was she losing the baby? With trembling hands, she turned on the lamp and the blood vanished. It was just a white sheet.

She remembered that time with Charlie, when she dreamed she left the baby in the drawer. "Come back to bed, you fruitcake," he'd said. "We don't have a baby."

He'd been so lovely to her. Look at him now, she thought sadly, stabbing her with a ski pole.

"Is it money?" asked Lyn one day. "Do you think you can't afford to bring up a child?"

"Yes, that's right," said Gemma. "I'm a humble serving wench who can't afford to keep my own child, so I'm giving it to the lady of the manor. Oh, m'lady, if you only knew what I'd been through!"

"Shut up. Dad said you were making a lot on the stock market."

"Well, I was showing off a bit for Dad's benefit."

"But you do invest in the stock market? How did you ever get into that?"

"I got some money when Marcus died. I didn't know what to do with it. Mum wanted me to see a financial adviser. Then, I read a story about how a blindfolded monkey throwing darts did just as well at picking stocks as a professional. So, I got the list of stocks in the newspaper, closed my eyes, and pointed."

"*Gemma!*"

"The next week that company made a big profit announcement and the shares went up by two hundred percent. I nearly fainted when I saw it in the paper. It was so exciting! I was hooked."

"So, do you still close your eyes and pick?'

"Well, actually," said Gemma, feeling a bit sheepish. "I'm more into technical analysis. I look at ratios. Trends."

Lyn looked quite scandalized. "You're kidding me."

"I always liked math and economics at school. Remember? I used to come first all the time. I always thought I was the sort of person who *shouldn't* be good at math. But, um, it seems that I am."

"So, why don't you ever have any money?"

"I don't spend it. I've never spent a cent of it. I just reinvest. And now I'll have a good little trust fund for Cat's baby."

"Your baby."

"Cat's baby."

As Gemma's pregnancy progressed, Lyn's tactics became nastier.

"You do realize," Gemma heard her say to Cat one day, "that this baby will actually be related to Angela? The woman who stole your husband?"

Cat said, "I couldn't care less. This is what Gemma wants! Not me."

"Are you frightened of looking after a baby? Is that what it is?" Maxine asked Gemma. "Because you know I will help you."

"Thanks, Mum. Cat will probably need your help," answered Gemma.

"Gemma! Are you even listening to a single word I say?"

"You and your sister should stick to your guns!" said Frank. "People are too narrow-minded. Can't think outside the square! I can think outside the square! I said to your mother, If this makes my girls happy, then I'm happy!"

"Thanks, Dad."

"That Charlie was a lovely fellow," said Nana Kettle. "I'm sure he would marry you if you told him! I'm sure he would! What does it matter if Dan is off being silly with his sister? I never liked that Dan much anyway."

Tchaikovsky and Guacamole

Oh him! His name was Alan. Ancient history.

One night the two of us went to Opera in the Park. There was a big family group sitting in front of us. You know how crowded it gets. Alan was getting annoyed because their picnic stuff kept encroaching on our area and they were sort of noisy. But you know, it's Opera in the Park, not opera at the Opera House!

But this family. They had, I don't know, charisma! There was a midget-sized little old lady bossing everyone and a teenage girl wearing headphones. They also had a little baby girl crawling around. Dark curly hair and dimples. Irresistible. She was such a cutie. Anyway, about halfway through the night, this little girl was standing up, clutching on to some guy's sleeve, when she suddenly started this sort of wobbly walk straight across their picnic blanket.

Well, obviously it was her first steps! Her family went wild! Clapping and pointing and grabbing for cameras. One woman started to cry.

The baby was beaming like a little show-off and somebody said, Watch the guacamole, and of course, her foot goes squelch in the dip and she topples sideways into somebody's lap.

One of them said something like, "Now there's a girl with style, she takes her first steps to Tchaikovsky." I said to Alan, "Did you see that?" And he said, "Yeah, do you want to move somewhere else? They're really ruining the night."

And I thought, Nah-ah.

I gave have him his marching orders during Beethoven's Fifth.

CHAPTER 22

Cat went with Gemma for her ultrasound. They sat opposite each other in the quietly murmuring waiting room and engaged in a brief, silent tug-of-war when both of them reached for the most salacious-looking magazine on the coffee table.

Gemma argued, "I need the distraction from my bloated bladder," which was true because after studying the Preparing for your Ultrasound instructions, Cat had made her drink four glasses of water that morning, instead of the required two. "The fuller the bladder, the better the picture. Drink up!"

Cat benevolently released her grip on the magazine. "Surely they can't keep us waiting long, when they know you're suffering." A woman sitting next to Cat looked up from her magazine with a strained smile. "Just watch them."

"That's ridiculous." Cat twisted around to glare at the staff behind the counter.

"I'm fine," said Gemma. "Just don't say anything funny."

Cat bit the inside of her cheek, and Gemma chortled painfully.

"What? I'm not being funny."

"I know, but you can tell it goes against all your natural instincts."

Cat sighed, picked up another magazine, and started flicking the pages a little feverishly. "Oh good, I can drop a dress size by Saturday night. I can't believe they still run this sort of article. It's no wonder Kara and her friends are so mixed up. You know what she told me the other day? She said she's been trying really hard to catch just a *little* dose of anorexia and felt like a real loser because she couldn't seem to manage it. She considered bulimia, but even the thought of it made her sick."

"Stop making me laugh!"

"It's not funny really. Anyway, now she's interested in some boy. I've been trying to remember all the relationship mistakes I made when I was a teenager. What mistakes did you make?"

Before Gemma had a chance to answer Cat was distracted by a headline. "Ten Ways to Change Your Life by Tomorrow," she read out loud. "What utter crap." She was instantly absorbed in the article, looking both scornful and hopeful, her crossed foot kicking rhythmically as she read.

Gemma looked down at her own magazine and wondered what relationship advice she would give Kara.

She saw Kara swirling a new dress for her boyfriend, flushed and silly, saying "I love you" for the first time. She saw the boyfriend suddenly slamming kitchen drawers, his face ugly with rage. She saw herself striding into the kitchen, ignoring the boyfriend (just a boy after all, a gigantic little boy throwing a tantrum, there was nothing complex or mysterious about it), and taking Kara firmly by the elbow and marching her right on out of the kitchen. *No, it's not normal. No, it's not your fault. Walk away now, young lady.*

"But I'm wearing a new dress!" Kara would whine. "I want to drink champagne!"

He's going to do it again, you silly little girl! He's going to do it again, again, and again until there's nothing left of you.

"Are you all right?" Cat waved a hand in front of Gemma's face. "What's the matter? You've gone all red." She lowered her voice. "You haven't wet your pants, have you?"

Gemma gave a yelp of laughter and Cat stood up decisively. "Right. I'm going to see how long this is going to take."

A few minutes later, thanks to Cat's stand-over tactics, Gemma was lying on her back, while a cheerful, blue-uniformed girl called Nicki rubbed a gooey cold gel across her stomach.

"It's my sister's baby," she explained to Nicki, so she'd treat Cat like someone important. "She's adopting it for me."

Nicki didn't even blink at that, which was nice of her. "O.K. then, Mum," she said to Cat. She gestured up at the TV monitor on the wall. "Keep your eye on that screen."

Cat smiled stiffly and crossed her arms awkwardly across her chest. She'll be wishing it was her and Dan here, thought Gemma, making their cool little jokes, holding hands while they watched their baby. Perhaps she should try and hold Cat's hand? Except Cat would be aghast, of course.

Nicki began to rub a little instrument back and forth over Gemma's stomach as if she were giving it a gentle polish. "In just a minute your baby will make his or her first public appearance!"

"We don't want to know the sex," said Cat sharply.

"My lips are sealed," said Nicki.

Cat dropped her arms by her side as a grainy, alien landscape emerged on the screen. "Oh look!"

"It looks like the moon," said Gemma, not really believing this picture had anything to do with her body; they probably showed the same picture to everyone. It probably *was* the moon.

"Let me give you the guided tour," said Nicki and she began to point out parts of the baby. The spine. The legs. The feet. The heart. Gemma smiled and nodded politely, fraudulently. It was nothing but fuzzy static. Change the channel, she imagined saying. Put something more interesting on. Cat on the other hand, seemed to genuinely believe she was looking at a baby. "Oh yes, I see," she kept saying, and her voice was all shaky and full of some lovely maternal emotion that Gemma definitely was not feeling.

"Only one baby," observed Nicki. "No twins."

"Or triplets," said Gemma.

"Heaven forbid!" chuckled Nicki.

That night, while Gemma did her house-sitting duties—chatting with the Violets, dusting dozens of tiny ornaments, listening to Mary Penthurst's unappealing older sister, Frances, deliver her weekly phone lecture—another layer of her consciousness continued to consider the suddenly very urgent relationship advice for Kara.

"I was only saying to my friend today," said Frances in her thin querulous voice, as if she were making this observation for the first time, "what an incredible amount of rent you must be saving!" It was a common complaint from the relatives of house-sitting clients, and Gemma knew exactly the right response—excessive gratitude.

"I know! I am *so* lucky! Every morning I think, I am *so* lucky!"

Frances grunted but was mollified and moved on to the garden. "You did plant Mary's sweet peas on St. Patrick's Day? She's been doing that religiously for the last twenty years, you know! It's a funny little ritual of hers." Gemma said, "I certainly did!" and imagined Kara cowering on a lounge, while her boyfriend raged about the way she'd flirted with one of his friends. *Everyone* saw it, said the boyfriend. Everyone was so embarrassed for me. You acted like such a dumb, stupid slut.

Gemma felt a white-hot flame of rage ignite like a blowtorch. *No, it's not proof of how much he loves you! Please, sweetie, I know it seems hard, but just leave. It's easy really. Stand up and walk out the door.* But Kara just sat there, in a stupor of fear and shame and apathy, and Gemma understood.

"You've been remembering to air that musty back room?" asked Frances.

"Absolutely," said Gemma.

When Frances finally wilted and hung up, Gemma called Kara.

"Have you got a new boyfriend?"

"*No.* Why are you asking that? Did Cat say something? She promised!"

"No, no! I just wondered. Look, Kara, it's really important if you do get a boyfriend, that he's really nice to you. O.K.? All the time. Not just some of the time. *All* the time."

There was silence. "O.K.," said Kara slowly. "Thanks, Gemma. Um. *Friends* is about to start."

"Oh! Sorry. Bye then."

She put down the phone and laughed out loud, imagining the condescending, "What a loony!" expression on Kara's face. She would have plunked herself in front of the television and not given her step-auntie's weird advice another thought.

Gemma sat down on the Penthursts' soft floral sofa, which made her knees slide up to her chin, and stopped pretending to talk to Kara.

You were nineteen. You didn't imagine it. You didn't deserve it. You didn't secretly like it. When he died, it was weird and con-fusing. Of course it was. You loved him as much as you hated him. I'm sorry for being so nasty about it for all this time.

"I forgive you," she said out loud. Who, Marcus? the Violets called out nosily from the windowsill.

No! I never *stopped* forgiving him! Me. I forgive me for staying with him. A pressure she didn't know she was feeling suddenly released. It felt like she was unclenching her fists for the first time in a decade.

Someone did a ladylike little fart during "Beginner Yoga for Mums-to-Be."

At the time everyone was lying flat on their backs, eyes shut, pinned to blue foam mats. The lights were dimmed and the cross-legged teacher was delivering gentle, melodic instructions: "Breathe in . . . one, two, three . . . and out . . . one, two, three."

Gemma's pupils danced behind her eyelids. That was not the slightest bit funny, she told herself sternly. You are not a schoolboy.

"Excuse *me!*" The frothy hint of a giggle in the culprit's voice was irresistible. All around her Gemma sensed the quivering vibrations of chortling, pregnant women.

"Breathe in . . ." continued the teacher reprovingly, but it was too late, the class united in a gale of warm laughter.

And at that moment, as Gemma laughed with them, she felt a small but unmistakable movement in her belly, like the delicate flutter of a butterfly's wings. It wasn't like those other peculiar tummy rumbles she'd been experiencing; this was separate from her, yet part of her. *Well, hello there, little butterfly baby! So, you really are in there! Do you think it's funny too?*

As the class pulled themselves together and the teacher resumed her chanting, a single tear slid down Gemma's cheek and straight into her ear, where it tickled.

Hello, sweetie! I'm your Auntie Gemma.

"It's absolutely gorgeous." Gemma stood in Cat's spare room surveying the exquisite nursery that was emerging. "You're so clever!"

"Yes, I am." Cat looked content in her yellow paint-splattered overalls, a glass of red wine, a bag of pretzels, and a portable stereo on the floor next to her. "I didn't realize home improvement could be so therapeutic. And check this out, I've been stocking up!" She opened the linen cupboard to reveal neatly stacked shelves of baby stuff—bibs, booties, disposable nappies, fluffy blankets. "Lyn's been giving me things."

"Oh, good! She must be coming around to the idea."

"I don't think so. Every time she hands something over, she says, "Don't think this means I approve!"

"She might need that stuff for herself if she gets pregnant."

"She told me yesterday they've revised the five-year plan. They're going to wait until Maddie is three. She wants to expand the business this year, set up a franchise operation."

"Gosh. She's so *driven.*"

"Michael told her he was leaving her if she didn't hire an assistant."

"Oh, that's so lovely of him!"

"Yes, I was pleased with him. What's your five-year plan, by the way? What are you going to do once the baby is born?" Cat gave her a sudden keen look.

"I work on five-minute plans," said Gemma. "But lately, I have been thinking about getting a real job. Maybe I'll go back to teaching. Or study again. Or maybe I'll travel for a bit!"

"Gosh, Gemma," Cat picked up her wineglass and grinned at her. "You're so *driven.*"

In August, when Gemma was seven months pregnant, Frank moved back into the family home at Turramurra.

A few weeks after, Maxine—not fooling anyone with her light-hearted tone—organized a "casual" family dinner. At the last minute Michael had to work, Nana got a better offer, and Kara offered to stay home and mind Maddie. So, for the first time in twenty-seven years, Frank, Maxine, and their three daughters found themselves sitting self-consciously around the dinner table.

"Well, I hope you girls all eat your vegetables these days!" Frank joked heartily, and then quickly jammed a huge forkful of food into his mouth, as if he'd heard his own words and realized how inappropriate they were, because the long-ago battles over vegetables hadn't really been that funny.

When they were in kindergarten, Cat developed a psychotic aversion to "green-colored food." "No *green!*" she'd cry passionately, as if it were a religious belief. In Gemma's memory there wasn't a dinnertime where Maxine hadn't raged, "You're not leaving the table until you've finished every scrap on that plate!" They'd argue violently back and forth until Frank would suddenly explode, "Oh for Christ's *sake,* leave the child alone!" and then it was no longer about Cat eating her vegetables, it was about Mum and Dad and hard, hating words and silent, vicious chewing and the cross clatter and scrape of cutlery across plates. "I'll eat them!" Gemma would offer desperately. "I *love* green!" Lyn, her plate cleared, would say in a tired, grown-up voice, "May I be excused?"

There was a moment's loaded silence around the table. "Of course they like their vegetables now. They all became *vegetarians* when they were teenagers," observed Maxine, who had never forgiven Cat for being the one to instigate that "ludicrous little phase."

"Can someone pass the broccoli?" asked Cat gravely.

"Will you make the baby eat vegetables?" Gemma asked Cat.

"Of course."

"Oh, *of course,* she says!" Maxine snorted. "As if it's easy! Tell her, Lyn!"

Lyn said, "Let her discover it for herself."

Gemma watched Cat's shoulders relax at this apparent acceptance of her soon-to-be-mother status.

"Cat will be a wonderful mum," said Frank, reaching down the table to refill wineglasses, "just like my beautiful Max."

Maxine rolled her eyes. "I'm sure I'm not her choice of role model."

"Of course you are, Mum," said Cat. "Look how brilliantly we all turned out!"

"Hear, hear!" said Frank while Maxine smiled a little dubiously and said, "I was just a silly young kid. So were you, Frank. Good Lord! Two kids trying to bring up three little girls."

That night Gemma put the headphones onto her stomach for the baby's nightly Mozart concert.

"Hello, there! How's life in the float tank?" she asked. Over the last few months, she'd been neglecting the Violets while she talked to the baby, but they didn't seem to be suffering. In fact they were fat and flourishing, as if they were enjoying the fertile atmosphere.

"Your mum's going to make you eat all your vegetables, you know," Gemma said. "I hope you don't mind the color green. Anyway, if you do, we can have a talk about it. There are other colored vegetables after all!"

She switched on the tape and began to compile a list of useful things to tell the baby—little tips for a happier life that Cat might forget, or might not know.

Never laugh when you don't really get the joke.

Stay right away from fireworks. Oh my goodness, stay *right* away from them!

TV sucks out your brain cells. Don't be a couch potato! Use the ad breaks productively for homework, housework, and other administrative tasks.

Avoid the lethal combination of bourbon and salt-and-vinegar chips.

Look both ways before you cross the road. *Both* ways.

Try not to saddle yourself with too distinct a personality too early in life. It might not suit you later on.

Say thank you to toll collectors. Your mum collected tolls once. Toll collectors are *human beings.*

She meant your Auntie Gemma, of course. Not your mum. Auntie Gemma.

CHAPTER 23

The birthday dinners had started in their mid-twenties. They were Lyn's idea. "No partners," she had said. "Just the three of us. Seeing as we never give each other presents, it could be our present to ourselves."

"How very sisterly," said Cat. "How very *triplety.*"

"It's a wonderful idea. I second it!" Gemma interrupted, as Lyn began to pinch her nose. "I know! We can each have our own birthday cake!"

And so the annual drunken Birthday Bash became an institution.

So you could say it was all Lyn's fault really.

This year they went to a new seafood restaurant in Cockle Bay, with shiny wooden floorboards, disdainful white walls, and sleek chrome chairs. The kitchen was a square box in the center of the room with narrow, horizontal windows revealing bobbing chefs' hats and occasional, rather alarming, fiery explosions.

"I hate it when you can see the kitchen staff," said Lyn. "It makes me feel stressed."

"You love feeling stressed," said Cat.

"You don't know me at all."

"Oh no. You're just a casual acquaintance."

A waitress with a blue-and-white-striped apron and a distressing row of silver studs under her bottom lip appeared at their table, her arms stretched wide around a giant blackboard. "Tonight's specials," she said, plunking down the board and flexing her fingers. "We're out of oysters and scallops, blue-eyed cod, and trout."

"Why don't you just rub out what you don't have?" asked Cat. "Is it just to torture us?"

The waitress shrugged, and her eyes flickered. "Ha-ha."

"Let's share the seafood fondue," interrupted Gemma.

"Could we get this opened soon, do you think?" asked Lyn pointedly, nodding her head at Michael's contribution to the evening—a bottle of Bollinger.

"What's the occasion, ladies?" sighed the waitress, sounding like a jaded hooker, as she lifted an expert elbow, popped the cork, and began to pour their glasses.

"It's our birthday," said Gemma. "We're triplets!"

"Yeah? Oh, yeah?" The hand holding the bottle hovered precariously off course as she looked at them. Lyn reached over and navigated the glass under the liquid.

"How cool!" The waitress grinned. "Hey! You two are the same, right!"

"Five bucks and you can get your photo taken with us," said Cat.

After their first sips of champagne, their moods became fizzy and frivolous. Lyn suddenly revealed a bizarre phobia about parking lots, at which Cat and Gemma howled with delight. "Thanks for your sensitivity," she said.

"*All* parking lots?" asked Cat. "Do they have to be like, I don't know, twenty-four-hour parking lots to be scary?"

"Actually, I'm sure I've got that phobia too," said Gemma.

"You do not," said Lyn. "*I'm* the interesting one."

"O.K., if we're doing secrets," said Cat and revealed that a few months after breaking up with Dan she'd gotten drunk and slept with her boss.

Gemma was genuinely shocked. "But I met him at your office. He was a gray-haired man in a suit and tie! I can't believe you slept with such a grown-up!"

"I sleep with a forty-year-old every night," commented Lyn.

"Oh, don't worry, *Michael's* not a grown-up."

"He'll be relieved to hear that."

"So what secrets have you got, Gemma?" asked Cat. "As if we wouldn't already know them."

Gemma, her mouth full of bread roll, considered sharing the secret she'd been lugging around for the last twelve years: My dead fiancé was . . . problematic.

"Look at her! Trying to look mysterious," giggled Lyn.

She was never going to tell them. It was too complicated and at the same time too simple.

She said, "Once I stole ten dollars from Mum's purse to buy cigarettes."

"That was *me,* you idiot!" said Cat.

"How are we doing? We ready to move on to that second bottle yet?" The waitress had become their good mate, Olivia, who lived at Padstow and was taking a massage course and had a pregnant sister-in-law and had never met triplets, although her best friend in primary school was a twin.

Olivia had clearly decided they were lovable freaks of nature, adorable madcaps. As a result, the three of them were starting to behave like, in Nana Kettle's words, "real *characters*!"

A waiter laden with seafood platters struggled by. "Triplets!" called Olivia proudly, pointing downward fingers at their heads. Obligingly, they all beamed and gave quirky waves.

The waiter smiled cautiously.

"Moron," said Olivia. "By the way, don't look now, but that man over there—*I said don't look!*"

They all turned back to look at her guiltily. "He asked if you could keep the noise down. I'm like, Take a chill pill, wanker! So, I reckon, crank up the volume! He needs to get a life."

They promised her they'd do their best to be even noisier.

She disappeared. "She's sort of cool, that Olivia," said Lyn. "I think I'm going to start being *cooler* now I'm thirty-four."

"Cool people, like Olivia, like me, are born cool," said Cat. "You can't change your fundamental dorky personality."

"That's not true!" cried Lyn. "You can be whoever you want to be!"

"Don't give me that self-help psychobabble bullshit."

"No fighting, please," said Gemma. "It's bad for the baby."

With the baby due in just three weeks, she was feeling superior and ladylike in her sobriety, carefully monitoring her first glass of champagne while Lyn and Cat were draining their third.

Cat and Lyn both looked at her stomach.

"Bad for Cat's baby," observed Lyn.

"Don't start," said Cat dangerously.

"I think I see our mains!" interrupted Gemma, even though she didn't.

"There's something I need to say about this," said Lyn.

"I *do* see our mains!"

"Just say it, Lyn," said Cat.

"Oh! I nearly forgot!" Gemma cried. "Guess what I brought tonight!"

She nearly lost her balance reaching down for her bag, which for some reason didn't want to be picked up.

The woman at the table next to them said something that Gemma couldn't hear.

"I beg your pardon?"

"She said the strap's caught around your chair leg. Here. Stand up."

The woman's dining companion reached over and dislodged her bag. He was short and broad, like Charlie, except fair, with a sunburned nose and a grin that scrunched his eyes.

"Thank you," said Gemma. "How does that always happen?"

"A mystery," agreed the man.

Cat rolled her eyes as the man sat back down. "The mystery is why there's always a good-hearted *bloke* around whenever Gemma does her damsel-in-distress thing."

Gemma pulled three crumpled stained envelopes out of her bag. "Do you remember when Miss Ellis made us write letters to ourselves to read in twenty years' time?"

Blank looks.

"Religion class. We were fourteen."

"That's right," said Lyn. "She was talking about achieving your dreams. It was a pointless goal-setting exercise! You need to set short-term, medium-term—"

"What? You've got all our letters? You managed to keep them for twenty years without losing them?" Cat reached out to grab them. "Let me see!"

"Nope. Not until after we sing 'Happy Birthday.' That's when we officially turn thirty-four."

The distraction was successful. Lyn and Cat began an impassioned argument about whether Miss Ellis's pink fluffy cardigans indicated latent lesbian tendencies, while Gemma sat quietly and wondered if the tiny person currently kicking her with such energetic determination was perhaps a boy.

Yesterday, she'd walked by a little boy and his father in the aisle of Woolies. They were buying globes.

"Dad? How does a light globe *work*?" the little boy asked, frowning with masculine concentration.

As Gemma walked by with her wagon, the father was squatting down, pulling a globe from its cardboard box.

Maybe the baby would be a little boy like that.

One of those sturdy, serious, *interested* little boys.

Freckles.

Long, curvy eyelashes.

Their three birthday cakes arrived with dozens of wildly crackling sparklers. The lights were dimmed, and Olivia led a choir of waiters and waitresses hollering three over-the-top renditions of "Happy Birthday." Eventually, the whole restaurant seemed to be singing. The final round of applause was ridiculous, Olivia shouting "Hip, *hip*!" and the restaurant responding *"Hooray!"* thumping their feet on the floor, as if they were in a raunchy theater restaurant, not a *Good Food Guide* recommendation.

Gemma watched her sisters' laughing faces illuminated by the fizzing sparklers, and remembered how excited their placid Nana Leonard used to become on their birthday.

"Make a wish, girls!" she'd say, fervently clasping her hands, as the three of them stood in a jostling row to blow out the candles on their shared cake. "Make a special wish!" It was as if she truly believed their birthday wishes could and would come true and as a result Gemma would construct elaborate wishes with multiple clauses: like school being canceled forever and living in a chocolate house and becoming a ballerina and Daddy finally coming back home.

The lights came back on and they blinked at one another. Olivia took their cakes away for cutting, promising to take some home for herself.

"Time to hear from our fourteen-year-old selves," ordered Cat. Her eyes were glassy. "Hand 'em over."

"We'll each read out our own letters." Lyn's words were blurring around the edges.

So that's what they did.

Cat went first.

Dear ME,

This is a letter from you in your past. You probably don't even remember it but once you had to do these STUPID, SHITTY things called religion lessons with this IDIOT teacher who PISSES ME RIGHT OFF. Glad you're finally FREE, I bet! I bet you're just laughing your head off remembering how boring school was and how you felt like you were in PRISON. (By the way, Gemma is sitting in front of me sucking up to the teacher like you would not believe. Meanwhile Lyn has got her arm wrapped around her page as if I'll try and steal her future for God's sake.)

So—I've got to tell you what I hope you've achieved. Here it is:

1. You should drive a red MX5.
2. You should have traveled EVERYWHERE..
3. You should have a LOT of money.
4. You should have a tattoo.
5. You should have your own really cool apartment.
6. You should go to any concert that you want. GO RIGHT NOW IF YOU WANT! COS YOU CAN, RIGHT? So just go!
7. You should be very SUCCESSFUL—I'm not sure in what. You are probably a famous war correspondent. (I hope they haven't got world peace yet. There are still wars, right?)
8. That's about it. I don't think you should be married yet. Wait till you're 35. You don't want to ruin your whole life like Mum did.

From, CATRIONA KETTLE, AGED 14.

Then Lyn:

Dear Me in Twenty Years' Time,

GOALS YOU SHOULD HAVE ACHIEVED BY NOW ARE:
1. Enough marks to do Hotel Management at uni.
2. Travel to exciting places.
3. Your own successful catering business.
4. A husband with a voice like Mr. Gordon's. (Husband should adore you and love you and be romantic and give you flowers.)

5. A big, beautiful house with views of Sydney Harbour.
6. Lots of beautiful clothes in a walk-in wardrobe.
7. One daughter named Madeline, one son named Harrison (after Harrison Ford. Mmmm, mmmm!).

Good luck and good-bye,

LYNETTE KETTLE.

And finally Gemma:

Ahoy there, Gemma!

It's me, Gemma!
I'm fourteen.
You're thirty-four!
Wow!
Anyway, here's what you should have achieved by now:

• A degree in something or other.
• A career in something or other.
• A HUNKY, SPUNKY husband whose name begins with either
    M, S, G, C, X, or P!
• Four children. Two girls and two boys. Order should be Boy,
    Girl, Boy, Girl (but I can be flexible).

So—have you done it?? I hope so! If not, why not?
Lots of love from Gemma.
P.S. Hey! You've had *sex*. What was it like???!!! AAAGGGGH!
P.P.S. Who did it first? You, Cat, or Lyn??? AAAAGGGGH!
P.P.S. Give that hunky, spunky husband a big kiss and tell
    him it's from your fourteen-year-old self!

"Wow," said Lyn. "We were so, so . . ."
"Exactly the same," said Cat.
"Different," said Gemma.
It wasn't so much the things that her fourteen-year-old self

wanted. It was the fact that she so blissfully, so completely, believed she had a right to want *anything*.

Ahoy there, Gemma! I'm sorry, but I seem to have stuffed things up. I forgot. I'm not sure what I forgot. But I forgot it.

She thought of her mother, the day of Cat's court case, watching Cat and Lyn obviously locked in some sort of vicious argument. "Those two need to let go!" she'd said. "What about me, Mum?" Gemma had asked frivolously. "What do I need to do?" "You're the opposite. You need to hold on, of course. Hold on to something. Hold on to anything!"

"So, Lyn, all you need is that little boy called Harrison and you've achieved everything you ever dreamed," said Cat.

"Yes, I know. I'm so *boring.*"

"You said it, not me."

"Oh, stop it! The two of you. Just stop it." Gemma could feel something indefinable inflating within her.

Cat and Lyn ignored her. They both took drowning gulps from their glasses.

"I note that your letter didn't even mention children," Lyn said to Cat.

"It wasn't a contract."

"It's just interesting."

"You know, Lyn, not everything is your business."

"It is my business! Gemma's baby is my niece or nephew. And I think children should be with their *parents.* That's why—"

She stopped, took a breath and brushed at some crumbs on the tablecloth with the back of her hand.

"That's why what?" asked Gemma.

"That's why I called Charlie to tell him you're pregnant."

Gemma nearly knocked over her glass. "What did he say?"

"He wasn't there," admitted Lyn. "I didn't leave a message. But I'm calling him again. I feel really strongly about this."

Gemma watched as Cat began to tremble.

"You bitch. You absolute bitch."

"Cat. It's not about you."

"It is about me. This is *my* baby!"

But it's not, thought Gemma, with surprise. It's my baby.

"Do you know how a lightbulb works?" she asked Cat.

"Oh, shut up, Gemma! This is serious!"

Charlie would know.

It seemed like the purest, most absolute truth of her entire life.

That Charlie would know how a lightbulb worked. And he'd pull a funny face. And he'd explain it so well that electricity would seem like something magical. And Gemma didn't want to miss it. She wanted to be there, loving them both in the bright, white light of Woolworth's.

"The thing is," she began.

She knew what she was about to say was unbearably cruel, but she said it anyway:

"I've changed my mind."

CHAPTER 24

She changed her mind. She just went right ahead and changed her mind.

"I'm sorry, Cat." Gemma looked across the table at Cat with wide-eyed sincerity. "I'm really, *really* sorry."

Cat almost laughed because she'd known this could happen. Maybe she even knew all along that it *would* happen.

But she'd given her every possible chance.

"Are you sure this is what you want?" she'd asked, again and again.

And again, again, Gemma had replied, "Absolutely sure! Deep down in my heart sure."

When Gemma had first suggested the plan, Cat had agreed in an almost lighthearted, fantastical way. It hadn't seemed possible that Gemma could really be pregnant, sitting in Cat's kitchen, in her cut-off shorts, looking normal and skinny. It felt like a game, an abstract distraction. It was the same as when she thought about the idea of going to a sperm bank. Yes, she was sort of serious, sort of *very* serious, but did sperm banks actually exist outside of comedy films? Did they have ads in the Yellow Pages?

Imagining Gemma's baby in her arms helped her to stop

thinking about Dan and Angela—and Angela's hair and Angela's breasts and Angela's underwear.

It helped her to walk by parents pushing their strollers, without wanting to stop and scream with savage rage at those smug, carelessly happy women, What makes you so special? Look at you! You're not that pretty or smart! How did you manage to have a baby? When I can't? When I've somehow failed to achieve this basic *boring* thing!

It helped her to sleep. It helped her get up in the mornings.

And that was why the violent opposition from Maxine and Lyn was so hurtful. They reacted as if it were all Cat's idea. As usual, evil Cat was exploiting fragile, helpless Gemma.

They never once said, We understand why you want to do this.

They didn't seem to notice that it was a miracle that Cat was still functioning, when she felt like she'd been fragmented into a million pieces. They weren't incredulous, like Cat still was on a daily basis, that Dan had actually gone, that he woke up in some other woman's bed.

Her hurt gave her a petulant resolve. Why not, after all? Why shouldn't this work, if Gemma wanted it? Why not?

She worked for hours on the second bedroom, painting the walls a buttery yellow. While she was scraping and painting, her mind was peacefully blank.

The nursery was beautiful. Everyone said so.

Just yesterday, she'd bought a white cane chair with blue cushions and put it by the window, where you could see the magnolia tree. She'd sat there in a pool of morning sunshine and imagined giving the baby its bottle and considered the possibility of happiness.

It was going to be her and the baby against the world. Just the two of them.

And now Gemma changed her mind.

All that softness and sunshine had been snatched away, and Cat was back out again in that bland wasteland of memos and office cubicles and divorce proceedings and *nobody waiting for her to come home.*

Better to have stayed cold all along than had this taste of warmth.

Cat sat there in the noisy restaurant with her head pounding from champagne, a huge nauseating triangle of chocolate mud cake in front of her, and for a few seconds she felt nothing, and then it came, all at once, a tumbling toxic torrent.

It was basic, childish disappointment.

It was "Ha ha! Who looks like a fool now!" humiliation.

It was the smug lift of Lyn's eyebrows.

It was tomorrow. And the day after that.

It was because fourteen-year-old Cat Kettle would have thought she was a loser.

Whatever it was, it sucked her down into a wailing vortex and afterward she never remembered how she came to be standing up, or what she was saying, or what she was holding in her hand until she threw it, screaming, "You have both fucking ruined my life!"

And then:

One day you'll go too far, Maxine always said.

She'd gone too far.

The fork protruding embarrassingly and impossibly out of Gemma's belly.

Blood!

Her first thought was, sweet Jesus, I've killed her.

And then, I'm going to be sick.

A roaring in her ears.

She was on the floor, with the most tremendous pain thumping down one side of her face and into her ear and something metallic filling her mouth.

Olivia was crouched down beside her, "It's O.K. You fainted. You all right? You hit your chin pretty hard against the table."

All around her, Cat could see the backs of people's legs. Their table was surrounded by a frenzied group of arguing strangers.

"Be calm! Tell her to be calm! Sweetheart, be very, *very* calm!"

"The ambulance is coming. Shhhh! Is that the siren I hear?"

"Has anybody called the police? Because I saw it! That was *assault*!"

"Did you hear? They're *sisters*! Unbelievable."

"Have I killed her?" she wanted to ask, but her mouth was full of marbles.

"Everyone is *freaking* out!" Olivia said happily.

"Um, Lyn?" It was Gemma's voice. She sounded perfectly alive, vaguely concerned. "I think, maybe, I just had a contraction."

Olivia's mouth dropped comically.

The crowd seemed to sigh and sway with the horror of it. Cat watched a pair of masculine shoes begin to shuffle discreetly away from the table. Then she heard Lyn, her voice slip-sliding into uncharacteristic panic, "Is there a doctor here?"

Cat prayed: frantically and obsequiously. *Please, God, Jesus, Holy Spirit, Mother of Mary, all of you, I'm begging you, don't let the baby die!*

"I've got my first-aid certificate," offered somebody.

"She doesn't need to be resuscitated," said somebody else.

"Of course I've never had a contraction before," continued Gemma thoughtfully. "So, how would I know?"

"Helsh me up," mumbled Cat, tasting blood. Olivia pulled on her wrists and heaved her to her feet.

"Here comes the boss." Olivia appeared to be having the time of her life. "Oooh! She'll be going ape shit over this! Afterbirth all over her floorboards."

It was the same elegant, all-in-black woman who had so graciously offered their table at the beginning of the night. She now gave Cat a look of appalled disgust and used the back of her hands to firmly flap the crowd back to their seats. "Could I ask everyone to move? The ambulance is on its way."

The grown-ups were coming. People hurried back to their

tables, looking slightly embarrassed, murmuring seriously to one another.

Ten minutes later, the paramedics walked through the restaurant radiating waves of drama and relaxed authority, like movie stars casually strolling into a press conference.

Lyn began to speak to them, but Gemma interrupted her, her tone succinct and urgent, even bossy.

"I'm due in three weeks. I saw my obstetrician just yesterday and she said I could expect to start feeling those pretend contractions. I don't know if that's what I just felt, or not. There's a lot of tissue around the uterus right? The fork couldn't have hurt my baby?

"It's unlikely," agreed the paramedic. "It would have to penetrate a very long way. It looks like it's just broken the skin. Let's take a look at your blood pressure."

"I think you should listen to the baby's heartbeat," snapped Gemma. "That's what I think you should do."

She sounded, Cat thought, exactly like Lyn.

Or maybe it was Maxine.

She sounded like somebody's mother.

Cat silently cradled her jaw and looked out the car window at the lights of the city. The guy who had been sitting at the table next to them, the one who had helped Gemma with her bag, was driving them to the hospital. Cat didn't know or care what had happened to the girl who was with him.

He'd introduced himself to Cat, but she hadn't bothered to listen. He didn't seem quite real. Nobody did. She felt as if she were separated from the rest of the world by a blurry membrane. Nothing really mattered, except that Gemma and the baby would be O.K. The pain down the side of her face was excruciating, and she felt strangely conscious of every breath that she took.

She could hear Lyn in the front seat, talking to Maxine on her mobile.

"Yes, I know it's our birthday. That's why—"

"Yes, I do know how old we—"

"No, Mum, we're not drunk—"

"O.K. Maybe a little tipsy."

"Yes, a fork. A fondue fork."

"A seafood fondue."

"Well, *we* liked it!"

"It was just a little argument, Mum. I'll explain—"

"O.K., maybe not so little. But—"

"Well, yes, actually. I think the whole restaurant probably saw. But—"

"Royal Prince Alfred."

"Fine. Bye."

Lyn pressed a button on her mobile and shifted around to look at Cat. "Mum says take care, she loves us, and she's coming right away."

Cat stared at her with incomprehension, and Lyn chortled. "I'm joking!"

The guy driving the car chuckled. Cat held her napkin to her mouth and looked back out the window. Now Lyn was sounding a lot like Gemma. The world had gone topsy-turvy.

At the entrance to the hospital, Cat got out of the car without speaking, slammed the door, and blinked at the bright lights and muted roar of activity: phones ringing, a child screaming relentlessly, clumps of people walking busily in different directions.

Lyn seemed to have made best friends with the man from the restaurant. Cat watched as she leaned back in the window and chatted enthusiastically, before straightening up and waving good-bye.

She held up a little fan of business cards. "He's a landscape gardener, a wedding photographer, *and* a personal trainer!" she said, as if this were interesting. "He was on a blind date but apparently it wasn't going too well."

Cat shrugged.

Lyn put the cards away in her purse. "Right, well, let's see what's happening with Gemma, and we'd better get someone to look at you. I wonder if you've bitten your tongue."

Cat shrugged again. Perhaps she would give up talking forever. It might make life less complicated.

"Is that you, Lyn? Um, Cat?"

They turned around. It was Charlie walking toward them. He was wearing muddy tracksuit pants, a T-shirt, and a black beanie. He looked sweaty and agitated.

"I'm on my way home from touch footie and your sister calls for the first time in six months," he said. "She asks me how a light-bulb works. So I start to explain it; I mean that's Gemma, right? She was always asking funny questions. But then she starts crying like her heart is going to break and says she's calling from an ambulance on the way to have a baby, and would I like to come and help her breathe, if I'm not too busy? Are you girls strange, or what?"

"No question, we're strange," said Lyn.

He held both palms upward in a very Italian gesture. "Man! She dumps me, she wasn't even going to tell me she's pregnant, and now suddenly she wants me to help her *breathe*?"

"It's quite presumptuous of her," agreed Lyn.

"And I don't how to do this!" An expression of pure terror crossed his face. "There are classes for this sort of thing. Books. Videos. I like to know how things work!"

Lyn beamed at him. "Just hold her hand. Do what they do in the movies."

"Jesus." He pulled his beanie off, ran one hand over the top of his head, and took a deep breath. "And is she O.K.?"

"Well, there was a little accident but they're looking at her now."

For the first time Charlie looked at Cat and her blood-soaked napkin. Cat looked at the ground and tried to pretend she was somewhere else.

"An accident?"

"Let's go inside and find out what's happening," said Lyn.

While Lyn and Charlie went off to find someone official, Cat sat down on a green plastic chair and began heavy negotiations with God.

All she wanted was for Gemma and the baby to be O.K. It didn't seem like too unreasonable a request. She simply wanted one particular action to be without consequences.

And if God would do that, Cat would give up alcohol and every other potentially pleasurable activity. She would graciously accept that she was never going to have children herself and live a quiet, nunlike existence, thinking only of others.

She might even consider some very unpleasant form of volunteer work.

After a seemingly endless discussion, Charlie and Lyn came back over to where Cat was sitting. She looked up at them wordlessly.

"Someone's coming to see us now," explained Lyn.

Charlie looked closely at Cat. "Are you O.K.? You don't look so good."

Cat nodded and mumbled, "I'm fine shanks."

"Gemma Kettle's family?" An efficiently frowning nurse appeared. "She's doing well. Four centimeters dilated. Who's going to be with her for the labor?"

"Just the father," said Lyn.

Charlie gave a little start. "I guess that would be me."

The nurse gave Cat and Lyn a meaningful and hugely unjust "Men!" look and said, "This way, please."

"Rightio." Charlie handed over a sports bag to Lyn and obediently followed the nurse without looking back, his shoulders in the dirty T-shirt very square.

Lyn sat down next to Cat and shook her head. "That man is a saint. If she doesn't hold on to him, I'll throw a fork at her!"

At that moment Maxine marched into the hospital waiting

room to find her daughters, propped up against each other's shoulders, laughing helplessly.

She held the strap of her handbag disapprovingly against her chest. "Well, *really*!"

At eight o'clock the next morning Cat held her nephew for the first time. A tightly bound eight-pound bundle with a wrinkly red face, matted black hair, and long eyelashes resting mysteriously against caramel-colored skin.

Cat and Gemma were alone in the room.

Charlie had gone home to change. Lyn was coming back with Maddie and Michael later that afternoon. Maxine and Frank were buying coffee in the cafeteria.

"I'm sorry, Cat." Gemma's face against the pillow was blotchy, puffy, and suffused with joy. "I did a terrible thing to you."

Cat shook her head and kept looking at the baby.

Some time last night, a doctor had informed her that her jaw was broken. Her back and front teeth were now wired together. If she tried to talk, her mouth started foaming with saliva.

She felt, fittingly, like a freak. It was her penance.

"I thought of the baby as yours," said Gemma. "All the way along. I swear to you. And then all of a sudden, I started wanting—I wanted the baby and I wanted Charlie. I wanted everything."

Cat placed her little finger in the palm of the baby's hand and watched his tiny fingers curl in a miniature grip.

Soap Bubbles on the Corso

It was a lovely day today, wasn't it? Did you have a lovely day? I bet you didn't move from that step, eh? I caught the bus down to the Corso, you know how I like to do that. I'm sure the sea air does wonders for my arthritis.

I sat on my favorite bench there and ate my banana sandwich, and watched the families. There were some lovely young girls sitting in the shade with their children. One was a toddler—oh, she was a terror that one! They had their hands full. And there was also the dearest little newborn baby! The girls were all taking turns holding the baby. I couldn't quite tell which was the mother but they were sisters, I'm sure of it. They each rocked the baby in exactly the same way, gently swaying their bodies. Tall, graceful girls. I always wanted to be tall.

Oh, and they had a clever way of distracting the little terror! They had one of those little bottles of detergent and they were blowing soap bubbles for her. She was running around with her hands outstretched, laughing, trying to catch them. Those bubbles looked so pretty floating and dancing in the breeze—like hundreds of tiny little rainbows. It made me cry a little. In a happy way.

But you know one of those young girls wasn't so happy. She was really down in the dumps about something. She was doing her best to hide it but I could tell. Something about the way she held her shoulders. As if she'd lost. You know what I mean? Defeated. That's the word.

I wanted to say to her, Oh, darling, don't be sad. Whatever it is that's worrying you will probably turn out to be nothing. Or eventually it just won't matter anymore. And one day all you'll remember is blowing soap bubbles on the Corso with your sisters. And how you were young and beautiful and didn't even know it. But she would have just thought I was a mad old woman, wouldn't she, Tabby? Yes, she would have.

CHAPTER 25

Cat got to the park a few minutes early and sat on one of the swings to wait for Dan.

It was a viciously cold Saturday morning, and the park was deserted. There was something a little spooky about all that empty play equipment, the chains of the swing rattling ghoulishly in the wind, like the laughter of ghostly children.

A wisp of a memory she felt like she was remembering for the first time floated across Cat's consciousness. Maxine pushing Lyn on a swing. A yellow dress.

"When's it *my* turn, Mum?"

Lyn flying high in the air.

She opened and shut her mouth like a fish, enjoying the glorious freedom of a fully functioning jaw.

It was six weeks since the night of the fondue fork.

Apparently the story was doing the rounds. Michael said he was at a work function when he overheard a guy tell a story about someone throwing a fork at a pregnant woman in a Chinese restaurant. The pregnant woman had then given birth to triplets on the restaurant floor.

Michael hadn't bothered to correct them. "I hope you're not embarrassed to know us," said Lyn.

"The opposite, my darling! I didn't want to show off."

Gemma and Charlie had called the baby Salvatore Lesley after both their grandfathers.

Little Sal was the baby from hell. He hadn't inherited his mother's love of sleep, or his father's saintliness. Gemma and Charlie had been walking around in dreamlike, sleep-deprived trances.

Fortunately, on Tuesday Sal cleverly chose to smile for the first time at both his parents, causing them to melt into adoring puddles at his bootied feet.

Cat kept the door to the yellow-walled nursery firmly shut and lived her life like a robot. *I feel nothing, I feel nothing* was her new mantra. She worked so hard at Hollingdale Chocolates that Rob Spencer felt the need to give her a smarmy little lecture on the importance of having "balance" in her life.

She gave up alcohol for a record four weeks before saying, "I think that'll do it, God," and returning to her faith as a devout atheist.

Dan had telephoned the day before and said he wanted to talk to her.

"Could we get together for a drink?"

"Tell me over the phone," she said, using the brittle, faintly mocking voice she seemed to have created especially for conversations these days with Dan.

"I'd rather we met, face-to-face." He had a new voice too. It was formal and restrained, as if he were in the witness box. It broke her heart.

I know the expression on your face when you come. I know how you clip your toenails, floss your teeth, and blow your nose. I know how your dad upsets you and spiders frighten you and tofu disgusts you.

"Fine. But not the pub." She didn't want to be surrounded by happy people talking in normal voices. "We'll meet in the park."

She kicked at the wood shavings under her feet and wondered what Dan wanted.

They'd been separated for seven months now. The law said you couldn't divorce until you'd been separated for a full year. No trial reconciliations were allowed during that time.

You had to prove to the government that it was more than just a little tiff, that your marriage vows were well and truly ripped to shreds.

And here he was.

She watched as he got out of the car and frowned up at the parking sign. He looked at his watch and then again at the sign, wrinkling his forehead. He always did have problems deciphering parking signs. You're fine, Dan. It's not after 3 P.M. or before 9 A.M.

Finally he came loping down the grassy embankment. He saw her, smiled, raised a hand in greeting, and it came to her in a matter-of-fact way that she still loved him.

"Hi."

"Hi."

"Cold."

"Very."

He moved toward her as if he was going to kiss her on the cheek, and she ducked her head and held a hand out at the swing next to her. "Have a seat."

He sat down, awkwardly stretching out his long legs.

He looked straight ahead. "How are you?"

"I'm fine."

Presumably, through Charlie and Angela, he knew everything about what had happened at the restaurant. Her humiliation was so complete it didn't really bother her. She had no more dignity left to lose.

He chose Angela. Gemma chose her baby.

"Cat."

And for one wild, heart-pumping moment she thought he was going to say that he'd made a mistake, he wanted to come back home, fix things up, try again.

"I'm going to France. We're going to France."

I don't feel anything.

"Did the Paris job come up again? I didn't know."

It was their dream. Angela was getting to live Cat's dream.

"They told me about a week ago."

He was doing his best to keep his voice flat, but she could hear the underlying ripple of excitement. The celebrations they must have shared!

"I didn't want you to hear it from anybody else."

"Gee, thanks."

He gave her a quick, sharp look.

"I don't know how to make you believe how sorry I am. About everything. I wish—I never meant—I'm just so sorry."

It occurred to Cat that Angela could one day have Dan's children. The little boy that Cat had always imagined, a miniature version of Dan, would now belong to Angela.

That woman was going to live her dreams and have her children.

And when Dan got home today, Angela would say, "How did she take it?" and Dan would say sadly, "Not good," and Angela would look sympathetic and pretty and large-breasted.

In a sudden rush of movement Cat leaped from her swing and positioned herself behind Dan. That woman would not hear about the tears in her eyes.

"Here, let me give you a push."

"Eh?" His shoulders stiffened.

She pushed him gently on his back and said, "Didn't your mum used to push you on the swing?"

"Yeah, I guess."

With her hands flat on his back, she rocked him forward. His legs dragged on the ground and he held on tight to the swing.

I don't feel anything. I don't feel anything. I don't feel anything.

"So, Paris! At last!" said Cat, like a charming girl at a cocktail party. "Have they got somewhere for you to live?"

"They put us in a furnished apartment for a month, and then we'll find somewhere for ourselves."

"And Angela? What will she do? Will she work?"

"She's not sure yet."

"Mmmm, and busy times, I guess! Are you selling your car? Putting things in storage?"

"I'm giving the car to Mel."

"Dan."

Because suddenly she couldn't do it anymore or bear it any longer.

She bent her head to his ear and spoke softly and urgently, in her own real voice, as if she only had a minute to pass on this dangerous message.

"Thank you for telling me. I'm fine. Really. But could you do something for me? Could you just go now, without talking, without looking at me? Don't say anything, don't look back. Please."

He sat very still. It wasn't his style to obey such a weird and melodramatic request. But then he put one hand up to hers and held it very tightly, and for a second she breathed in the smell of his hair. He squeezed her hand, stood up, and walked away, back to the car.

It was nearly an exquisitely tragic moment except that as he got to the embankment, he tripped, one foot sliding clumsily out behind him.

Well, exquisitely tragic moments weren't really her thing. Farce. That was more her style.

Cat applauded. *"Au revoir!* You big klutz!"

Without turning around, he gave her an ironic thumbs-up signal and kept walking to the car.

CHAPTER 26

At around 9 P.M. the night before Cat met Dan in the park, while Nana Kettle was eating a little snack of grilled cheese on toast, with a nice cup of tea and watching her favorite recorded episode of *Who Wants to Be a Millionaire,* a brick came smashing through a glass pane on her back door and landed with a thud on the floor.

Nana heard a strange noise and naturally assumed it was Pop's bloody dog. She enjoyed being cross with the dog and immediately put the video on pause.

"What have you done this time, you silly, no-good animal?" she called out querulously, as if for Pop's benefit. Yelling at the dog made her feel like Les was still alive, working away on some project in the back room. She could almost hear him calling back, "I'll see to it, love! You stay where you are."

It used to drive her mad the way Les spoiled that damned dog.

She was on her feet, at the TV room door, muttering crossly to herself, when she heard footsteps.

"Who's that?" she called out, annoyed rather than frightened, as she walked down the hallway. Frank and her granddaughters all had keys. But, really, it was polite to knock.

That's when a strange person pounded toward her, somebody

she didn't know, in her own house, and a tremendous wave of fear shot vertically through her body, from the soles of her feet and into her mouth.

He came straight for her, without hesitating, as if he'd been expecting her, and punched her in the face.

She fell. Her shoulder banged painfully against the wall.

For a few seconds, her world turned misty red. Her eyes blurred with tears. She could feel blood coming out of her nose.

In the TV room, the video came back on. "What do you want to do? Have a go or take the dough?" Eddie McGuire asked the contestant.

She could hear the boy in her bedroom, pulling out drawers, touching her things.

I bet you think I'm one of those stupid old biddies who keeps all her money under the bed, she thought to herself. Well, too bad it's all safe and sound in the Commonwealth Bank, matey!

Later, she found that he took her purse, her best jewelry, her jar of two-dollar coins for the slots, and a crisp $10 bill she had ready on the dining room table to include in Kara's birthday card. He also took the brand-new camera that she'd won in a late night talk-back radio competition for knowing how much the colt was worth in *The Man from Snowy River*.

He spent twenty minutes walking through her house, picking and choosing what he liked, as if he were bloody shopping.

Then he walked straight out the front door, without looking at her.

The dog appeared from wherever he'd been skulking and for a full five minutes, did nothing but run around and around in distressed circles, before stopping to lick the side of her face, panting and whimpering.

She tried to get up, but her arm wouldn't work.

She tried again and gave up. "Les," said Nana into the carpet.

Around ten o'clock the next day, Bev told her husband, Ken, that it was a bit funny that Gwen Kettle hadn't been out to water her garden yet. She always watered her garden on a Saturday, and she hadn't mentioned that she was doing anything special this Saturday. Perhaps Gwen had a visitor? Although there were no strange cars out the front. What did Ken think?

Ken didn't think anything. So finally, with a little "tsk" sound—it was impossible to have a conversation with a man—Bev went over to investigate, pushing tentatively on her neighbor's open front door.

When she saw Gwen lying there in the hallway, she went back out onto the front porch and screamed Ken's name so loud that he nearly put his back out jumping over the retaining wall and running over to see what was the matter.

"For heaven's sakes, Bev, you took your time," said Nana.

There was a messy blot of dried blood under her nose.

Bev bent down on arthritic knees to pluck uselessly at Nana's sleeve and for the first time in her life was entirely incapable of speaking.

Cat caught a cab to the hospital. She sat in the backseat with her hands jammed hard between her knees and imagined a parallel existence where by lucky chance she'd popped by to visit Nana Kettle just at the same time that lowlife prick broke into her house.

Oi! Fuckface! she would have yelled.

When he turned around, she would have kicked him hard in the balls.

As his head bent forward she would have grabbed him by the ears and driven her knee into his face. And then, while he was moaning pathetically on the ground she would have kicked him again and again in the kidneys.

Pick on someone your own size!

Cat saw her family before she saw Nana. They were sitting very straight and still in a little semicircle of chairs around Nana's bed.

"Oh, good, you're here," said Maxine.

Frank didn't say anything, just held up a hand in acknowledgement. He looked like a man suffering from a fever. His neck was covered in splotches of red.

Gemma, in contrast, was deadly pale. Sal was in her arms, sucking frantically on a pacifier, dark eyes darting back and forth. "Look, Nana, it's Cat!" said Gemma.

"Hey, Cat," said Lyn, with a weird contortion of her lips that was presumably meant to be a smile. She was arranging flowers in a vase, her eyes red and watery.

"Nana." Cat couldn't finish her cheery hello. Now she could see why everyone looked frozen with shock, as if their faces had just that instant been unexpectedly and painfully slapped.

Seeing Nana was like seeing the attack happen in front of their very eyes.

There was a large bluish bruise smeared across her mouth and a bloody scab on her bottom lip. One arm was in a sling. Her hair was especially distressing. Normally, Nana took a lot of time with her hair, using hot rollers to create a neat cap of snowy white curls. Today it was limp and greasy, flat against her head.

She looked like a frail, ugly old woman. Someone else. Not Cat's annoyingly spry grandmother.

"Did you hear?" Nana said to her, clutching her hand, as Cat kissed her on the fragile, wrinkled skin of her cheek. "He took the camera I won on the radio. I waited over an hour to get on!"

"We're going to get you another camera, Gwen," said Maxine. "An even better one."

Nana didn't seem to hear her. She clutched on tight to Cat's hand. "It was only last week, I got one of those little green cards in my letterbox. And I said to Bev, now what could this be? It says there's a parcel at the post office for me! I'd forgotten all about winning that competition you see. So Bev said—"

Suddenly, she stopped and looked up at Cat, and her pale blue eyes filled with tears.

"I got quite a fright last night, darling."

Her voice quavered.

"Yes. I can imagine you did, Nana," managed Cat.

Frank scraped back his chair and stood up.

"This is bloody—I can't bloody—this is—*Jesus!*"

He slammed both his fists violently on the back of his chair.

Nana dropped Cat's hand and became instantly peremptory. "Calm down, Frank! There's no need to behave like that. It's life! Bad things happen!"

They all looked silently at the bruise across her face.

"Hello, Mrs. Kettle!" A nurse broke through their silence, breezing efficiency. "Lots of lovely visitors I see! And look at all those flowers!"

"My back is killing me," said Nana.

"Well, let's see what we can do to make you more comfortable. Perhaps you could all come back in a few minutes?"

The nurse looked at them brightly and firmly.

"We'll go and get some lunch downstairs," pronounced Lyn. "We won't be long, Nana."

"Take your time," said Nana. "Don't know about lovely visitors. You're all such misery heads."

Gemma went to put Sal in his pram.

"Let your father carry the baby." Maxine's eyes were on Frank.

"You want him, Dad?"

"What? Oh yes, of course." He took the baby into his arms. "Hello, little mate."

Cat looked at Sal in a bright orange romper suit, a chubby fist clinging to Frank's shirt. It had become like an old sporting injury: this familiar, reflexive twinge of pain whenever she saw Sal.

"What did Dan want?" asked Lyn as the three of them walked ahead to the elevator.

"He got the job in Paris. He and Angela are going."

Both Lyn and Gemma turned to look at her with stricken faces.

"I didn't know," said Gemma immediately. "Charlie never said anything."

"You're not responsible for everything Angela does," said Cat.

"I thought—" Lyn bit her lip. "Sorry."

"Yeah. I thought it too," said Cat as the elevator bell dinged and their parents caught up with them. The doors closed, and Frank suddenly handed Sal over to Gemma and buried his face in his hands. His shoulders shook. It took Cat a confused second to realize that for the first time in her life she was seeing her father cry. He lifted his face and wiped the back of his hand across his nose. His mouth twisted with violent hatred. "I want to *kill* that bloke."

At the exact moment that Dan and Angela's flight was due to leave Sydney, Cat was heaving a giant green garbage bag of junk out onto her grandmother's front porch, her nose twitching and eyes streaming from the clouds of dust.

Would they hold hands? Make nervous jokes about their new lives together as Sydney rolled away beneath them?

Cat and Maxine were cleaning out Nana's house: the house she had lived in for over fifty years. Nana was moving into a "lifestyle resort exclusively for over fifty-fives."

"Of course, it's a retirement village," said Nana, showing them the glossy brochure with its pictures of white-haired couples ecstatically clinking champagne glasses on their "spacious balconies." "I'm not stupid. Full of silly old biddies. But I'll feel a lot safer and really what do I need this big old house for? I don't know why none of you ever suggested it. Probably worried about me spending your inheritance, I bet!"

The family heroically refrained from mentioning that they'd been suggesting it for the last ten years. Now, it was Nana's idea—and an extremely clever and sensible one.

She had said from her hospital bed that she was too frightened to spend another night in that house alone.

"Of course not, Mum!" said Frank. "You can live with Max and me!"

Cat saw her mother's eyes flicker, but Nana interrupted him. "Don't be stupid, Frank. Why would I want to live with you? I want to live in a *lifestyle resort.*"

Since the attack, Nana Kettle seemed to have developed two conflicting new personality traits.

She had moments where she seemed to Cat heartbreakingly frail and frightened, like a child waking up still in the grips of a nightmare. Describing the attack, her voice would quiver with surprised tears. It was as if her feelings had been hurt. "He didn't look at me," she kept saying. "Did I mention that? He never once looked at me." But at other times, she seemed sharper than ever before. She had a new way of lifting her chin, a determined new edge to her voice.

It helped perhaps that she had become something of a minor celebrity.

A story appeared in the *Daily Telegraph* with the headline OLYMPIC VOLUNTEER ATTACKED! Lyn had given them a photo she'd taken of Nana marching in the Volunteers' Tickertape Parade. Nana grinned cheekily up from the page—a charming, innocent old lady who could recite all the words to *The Man from Snowy River,* whose husband was a World War II soldier!

Sydney threw up its arms in horror. Nana was inundated with letters of support, flowers, teddy bears, cards, checks, and close to a hundred brand-new cameras. People wrote letters to the paper and rang up talk-back radio stations. It was un-Australian, it was appalling, it was plain wrong.

The attacker was arrested after his girlfriend recognized the Identikit picture Nana had helped create. "When I saw that sweet little old lady in the paper, I just thought, Nah, that's it," said the girlfriend self-importantly to the television crews.

"Sweet little old lady, my foot," said Maxine now, as she joined Cat out on the veranda, dragging another green bag of rubbish behind her. "She's driving me up the wall."

"Me too." Cat wiped the back of her hand across her nose and looked down at her T-shirt and jeans. They were covered in dust.

Her mother, naturally, looked neat as a pin.

"The last time she threw something out," sighed Maxine, "must have been 1950."

Nana Kettle was bossily insisting that before any object could be assigned as "rubbish," "Smith family," or "new place," she first be approached for authorization. She then wanted to chat at length about the history of each item and after finally making a decision, would more often than not change her mind, demanding that Cat and Maxine rummage through the rubbish bag and re-present the item for another lengthy discussion.

Neither Cat nor her mother had the right personalities for this sort of work.

"We need Gemma," said Cat. "She could sit and talk to Nana while we just throw the lot out."

"She's doing something with Charlie's family," said Maxine and then compressing her lips at her mistake, quickly changed the subject, producing some creased and faded sheets of paper. "Look what I found!"

Cat smiled as she recognized her own childish handwriting. "Another blast from my past."

It was the *Kettle Scoop,* a weekly family newspaper that Cat had produced when she was around ten. There had been four issues before she got bored.

"I'm really pleased," said Maxine. "This is the missing issue! I was convinced Gwen had it!"

"You would come in and present it to me with this stern little frown on your face," said Maxine. "And I had to sit there and read it without laughing. It nearly killed me. Then you'd leave the room and I'd laugh myself silly. You were such a funny, passionate kid."

"I thought I was producing a serious publication!"

Cat read the front page:

INTERVIEW WITH POP KETTLE!

Mr. Les Kettle (sometimes known as Pop Kettle) is a tall, very elderly man aged approximately sixty years old. His hair is gray and his favorite foods are baked dinners and Tooheys beer. His favorite hobbies are reading the paper, betting on the doggies, and doing his wife's nails. His least favorite things are mowing the lawn and broccoli. This reporter has sometimes seen him sneaking broccoli to his dog under the table. Pop Kettle has three granddaughters (they are triplets) and when they're all together he calls them all by the same name, which is "Susi." He doesn't know why he does this. Our undercover reporter asked which Susi was his favorite. His answer was "CAT." "But don't tell your sisters," commented Mr. Kettle quietly and under his breath. Mr. Kettle did not know that he was speaking to an undercover reporter at the time but this is what he said. This is an example of FREEDOM OF THE PRESS.

Next to the article was glued a blurry photo of Pop Kettle that Cat remembered taking herself. At the bottom of the page was a star: *Look out for next week's issue of the* Kettle Scoop *when we reveal who are Gemma's* real *parents! As everyone knows, Gemma Kettle is adopted.*

Maxine wiped tears of laughter from her eyes.

"Give it to me," she demanded. "I'm not letting it out of my sight again."

Cat handed it over. She liked hearing herself described as a "funny, passionate kid."

"So," Maxine folded the page neatly in two and tapped it against her hand, "just what are you going to do with your life?"

"Sorry?"

Typical. The very moment she became the slightest bit likable, she had to repair the damage by reverting to bitch mode.

"Well? Not many people get a chance like you've got. I hope you're not going to mope around forever, throwing cutlery at people whenever you don't get your own way."

Cat stared at her. She couldn't believe it. And here she was helping move out Nana's stuff while Lyn and Gemma spent the day with their happy little families. Cat had been feeling like the old maid daughter, the saintly one, Beth in *Little Women*—except she wasn't dying, unfortunately.

"What do you mean?" Heavy, resentful bitterness filled her voice. "Not many people get the chance to enjoy a miscarriage and a divorce? How unfortunate for them."

"Not many people get the chance to choose a new life," said Maxine. "You're young, smart, talented, you've got no ties, you can do whatever you want."

"I'm *not* young! And I want ties! I might never get the chance to have children!"

"You might not," agreed Maxine. "Would that really be the end of the world?"

"Yes!" It came out like a self-pitying sob of fear.

Maxine sighed. "Look. When I was your age I had three teenage daughters who were all convinced I was trying to ruin their lives. I had a dead-end job and an ex-husband with a bizarre habit of introducing me to all to his new girlfriends. I felt trapped, depressed—and now I think about it, a little bit insane. I would have given anything to be you with all those choices."

"But I don't have any choices. Not any that I want."

I want to be sitting on a plane next to Dan. I want my baby. I want Sal. I want to be somebody else.

"But you *do,* you infuriating child."

Nana's voice trilled imperiously down the hallway. "Maxine! Cat! Where are you both?"

"Look at your grandmother," said Maxine.

"What about her?"

"Oh, well, now you're just being obtuse."

Nana called again, "Maxine!"

"Just a minute, Gwen!"

At that moment a plane flew overhead, and Cat put her hands on the balcony fence and watched it turn into a speck on the horizon.

Maxine opened the screen door to go back inside.

"France was Dan's dream," she said, her hand on the door. "Why don't you come up with some of your own?"

"That's not true," said Cat furiously, but her mother was gone, the screen door slamming behind her.

It was pride that was holding her back. There was something pathetic about the rejected wife bravely pulling herself together, joining a tennis club, doing a photography course, cutting her hair, venturing timidly back out onto the single scene. It was like *accepting* the punishment handed over by the malevolent forces of fate. She wasn't going to be a good little girl stoically picking up the pieces.

While her personal life was being pulverized, her professional life had been ticking along nicely. The "Seduce Yourself" Valentine's Day campaign had been an unqualified success, with sales rocketing. There were even complaints! She'd always wanted to do a campaign that generated complaints. ("It was certainly not our intention to offend anyone," said Marketing Director Catriona Kettle.) Breakfast show DJs made risqué jokes about Hollingdale Chocolates. "What are you going to do next, Cat?" asked Rob Spencer. "Give away a vibrator with every box of chocolates?" "Now you're talking," said Cat.

Rather than being embarrassed about their night together, Graham Hollingdale seemed to find it all rather delicious. He gave her twinkly little nudge, nudge, wink, wink looks in meetings. Sometimes she twinkled back. He was too dorky to be lewd. Polyamory was just a really interesting new hobby he'd taken up.

One day, he called her into his office and told her that he was giving her a promotion. Her lengthy new title would be "General Manager—Marketing and Sales, Asia-Pacific Region." Rob Spencer and his team would report to her. (Rob Spencer would rather be savaged by a rabid dog.) She'd receive a twenty percent increase in her salary.

Graham grinned, and Cat thought, Did I just sleep my way to the top?

"Twenty percent?" she said.

"Yes," said Graham fondly. "The Board is over the moon about the last quarter results. Your new strategy is so powerful!"

How far could she push this? Could she get more? Could she double it?

"Triple it," she heard herself say.

"You want a sixty percent increase?"

"Yes."

"All right."

Bloody hell!

She sighed and thought of her mother telling her to come up with some dreams of her own.

"The thing is," she said to Graham. "I don't really want to sell chocolates anymore."

He looked at her with doleful sympathy. "No. No, neither do I. What do you want to do instead?"

"I don't know."

"Neither do I."

They laughed guiltily, like two teenagers sitting outside the careers adviser's office.

"Wednesdays still no good for you?"

"No, Graham."

It was a Sunday afternoon, and Cat was legally behind the wheel for the first time in seven months. Driving again after so long was an enjoyable sensation. It reminded her of that flying-free feeling of her first solo drive as a teenager. Not nearly as good but then, all her adult emotions felt like shadows, self-conscious imitations of those intensely real feelings from her childhood.

She had passed her driving test the first time, at 9 A.M. on the morning of her seventeenth birthday—the earliest possible moment she was allowed to try for it. Her sisters didn't bother. Lyn wasn't in a hurry, and Gemma couldn't stop driving into things.

Frank had been waiting for her in the registry office, his head down reading the newspaper. When he glanced up and saw the expression on her face, he grinned, folded the paper in half, and tucked it under his arm. "That's my girl."

He let her take his brand-new Commodore for a drive. "Please don't kill yourself. I'll never hear the end of it from your mother."

She drove all the way to Palm Beach. No alert-eyed grown-up in the passenger seat, the car felt so empty! Accelerating around each new swoop of the road made her delirious with freedom. She could do anything! If she could parallel park—she could take on the whole world!

Her future back then, thought Cat now, was like a long buffet table of exotic dishes awaiting her selection. This career or that career. This boy or that boy. Marriage and children? Maybe later—for dessert, perhaps.

She didn't realize they'd start clearing the plates away so soon.

Somebody pulled into the lane in front of her without signaling, and Cat slammed on her brake and her horn simultaneously. That was it. The novelty of driving had taken approximately four minutes to wear off.

She was going over to Lyn's place for coffee.

The famously gorgeous Hank, Lyn's American ex-boyfriend, was in Sydney, and Lyn, for some unfathomable reason, wanted Cat to meet him.

"You're not trying to set me up with him, are you?" asked Cat. There was a suspicious breathlessness in Lyn's voice.

"No!" said Lyn. "And anyway—well, you'll see. Just come. Bring a cake."

Cat pulled over across the road from the bakery and hopped out of the car. The traffic was beginning to slow and a truck pulled up beside her. The passenger, his arm resting along the windowsill and his feet up on the dashboard, glanced down at her and gave a relaxed wolf whistle.

Cat looked up and met the guy's eyes. He grinned. She grinned back. The traffic moved and she ran across the road, the sun warm on the back of her neck.

As she waited in the bakery for her turn, Cat the sneering sideline observer popped into her head. You do know why you're feeling a little bit happy, don't you? It's because that guy whistled at you! Instead of feeling objectified like a good feminist should, you're actually feeling flattered, aren't you? You're feeling *pretty*! You're even feeling *grateful*! You must be getting old if you feel good when some guy in a truck whistles at you. You make me sick!

"What can I do for this beautiful young lady?"

The little man behind the counter gave her a big flirtatious wink.

"Mmmm. I don't know. What are you offering to do for me?" said Cat, and the little man roared with appreciative laughter, slapping his hand on the counter.

"Hoo-eee! If I was twenty years younger!"

Bloody hell. Now you're getting off flirting with old men.

Shut *up*, you boring cow! Get off my back!

As she drove toward Lyn's place, the cake in its white paper bag on the seat next to her, together with a free chocolate éclair—"Don't you be telling my wife!"—she remembered how Nana Kettle always flirted outrageously with the butcher and the man in the fruit shop. When you went shopping with Nana it was like shopping in a village. "Here comes trouble!" people would call out as she approached.

Cat reached over for the chocolate éclair and took a gigantic bite. Chocolate, pastry, and cream exploded sweetly in her mouth.

Nana would have to make all new friends in her new local shopping center. She would too. She'd probably know all their names after the first week.

Cat was there when Nana had walked through the empty rooms of her house for the last time. Her bruises had faded to dirty yellow. Her hair was bouncy and curly again. "Looks much bigger now, doesn't it, darling?"

Then she took a big breath, turned on her heel, and walked out the front door.

"That's that," she said firmly.

Cat drove with one hand on the wheel and licked cream from her fingers.

She pulled into Lyn's street and took another gigantic mouthful of éclair.

The sun really was quite warm. The éclair really was quite delicious.

She parked the car and peeled off her sweater as she got out of the car and walked up the driveway to knock on Lyn's door; she listened for the sound of Maddie's footsteps pattering excitedly down the hallway, about to catapult herself into Cat's arms.

Maybe it wasn't that hard to be happy.

Maybe tomorrow morning, she would walk into Graham Hollingdale's office and hand him a letter of resignation, launch herself free, and see what happened.

Maybe she'd sell the unit.

Fuck it, maybe she'd even get her hair cut.

Steady on, girl, said sideline Cat.

Maybe it wasn't giving in. Maybe it was fighting back.

Approximately two hours later Cat came back out to her car. She put on her seat belt, and turned the keys in the ignition.

There were goose bumps of possibility on her arms. Her fingers danced a celebratory jig on the steering wheel.

CHAPTER 27

Hank was about to arrive, and Lyn went into Kara's bedroom to ask her whether her new shirt looked better buttoned or
unbuttoned with a camisole underneath. One of Lyn's new goals
was to ask the people in her life for help more often ("*Make at
least two requests per week, whether needed or not*"). So far, it
was working surprisingly well. Everyone was so pleased to be
asked (her mother-in-law almost cried with joy when Lyn asked
her to bring a dessert to dinner), and occasionally their help
actually was somewhat helpful.

She'd also enrolled in a meditation course. It was true that
she gave up after one class (she couldn't stand the way the
teacher spoke so very, very slowly), but as she explained to
Michael, the old Lyn would have forced herself to finish it, so that
was definite progress.

Her battle with parking lots and panic attacks wasn't quite
over yet, but she was confident she would win. She *would* take a
calmer, more relaxed approach to life—even if it killed her.

Lyn knocked on Kara's door. "I need some fashion advice. Your
father is useless," she told Kara. "He just grunts. What do you
think?"

Kara pushed her headphones down onto her neck and sat up

on her bed. "I think unbuttoned but *without* the camisole. Show your ex your sexy stomach."

Lyn unbuttoned the shirt to reveal her midriff and looked at herself in Kara's wardrobe mirror.

"I'm too old for that, don't you think?"

"No way. You look hot. Dad will freak."

Lyn smiled and swung her hips.

"All right." Michael probably wouldn't even notice. She just wanted to please Kara really. "Thanks."

The doorbell rang.

"Ooh! You'd better go quick before Dad punches him in the nose!" said Kara, in a tone of mild condescension, as if the affairs of Lyn and Michael could never hope to be that interesting.

Lyn met Michael in the hallway going to answer the bell, pulling rather sternly at his shirtsleeves, while Maddie ran ahead of him.

He blocked her way. "Cover your stomach, woman!"

Lyn did a netball feint and easily dodged around him.

She opened the door to reveal a rosy, double-chinned, smiley face.

"Hank?"

"Hey, Lyn!"

She peered at him. The boy from Spain was still there. He'd just been inflated like a balloon.

"I've packed on a few pounds as you can see."

"Haven't we all!" Lyn pushed open the door with one arm and rapidly buttoned up her shirt with the other.

"Not you! You look great! Wow!"

"Hank!" Michael crowed, his dimple creasing his cheek as he held out his hand. "Pleased to meet you, mate!"

In fact, thought Lyn, he sounded excessively pleased to meet him.

"Who you?" asked Maddie suspiciously, pulling at his trouser knee.

"I'm Hank, honey!"

Maddie observed him doubtfully and suddenly her face broke into a smile of delighted recognition. "Teletubby!"

"Come in!" cried Michael and Lyn simultaneously and loudly, studiously ducking their heads to avoid each other's faces.

They entertained Hank with a barbecue on the balcony. He was pleasingly enthralled with their harbor views and Australia in general.

"This is the life!" he kept saying, as he sipped his beer and Lyn and Michael, who after all, *lived* the life, became expansive and smug.

After awhile, Hank's fatness seemed to wear off, and when he laughed, Lyn could just catch a sliver of his former sexiness. It seemed unlikely however, that he would be making any more erotic appearances in her dreams. She blushed at the thought of eating mangoes in the bath with Hank, juice dripping from his double chin. "This is the life!"

Kara came down and ate lunch with them and was chatty and intelligent, asking Hank interested questions about America. She even cleared away the plates, as if it were her normal practice.

"What a charming girl!" said Hank after she'd gone back up to her room. "My teenage daughter won't talk to me. She just sneers from her bedroom door."

"Oh, Kara won't talk to me either," said Michael. "She thinks I'm an idiot."

"Teenagers!" said Hank. "All the parenting articles say, Talk to them, listen to them! But how can you when they seem to find it physically painful to even *look* at you?"

"Kara walks ten paces behind me," said Michael dolefully, refilling Hank's glass. "She says I shouldn't feel insulted—it's just in case she sees somebody she knows."

"And there's so much to worry about! Suicides! Drugs! Boys!" continued Hank. "Those kids who go on shooting rampages. I can't even imagine the guilt their parents must feel."

"Oh, I don't think Kara would shoot anybody," said Michael worriedly.

"This year, we want to publish a sort of self-help title for teenagers," said Hank. "Something funny. Not preachy. Speaks their language. I'll tell you, though, we're having a helluva job finding a good manuscript. Proves my point—nobody can talk to teenagers!"

"I'll get us another bottle of wine," said Lyn.

She went upstairs to Kara.

"That newsletter Cat's been writing for you and your friends. Can I show some of them to Hank? He's a publisher and he's looking for an author. I think Cat could do it."

"As if," said Kara, dismissively.

"This could be good for Cat," wheedled Lyn. "And I'll let you borrow my leather jacket for Sarah's birthday."

Kara gave her a shrewd look. "And your new boots?"

Lyn squirmed.

"I haven't even worn them yet myself! But O.K. Deal."

"Don't let Dad see it!" shrieked Kara as Lyn went back downstairs.

"Here's something that might interest you," she told Hank. "You can read it now, while Michael helps me with dessert."

"Oh," said Hank, looking disappointed. "Sure." From the roar of laughter as she came down the stairs, he and Michael had obviously been doing some male bonding.

"Are you sure fruit and cheese are enough?" chortled Michael in the kitchen. "He probably eats pumpkin pie or, I don't know, hotcakes. I didn't know you liked your men so . . . tubby."

Lyn shoved a piece of Brie into his mouth and a colander into his hands. "Shut up and wash the strawberries."

"Who is the author?" asked Hank, when they went back out on the veranda. He looked thinner now he was talking in his professional voice.

"It's my sister," said Lyn proudly.

"Who hates self-help books," contributed Michael.

"Well, I'd sure like to meet her while I'm here." Hank cut himself a piece of cheese and looked fat again. "I think she could write in exactly the right sort of tone. This could be a winner."

"I'll get her," said Lyn. "I'll get her to come now."

"Oh, that's not nec—"

But Lyn was already rushing for the phone.

When Cat arrived, she presented her to Hank, dragged Michael away to help put Maddie to bed, and stayed in the kitchen. About twenty minutes later, Hank came inside looking for the bathroom.

Lyn took a pot of coffee outside and sat down in front of Cat. She put her elbows on the table.

"That man," said Cat slowly, looking at her fingernails, "wants me to do a proposal for a book. He seems to think there could be some money in it. Potentially quite good money."

"So are you going to do it?" asked Lyn.

Cat smiled. It was the wicked wide grin of ten-year-old Cat, hatching up another plan to swap classes or skip school or get around Maxine. Lyn hadn't seen her smile like that since before she lost the baby.

"You bet I am."

"Dad. How are you?"

It still gave Lyn a little start, seeing her father open the door to the house in Turramurra. There was a tea towel over his shoulder.

"Never better, love."

In fact, thought Lyn, he had never looked older. His cheerful grin hadn't changed, but his cheeks seemed to have sagged and there were two deep crevices on either side of his mouth. Her eternally youthful father suddenly looked his age.

The attack on his mother had deeply affected Frank. He couldn't read the paper or watch the news without winding himself into a frenzy. Maxine said that he'd been having nightmares. He kept leaping out of bed and abusing various pieces of furniture.

It seemed that at the age of fifty-four, Frank Kettle experienced a terrible revelation. All those bad things that happened on the TV news—knife attacks, terrorist attacks, sniper attacks—actually happened to real people. They could happen to anybody. They could happen to *his* family. He wrote letters to his local MPs. He talked at length about "sick lunatics" and "murderous bastards." He wanted capital punishment. He wanted longer jail sentences. He wanted the lot of them bombed.

"He's experiencing empathy for the first time in his life," said Cat, with a noticeable lack of empathy. "About time."

"He's just surprised, poor Dad," said Gemma, who had always suffered from excessive empathy. Lyn had seen her walking down a street of parked cars, wincing each time she saw a parking ticket on a windshield.

Lyn was surprised at her own reaction. All her life she had thought her father didn't take life seriously enough, and now that he was, she wanted him to stop it. She wanted to shield his bewildered eyes from the world and bring back silly Dad; Dad who used to be so absurd that Nana would say to him, "Stop being such a *ham*, Frank!" One day Cat changed it to: "Yeah, Daddy, stop being such a ham sandwich!" which Gemma thought was so incredibly funny that she literally fell off her chair laughing. After that they'd always be saying, "Daddy's being a ham sandwich again!" while he pranced around, doing the most stupid, slapstick things; anything for a laugh.

She remembered their trips to Manly Beach and how they always had to run to catch the ferry. It drove her mad. She'd look back and see him staggering along, carrying Cat and Gemma under each arm, making grunting sounds and wobbling his head, because he was pretending to be a *gorilla*, for goodness' sake! Lyn would scream, "Come *on*, Dad!" What an uptight child she'd been.

"Sleeping better?" she asked now, as she followed her father down the hallway.

"Max tells me I had it out with the wardrobe last night," said Frank. "I don't remember a thing. I think she's making it up."

"Why is there a tea towel on your shoulder?"

"My turn to cook," said Frank. "I learned it from your mother. The first rule of cooking—carefully drape tea towel over left shoulder."

Maxine was sitting in the living room drinking tea and doing the crossword. "Maddie hasn't woken up from her nap," she said, taking off her glasses. "Have a cup of tea with me? I've just made a pot."

"I'll just get back to slaving away in the kitchen," said Frank.

"You do that, dear."

"You take turns to cook?" asked Lyn.

"Of course!" Maxine poured tea for her. "We're a new-age couple."

Lyn raised her eyebrows and didn't comment. "How was Maddie today?"

"Dreadful." Maxine waved a dismissive hand. "I wanted to ask you something. How do you and your sisters feel about us being back together now?"

"Um," said Lyn. She wasn't ready for the question. Her mind was feeling pleasantly stimulated by her day's work. Her new assistant wanted to introduce a "Frequent Brekkie Buyer" program. She was very professional and not annoyingly enthusiastic, but quite funny and nice. Actually, Lyn thought, she was probably going to be a new friend. It had been years since she'd made a new friend— it was a little bit like falling in love, except without the stress.

"At Christmas lunch when you went off in a huff," began Maxine.

It felt like centuries had been and gone since Christmas.

"It was a very stressful day," said Lyn. "I thought my head was going to explode. I shouldn't have reacted like that. Sorry."

Maxine looked irritated. "No, don't say sorry. Tell me what you felt. I don't think we do enough of that in this family."

"Are you kidding? I think we do far too much of that in our family!"

"I meant in a calm, rational way."

"All right."

Lyn lowered her voice. She could hear Frank whistling "Rhinestone Cowboy" in the kitchen, accompanied by clattering pots.

"I always thought that Dad treated you badly," she said quietly.

"Speak up! He can't hear a thing! He gets deafer every day."

"Dad treated you badly. I remember. So, when he made his announcement, I just felt—"

Maxine interrupted her, and Lyn smiled into her teacup.

"He did treat me badly. I treated him quite badly too. But we were different people! That's what you girls don't understand! Do you remember when I was seeing that orthodontist? He admitted that he'd been *dreadful* to his ex-wife. I didn't care! He was an extremely uninteresting man, as you know, so that was the end of that, but my point is that when I think about Frank's ex-wife, she seems like a stranger! I don't think about her as being me! He has mistakes in his past. I have mistakes in mine. The fact that we actually *are* each other's mistakes is irrelevant!"

"O.K. then," said Lyn.

"Of course, your father likes to pretend that we are the same people and he never stopped loving me." Maxine rolled her eyes but couldn't hide her pleasure. "But that's Frank."

"As long as you're happy," Lyn was beginning to wonder where all this was leading.

"So. I've been worried about him lately."

Lyn put a finger to her lips.

"I'm telling you, he can't hear. I thought of something nice to cheer him up."

"Yes?"

Her mother laced her hands across her stomach and looked slightly bashful.

"Tomorrow night I'm going to propose to him."

"You're going to ask him to marry you?"

"That's what proposals are generally for, Lyn, yes. What do you think?"

"I think." Lyn put down her teacup and wondered what she did think. "I think it's a . . . lovely idea." There were worse ideas, after all.

"Good!" said Maxine in a "that's settled" tone. "I'll go and check if that little horror is showing any signs of waking up."

Lyn could hear her father still whistling in the kitchen. The tune wasn't "Rhinestone Cowboy" anymore.

She picked up the empty cups and carried them into the kitchen.

Frank looked up from the saucepan of pasta sauce he was stirring and gave her an innocent look, as he continued to whistle.

Now she recognized the tune. It was a rather upbeat version of the Wedding March.

"You're such a ham sandwich, Dad."

And to her surprise Lyn found herself reaching up to plant a kiss on her father's cheek.

"What a lucky fellow I am," said Frank.

CHAPTER 28

Bottles. Nappies. Wipes. Lotion. Baby powder. Bedtime book. Pajamas. Overalls for tomorrow. Spare clothes for tonight. Funny bathtime toy. Cuddly, sleepytime toy. Noisy, quick-distract-him-with-this toy. Keep-for-full-on-wailing-emergency toy. Oh! What about one of the toys *they* gave him? That would look good. Favorite apple and pear baby food. Package of rusks.

What else?

Gemma was packing a bag for Sal's first overnight trip. He was going to stay with Charlie's parents while Gemma and Charlie went to the wedding.

His parents didn't approve of Gemma. They found the whole business of their son becoming an instant Daddy upsetting and suspicious. Plus, they unfairly connected Gemma to Dan—their youngest daughter's highly unsuitable new boyfriend who had taken her off to France before she finished her law degree.

On visits, Gemma sat stiffly and smiled inanely, while Charlie and his parents spoke in rapid-fire, angry-sounding Italian. His nonsmiling mother kept pushing plates of food in Gemma's direction, while his father punched the tabletop a great deal. It was stressful. Gemma was used to people liking her.

"Well really, Gemma," said Maxine. "What do you expect? I wouldn't approve of you either!"

But his parents did approve of Sal and Sal approved of them, virtually shot-putting himself out of Gemma's arms whenever he saw them.

Gemma zipped up the bulging bag and went through her mental checklist one more time. She'd probably forgotten something fundamental that would show her up as an unhygienic, unfit mother.

What if they just refused to give Sal back? What if they called the Department of Community Services and said, "Take a look at this overnight bag. Can you believe it? Calls herself a mother!"

She felt cold with fear at the thought. And then they'd find out that she had been planning to have Sal adopted, planning to abandon him. "You never wanted him in the first place," they'd say.

During those first few months, when Sal would cry and cry for no reason, it sounded to Gemma like a cry of grief. "You never wanted me! You were giving me away!"

As she paced back and forth down the hallway of Charlie's little flat, rocking and patting and begging him to please, please, please stop crying, guilt would knot her stomach.

One night at 3 A.M., after Sal had cried for two hours straight, Charlie, with red-rimmed eyes, said, "Why don't we get Cat on the phone? Tell her we've changed our minds. She can have him after all."

Gemma burst into tears.

"I was joking!" said Charlie, and the genuine distress on his face made Gemma cry even harder because he was so sweet, so wonderful, and she'd abandoned him too. ("So you're the girl who broke his heart," said Charlie's best friend when he met Gemma for the first time.)

"Maybe you've got that postnatal depression," said Charlie, while Gemma and Sal wailed into his chest.

"I've got post-*me* depression," said Gemma.

The next day Charlie phoned Maxine, and she appeared like the cavalry.

"Three!" exclaimed Gemma, watching her rock the baby. "You had *three* Sals, all at once! And you were twenty-one!"

"It was a nightmare of truly epic proportions," said Maxine grandly. "It was the worst time of my entire life."

"It must have been," breathed Gemma. "My God."

"Your sister said exactly the same thing a few months after Maddie was born," said Maxine. "I'm looking forward to when Cat has a similar revelation. That will be especially satisfying."

Sal's head lolled drunkenly in the crook of Maxine's arm.

"There was always one of you crying." Maxine brushed a fingertip along the length of Sal's eyelashes. "Always. I used to long for just one moment when all three of you were simultaneously happy."

Now Gemma gave up trying to think of anything else that Sal could possibly need and carried the overnight bag out beside the front door.

"We need to leave here in twenty minutes if we're going to make it," called Charlie from the bedroom, where he was dressing Sal. "Did you hear me? Twenty minutes."

He sounded slightly irritable.

In a funny way, Gemma quite liked it when he was annoyed with her. He didn't become someone else. He didn't frighten her. He didn't make her feel ashamed.

He just got in a bad mood every now and then. Like people did.

Sometimes, she still felt the beginning of that icy breeze whistling around her bones, but now she had a cure. She simply thought back to the night when Sal was born and she was in the ambulance listening to Charlie's voice on the mobile telling her how a lightbulb worked. "There's a thin little piece of wire and it resists the flow of electricity. That's why the filament glows . . . Everything has to flow back to earth, you see . . . Look, Gemma, you're not planning on *rewiring* or something like that, are you?"

It was like remembering the words to a beautiful poem. ". . . *It resists the flow of electricity . . . That's why it glows . . .*"

She put her head around the door. Sal was chortling up at his father, his legs windmilling wildly while Charlie attempted to hold him still to dress him.

"I love you," she said.

Charlie said crossly, "I should think so."

Frank and Maxine were married for the second time in the little white gazebo on the grassy area opposite Balmoral Beach. Picnicking families and hand-in-hand couples all watched the event with interest from behind their sunglasses.

Maddie was flower girl and was so entranced by her own prettiness that she managed to be good for the entire ceremony, swaying the silky skirt of her dress. Kara brought along a tall, skinny boy, who actually looked a lot like her father but fortunately nobody was foolish enough to mention it. Nana Kettle wore hot pink and spoke at length about her charming new neighbor, George. George's wife, Pam, was very ill. Nana hoped Pam wouldn't be in pain for too much longer.

Before they went off to dinner, the photographer that Lyn had organized took some spectacular shots of the family with the sun setting behind them.

But the best one, the one they got framed and blown up afterward, was one that he took without their even noticing.

It's when they were all walking toward the restaurant. Nana Kettle has stopped to give a demonstration of her newly acquired tai chi skills and is squatting slightly at the knees, her hands curled in the air. Cat, Gemma, and Lyn are all doing their own untrained, unbalanced versions of tai chi moves, and Gemma is in the process of toppling over toward her sisters. Charlie and Michael are walking behind them, their heads thrown back, laughing. Maddie has stopped to admire her new shoes. Kara and her new boyfriend are also looking at their shoes and secretly holding hands.

Frank and Maxine are holding hands too. Frank is striding ahead, looking at his watch. Maxine has turned back to watch her daughters. One hand is shading her eyes. She's smiling.

Epilogue

But wait, I'm not finished!

Listen to this! About six months later, I go and meet Cheryl from school one Saturday afternoon. She's all la-di-da at Mosman now, so we go down to Balmoral Beach for coffee. Anyway, we were watching this wedding party come back from having their photos taken. These two old people had got married, which was sort of cute.

All of a sudden, this girl in the party calls out to me, Olivia! And it's them! The weird triplets from the restaurant! I was like, oh my God, I don't believe it! I was really flattered that they remembered my name!

So the three of them come over for a chat and turns out it was their parents getting married, for the second time! Seems like the whole family is pretty wacko tobacco.

The one who'd been pregnant was all skinny again and I'm freaking out, thinking, Oh no, what if the baby died from the fork? I didn't like to ask. But then she said she'd had a little boy and he was fine and showed me photos. So that was a relief. I hate trying to work out what to say with, you know, tragedies and that sort of stuff.

The one who threw the fork, she seemed different. I couldn't tell why. I think maybe she got her hair cut.

They asked me if I recognized the photographer—and I said, hey, he was there that night at the table next to you, wasn't he? And they said, Yeah. Then the fork-thrower, she goes to me, Do you think he's cute? When she said that, her sisters just went off! They're going, Oooh, she likes him, she likes him! You know, even though they're in their thirties, they still act really young and normal. Cheryl could not believe it when I told her how old they were! I'm going to be like that when I get old.

Anyway, the fork-thrower gives me a wink and says, I'm going to ask him on a date, what do you think? I said, I think you should. I thought her sisters were going to have heart attacks they were so excited.

So she went off to talk to the photographer.

By the look on his face, I reckon he said yes, for sure.

A Reading Group Guide

to

Three Wishes

Questions for Discussion

1. Told from the perspective of spectators, the prologue begins with a fight between the sisters that ends with a fork protruding from the pregnant sister's belly. How does this event as the opening affect the way in which you read the rest of the novel? How does hearing the story from a variety of viewpoints affect you?

2. Short vignettes of people who have observed the triplets throughout their lives are interspersed throughout the novel. What was the author trying to achieve with this technique? Was it successful? How does it remind you of the film *It's a Wonderful Life*?

3. Why did Gemma never tell her sisters, with whom she shared everything, about the abuse from her fiancé? What would her sisters have done had they known? Why didn't Lyn and Cat notice the abuse? We don't learn of the abuse until well into the novel. How does this affect your understanding of why Gemma lives her life the way she does?

4. Ultra-organized and efficient, Lyn begins to experience panic attacks. Why does she hide them from her sisters and her husband? How are the panic attacks a message to Lyn about changes she needs to make?

5. Cat learns that her perfect marriage to the perfect husband is not so perfect after all. She believed that she and Dan had great communication and love, but Dan has an affair. How could her understanding of their relationship be so wrong? How does Lyn and Dan's secret relationship prior to Cat and Dan's affect Cat's relationship with her husband and her sister?

6. Coincidentally, the woman Dan has an affair with is also the sister of Gemma's new boyfriend, Charlie. How does this affect the tension of the story?

7. When Cat learns that Charlie's sister is Dan's "other woman," she demands that Gemma break up with Charlie. Why did Cat think she had the right to ask this of Gemma? Describe the sisters' relationships with men. How are they manifestations of their personalities? How does sibling rivalry affect the decisions they make about their lives, including the men they choose?

8. How do each of the sister's relationships with their mother and father differ? Do you think the rekindling of their mother and father's relationship will last? Why?

9. How do your opinions of Lyn, Cat, and Gemma change from the beginning of the novel to the end? Are you surprised by their transformations?

10. Humor runs throughout *Three Wishes*. It endears us to the characters and provides a buffer to some of the "heavier" issues that arise in the story. How would this story be different if the author had not used humor as effectively?

BOOKS BY LIANE MORIARTY

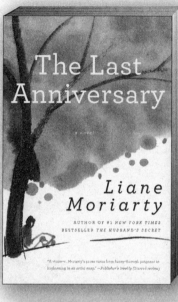

THE LAST ANNIVERSARY

Available in Paperback and eBook

Sophie Honeywell always wondered if Thomas Gordon was the one she let get away. He was the perfect boyfriend, but on the day he was to propose, she broke his heart. A year later, he married his travel agent, while Sophie has been single ever since. Now Thomas is back in her life because Sophie has unexpectedly inherited his aunt Connie's house on Scribbly Gum Island—home of the famously unsolved Munro Baby mystery. Sophie moves onto the island and begins a new life as part of an unconventional family where it seems everyone has a secret. Grace, a beautiful young mother, is feverishly planning a shocking escape from her perfect life. Margie, a frumpy housewife, has made a pact with a stranger, while dreamy Aunt Rose wonders if maybe it's about time she started making her own decisions.

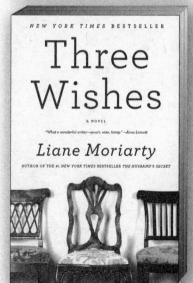

THREE WISHES
A Novel

Available in Paperback and eBook

Australian triplets Lyn, Cat, and Gemma Kettle are about to turn thirty-three and one is pregnant, one has just had her life turned upside down, and one is only just keeping hers from skidding off the fast lane. Meanwhile, their divorced parents have been behaving very oddly indeed. In this family comedy by Liane Moriarty, we follow the three Kettle sisters through their tumultuous thirty-third year—as they deal with sibling rivalry and secrets, revelations and relationships, unfaithful husbands and unthinkable decisions, and the fabulous, frustrating life of forever being part of a trio.